The Child and Adolescent Stuttering Treatment and Activity Resource Guide

DEDICATION

We dedicate this book to the hundreds of children, teens, and adults who have taught us so much about the courage required to live with a stuttering disorder and who have shared with us their hopes and dreams. We thank them for challenging us to be better clinicians and for providing the lessons and understanding we needed to help others become more fluent speakers. We also thank the caring clinicians who helped us become more fluent speakers and who provided role models to which we could aspire. Finally, we dedicate this book to Drs. Charles Van Riper, Joseph Sheehan, Hugo Gregory, and Dean Williams, and to Malcolm Fraser (founder of the Stuttering Foundation), individuals who through their own personal experiences and struggle with stuttering went on to develop and promote effective treatments for many who stutter, while enabling thousands of students and clinicians to better understand its impacts.

The Child and Adolescent Stuttering Treatment and Activity Resource Guide

Peter R. Ramig,
Ph.D., CCC-SLP

Darrell M. Dodge,
M.A., CCC-SLP

THOMSON

DELMAR LEARNING

Australia Canada Mexico Singapore Spain United Kingdom United States

THOMSON

DELMAR LEARNING

The Child and Adolescent Stuttering Treatment and Activity Resource Guide

by Peter R. Ramig, Ph.D., CCC-SLP and Darrell M. Dodge, M.A., CCC-SLP

Vice President, Health Care Business Unit:
William Brottmiller

Editorial Director:
Cathy L. Esperti

Acquisitions Editor:
Kalen Conerly

Developmental Editor:
Juliet Steiner

Marketing Director:
Jennifer McAvey

Marketing Coordinator:
Chris Manion

Project Editor:
John Mickelbank

Art & Design Specialist:
Robert Plante

Production Coordinator:
Kenneth McGrath

Library of Congress Cataloging-in-Publication Data
Ramig, Peter R., 1946-
The child and adolescent stuttering treatment and activity resource guide / Peter R. Ramig, Darrell Dodge.
   p. ; cm.
 Includes index.
 ISBN 1-4018-9719-3
1. Stuttering in children—Treatment.
2. Stuttering in adolescence—Treatment. 3. Speech therapy for children.
 [DNLM: 1. Stuttering—therapy. 2. Speech Therapy—methods. WM 475 R173c 2005] I. Dodge, Darrell. II. Title.
 RJ496.S8R35 2005
 618.92'855406--dc22
                               2004031002

NOTICE TO THE READER

Publisher does not warrant or guarantee any of the products described herein or perform any independent analysis in connection with any of the product information contained herein. Publisher does not assume, and expressly disclaims, any obligation to obtain and include information other than that provided to it by the manufacturer.

The reader is expressly warned to consider and adopt all safety precautions that might be indicated by the activities described herein and to avoid all potential hazards. By following the instructions contained herein, the reader willingly assumes all risks in connection with such instructions.

The publisher makes no representations or warranties of any kind, including but not limited to, the warranties of fitness for particular purpose or merchantability, nor are any such representations implied with respect to the material set forth herein, and the publisher takes no responsibility with respect to such material. The publisher shall not be liable for any special, consequential, or exemplary damages resulting, in whole or part, from the reader's use of, or reliance upon, this material.

TABLE OF CONTENTS

PART I

CHAPTER 1:
Helping Parents Learn about Stuttering in Children: Information for Clinicians, Students, and Parents

CHAPTER 2:
Strategies for Counseling Parents of Children Who Stutter

CHAPTER 3:
Strategies for Assessment of Fluency Disorders

PART II

This resource manual was written primarily for certified speech-language pathologists and for students working toward degrees in communication disorders who are striving to effectively intervene with preschool children, school-age children, and teens who stutter. In addition, this book provides valuable information for parents, teachers, and day care providers—important people who often play an influential role in the life of the child who stutters. Above all, it is our hope that this resource manual will assist the thousands of clinicians who may feel uncomfortable working with children and adolescents who stutter. We know from many years of experience, as well as from our own personal experience as recovering stutterers, that intervention by a caring, knowledgeable speech-language pathologist can make a significant and lasting difference in the lives of most who stutter.

Why This Book Is Unique and Beneficial to Clinicians

Among the unique aspects of this book are the hundreds of specific and detailed how-to activities and ideas that can be used in the treatment room and classroom to help children and adolescents who stutter. Specifically, in Part II we provide activities to achieve many goals important to consider in working with dysfluent children. Under each goal or focus area is a list of citations that explain why attention to that particular area is important. We then provide scores of activities pertinent to a clinician or student in training. To date, no texts on stuttering offer the vast number of detailed intervention ideas found in this book, nor do any other sources offer usable activities and strategies that can be implemented regardless of what the clinician's training or treatment bias might be. Another important and unique aspect of this book is the detailed handouts for parents, teachers, and clinicians found in the appendix; we encourage clinicians and teachers to copy and distribute them. This appendix is a source of a great deal of specific intervention-related information for every working clinician and student who wishes to increase his or her knowledge and understanding of preschool, school-age, and teen stuttering.

How This Book Is Organized

To support the clinician's use of the hundreds of treatment activities listed in Part II, we begin Part I by outlining many of the basic principles about stuttering and its treatment that all people need to know about this disorder. Though Chapter 1, "Helping Parents Learn about Stuttering in Children: Information for Clinicians, Students, and Parents," implies a focus on helping only parents learn about stuttering, the information therein is also crucial for professional clinicians, students, and teachers. In Chapter 2 we suggest ways to counsel parents of children and adolescents who stutter. Chapter 3 presents detailed information on fluency assessment and ends with ways to use that information to determine who needs treatment.

Another unique aspect of this book is the information in Chapter 4, "Strategies for Developing Individualized Education Programs," pertaining to developing and writing IEPs. Here we provide sample goals to the school clinician who is concerned about the impact of dysfluency on the educational needs of the child.

Chapter 5, "Working with Teachers," presents very important information on how to positively and constructively react to and interact with the stuttering child in the classroom. Possible solutions to commonly asked questions are presented. In addition, the chapter includes a list of available resource materials that is a must-see for every teacher of a student who stutters.

Chapter 6 contains information on basic principles underlying clinician interaction with children who stutter, and a generic breakdown of game activities and rewards designed to develop and maintain the child's and adolescent's interest and motivation in the intervention process. Specific and more detailed step-by-step ideas and activities are outlined in Part II of the text, while this chapter describes these generically in a way that may help the reader understand why this topic is important.

Chapter 7, "Direct and Indirect Therapy for Preschool Children," both describes and outlines indirect and direct therapy approaches. In Chapter 8, "Strategies for Teaching Normal Speech Production and Fluency-Enhancing Techniques," we focus on why it is necessary to teach clients the components or "ingredients" that help them generate fluent and stuttered speech. Examples of exercises to accomplish this are described. Next, in Chapter 9, "Strategies for Desensitization and Teaching Stuttered Speech Production," we apply information to help the client learn specifically where in his vocal mechanism he is pushing and forcing in ways that can trigger or exacerbate stuttering episodes.

In Chapter 10, "Strategies for Modifying Stuttered Speech," we describe and give examples of ways the child can manifest his stuttering in an easier, more forward-flowing, less struggle-related manner. In Chapter 11, "Transfer and Maintenance," these complementary issues are discussed as an ongoing process. The text addresses the importance of these issues and ways to deal with them in the various stages of treatment.

Cluttering is too often ignored, resulting in ineffective or incomplete treatment regimens. In "Strategies for Cluttering Evaluation and Therapy" (Chapter 12), cluttering is defined, assessment factors are outlined, and guidelines for deciding treatment directions are described.

Chapter 13, "Explaining the Progress of Treatment and Recovery to Children and Parents," explores ways of discussing the therapy and recovery process with parents and children, providing possibilities for integrating the observations and experiences of those undergoing therapy with experimental findings.

Part II incorporates hundreds of therapy activities and strategies. We developed most ourselves, but, some were contributed by our colleagues and graduate students. These more than 150 pages of specific therapy activities are listed under 16 global intervention goals or components, such as "Establishing Light Articulatory Contacts and Movements" and "Working with Young Children."

The appendix includes numerous handouts written in both English and Spanish for clinicians, parents, and teachers; all of these handouts can be reproduced and used or distributed as needed. We hope that after reading the wealth of information in this resource book, clinicians will be less likely to view stuttering as the pathology of speech they fear and know little about; in contrast, they will begin to develop confidence in their ability to assess and effectively treat children and adolescents who stutter.

Note to the Reader: When referring to mistakes in speech that are considered normal, we often refer to them using the spelling "disfluency" or "disfluencies." However, when referring to actual stuttering, we often use the spelling "dysfluency" or "dysfluencies."

CONTRIBUTORS

Some of the activities provided in Part II were derived from *Treating the School-Age Child Who Stutters: Some Intervention Ideas and Resources*, an earlier, unpublished manuscript by Ramig, Stewart, Ogrodnick, Bennett, Dodge, and Lamy (1988).

Additionally, approximately 35 of the several hundred activities listed in Part II of this book were developed by students in the senior author's graduate course in stuttering. Both authors wish to thank each and every one for their creative thinking and dedication to helping children and adolescents who stutter.

Teacher and Peer Education
Andrea M. Dewan
Meghan Morley
Sharon Worthman

Working with Young Children
Kari Hickman
Amy Acres Rivera

Normal Speech Production
Jill Cornforth
Helen Oesterle

Facilitating Adequate Breath Support
Angela Runyon

Controlling Speaking Rate
Kari Hickman
Laura Montesano
Castara Stroman

Light Articulatory Contacts
Cynthia Audo
Laura Montesano
Julie Pellet
Megan Bradley Wood

Desensitization
Charni Laura
Leigha Topol-Monaghan
Meghan Morley
Melinda Pampush
April Parmley
Megan Bradley Wood
Courtney Yurow

Reduction of Avoidance Behaviors
Amy Nugent
Castara Stroman
Sharon Worthman

Modification
Charni Laura
Meghan Morley
April Parmley

Self-Awareness and Self-Monitoring
Nicole Phillips

Transfer and Maintenance of Fluency
Jamie Galbari
Irene Kim
Leigha Topol-Monaghan
Amy Nugent
Melinda Pampush
Amy Acres Rivera
Angela Runyon

ACKNOWLEDGMENTS

Our Sincerest Thank-You to John B. Ellis

The authors wish to extend their deep appreciation and thanks to John B. Ellis, certified speech-language pathologist, for his important contribution to the editorial work and content included in this book, as well as his expertise in the graphic design and layout incorporated to enhance the appearance and content of the entire text. His contributions are significant, appreciated, and invaluable.

We also wish to thank our colleagues, all of whom are respected authorities on stuttering who influenced our thinking, contributed to our knowledge, and supported our personal and professional endeavors in one important way or another. They include Professors Emeritus Marty Adams, Hal Homann, and Lois Nelson. We also wish to thank our colleagues and clinicians of stuttering, Joy Armson, Ellen Bennett, Gordon Blood, Charlene Bloom, Dorvan Breitenfeldt, Lee Caggiano, Tony Caruso, Roger Colcord, Kristin Chmela, Edward Conture, Donna Cooperman, Doug Cross, David Daly, Carl Dell, Susan Dietrich, Judith Eckardt, John Ellis, Sheryl Gottwald, Carolyn Gregory, Hugo Gregory, Barry Guitar, Tom Gurrister, Susan Hamilton, Mick Hanley, Charlie Healey, Diane Hill, Steve Hood, Deborah Kully, Judy Kuster, Marilyn Langevin, Lisa LaSalle, Jeff Lewis, Ken Logan, Walt Manning, Catherine Otto Montgomery, Ann McKeehan, Larry Molt, Bill Murphy, Fred Murray, Florence Myers, Marilyn Nippold, Libby Oyler, David Prins, Bob Quesal, Nan Bernstein Ratner, Nina Reardon, Gary Rentschler, Gyndyn Riley, Jeanna Riley, Bill Rosenthal, Betsy Runyan, Chuck Runyan, George Shames, David Shapiro, Vivian Sheehan, Vivian Sisskin, Woody Starkweather, Lisa Scott, Meryl Wall, Karen Wexler, Dale Williams, Scott Yaruss, and Tricia Zebrowski.

We list these friends and colleagues because most are contemporaries who have contributed significantly to our knowledge of stuttering through their writings and publications; they are also dedicated, ethical, caring specialists in stuttering who continue to work with children and adults who stutter. In addition, they are all people who understand the importance of acknowledging and addressing in their treatment the very important factors of embarrassment, fear, shame, and avoidance—those behaviors that often maintain and exacerbate existing stuttering.

Last, but far from least, Peter Ramig wishes to thank the most wonderful family a man could have: daughter Caroline Susan Ramig, and wife, Lorrie Scott. Darrell Dodge wishes to thank Michael Hartford; John Ahlbach; Annie Bradberry; Rho Vidal; and, most importantly, Loraine Kreznar, without whose loving support it would have been impossible to negotiate the career change that enabled him to cowrite this book.

"The Child and Adolescent Stuttering Treatment and Activity Resource Guide is exactly the publication I've been waiting for!

"Reader-friendly and practical, Ramig and Dodge eliminate much of the mystery out of assessment and treatment for children and adolescents with fluency disorders. From assessment strategies to developing an appropriate IEP to working with parents and teachers to providing basic treatment strategies explained in Part 1, this book is already worth its weight in gold. But even more exciting is Part 2, where the authors supply references to the research data and share hundreds of treatment ideas from their own and other clinicians' experience, providing the rational and support from experts in the field of fluency disorders for each treatment goal.

"Students in practicum and beginning clinicians will be able to adapt an appropriate treatment plan for their clients, and experienced clinicians will find a wealth of new ideas and creative approaches.

"This book is a gem and belongs in every clinician's library."

—Judith Kuster, Associate Professor
Minnesota State University, Mankato

"The Child and Adolescent Stuttering Treatment and Activity Resource Guide is a gold mine of therapy techniques and activities in which to teach them. The authors' clinical experiences shine through in their clear explanations of why, when, and how to employ a multitude of tools to increase fluency and make stuttering easier and more like normal speech. Anyone working with children or adolescents who stutter—using almost any treatment approach—will find Ramig and Dodge's book to be a resource brimming with ideas for evaluation, treatment planning, and report writing."

—Barry Guitar, Professor
University of Vermont

"Authors Peter Ramig and Darrell Dodge have created an outstanding resource for therapists and parents alike, one that is thorough yet readable, detailed yet practical, and helpful without understating what a complex and encompassing disorder stuttering can be. Packed with sound advice, useful information, therapeutic activities, and other diagnostic and treatment resources, *The Child and Adolescent Stuttering Treatment and Activity Resource Guide* should be regularly consulted by every speech-language pathologist treating children who stutter."

—Dale Williams, Associate Professor
Florida Atlantic University

"We have a crisis need for helping SLPs work with children and adolescents who stutter and their families and teachers. This need is especially strong in the schools.

"This book will be very useful for practicing SLPs or graduate courses in stuttering. It will enhance knowledge about stuttering and improve skills in diagnostics, treatment, counseling, and goal writing.

"The book is well organized, is rich in practical material for diagnostics, therapy, and counseling, has 'state of the art' information for goal writing, and has excellent references for additional learning."

—Judith Eckardt, M.S., CCC-SLP
Board Recognized Fluency Specialist

"I would recommend this book to all clinicians who work with children and adolescents who stutter. It is packed with information and practical activities that will give clinicians confidence and competence in working with this often complex disorder of communication. The authors' writing style ensures that the reader is offered clear guidance as well as choice about the range of therapy options. In addition to the direct speech modification and fluency shaping aspect, clinicians will gain skills in managing the cognitive and affective components of the problem and discover the importance of involving parents and teachers throughout the therapy process. It is an excellent book."

—Frances Cook
Principal Speech and Language Therapist
The Michael Palin Centre for Stammering Children

Speech-language pathologists rank stuttering as the disorder that they feel least capable in treating. Many clinicians suggest that their academic training neglected the treatment aspect of fluency disorders. Some say they were trained to treat the speech-motor symptom of stuttering but not the emotional issues that affect their clients. Others report success in helping their clients reduce communicative anxiety but say they need more information to combine counseling with other techniques. Finally we have a book that focuses on taking our understanding of stuttering into the actual therapy room.

The Child and Adolescent Stuttering Treatment and Activity Resource Guide is an invaluable resource that is written especially for practicing clinicians and for parents of children who stutter. The book is masterfully organized, allowing the book its delightful readability while preserving its reputation as a scholarly text. It offers practical information on stuttering and detailed assessment protocols with suggestions in interpreting the diagnostic findings. It clearly differentiates the two primary types of treatment—fluency shaping and stuttering modification—with explanations enhanced by a variety of examples and guidance for combining these approaches. It also gives a broad list of therapy goals with detailed rationale and research support for each. This book does not promote a canned program, suggesting that one approach will serve the needs of all clients. It does not sell a device or promote a singular philosophy. Instead, *The Child and Adolescent Stuttering Treatment and Activity Resource*

Guide offers treatment strategies and procedures that can be used in combination, allowing the clinician freedom to individualize treatment for the client. It also includes clinical insights into working with parents and teachers of children who stutter, supplying necessary materials such as the examples of IEPs. In the appendix they include many detailed reproducible handout forms for distribution to parents and teachers in English and Spanish. For all its strong attributes, indeed the most outstanding feature of this book is its precision of explanation in teaching therapy techniques through clear description and by listing an abundance of effective activities and resources to implement these skills.

The Child and Adolescent Stuttering Treatment and Activity Resource Guide is a true collaboration between acclaimed author, professor, and clinician Peter Ramig and his former client, graduate student, and now friend, fluency-specialist and university colleague, Darrell Dodge. Both skilled fluency clinicians, these authors compiled activities and handouts for clients, parents, and teachers that they found to be most clinically effective through their own clinical practices, and through teaching graduate student clinicians at the University of Colorado, Boulder. Ramig and Dodge share literally hundreds of effective ways to bring therapy skills into the therapy room and to the home of the child who stutters. This book is a long-awaited answer to the need of many speech-language pathologists working with fluency disorders.

Susan Dietrich, Ph.D.

Harvard University

Peter Ramig is Professor and Associate Chair in the Department of Speech, Language and Hearing Sciences at the University of Colorado in Boulder, where he teaches and specializes in stuttering issues in children, teens, and adults. He is also a member, fellow, and board-recognized fluency specialist of the American Speech-Language-Hearing Association. The majority of Dr. Ramig's professional publications include work on the aerodynamic aspects of dysfluent speech in conditions that reduce stuttering, as well as various treatment and efficacy issues related to intervention with persons who stutter. As a working therapist and respected authority on stuttering, he annually presents many workshops and seminars pertaining to the treatment of children, teens, and adults, and continues to consult for the Stuttering Foundation with a team of respected stuttering specialists in developing numerous education/demonstration treatment videos now marketed worldwide.

Darrell Dodge is a certified speech-language clinician and private practitioner working as an associate in the Denver area private practice offices of Peter R. Ramig, Ph.D. and Associates, specialty clinics focusing in the evaluation and treatment of children, teens, and adults who stutter. Mr. Dodge received an M.A. in English literature from the University of Cincinnati in 1973 and had a long career in advertising, writing, wind energy research and development, and Web site development. Following successful therapy for stuttering with Peter Ramig that commenced at age 45, he returned to graduate school to obtain a masters degree in speech-language pathology at the University of Colorado at Boulder. Since 1998, Mr. Dodge has treated more than 150 children and adults who stutter. He has also facilitated adult stuttering support groups for many years and is a past National Stuttering Association Member of the Year. He is the developer of a Web site that explores many aspects of stuttering and includes the essay "The Veils of Stuttering."

PART I

What Every Speech-Language Pathologist and Student Should Read and Believe

We begin our book in a somewhat unusual way by citing Dr. Carl Dell, from an excellent reprinted publication by the Stuttering Foundation, called *Treating the School Age Child Who Stutters: A Guide for Clinicians* (2000). This quotation says so much that is important for the clinician to carefully read and remember. Even though Dr. Dell continued to stutter during and after the years of stuttering therapy he received in the schools, it was the caring, warmth, and understanding he received from his clinicians that helped him manage and cope at the time. More importantly, he goes on to state that the significant role his clinicians played during his school years led to his eventual mastery of his stuttering in his adult years. One of the authors of this book, Peter Ramig, had an experience identical to that described by Dell. Although his stuttering was not significantly changed at the time, it was the caring and understanding he felt from his school clinicians, and the strategies and techniques they taught him as a child and adolescent, that led to the very significant changes he was able to make in his mid-twenties.

Let me tell you about some of my own personal feelings as a young stutterer going to speech class, for I have been on both sides of the therapy room table. Although my stuttering was not cured during my school years, the school clinicians did accomplish several very important things. They provided a place where I could come and talk, where no one would laugh at me or scorn me, where I felt free to communicate even if I did stutter. What a great feeling that was! My dog was the only other living creature with whom I felt that way. Here was a place where I could learn something about my stuttering, that mysterious thing no one else ever mentioned. I needed a safe place where I could touch it and confront it. All of these benefited me a great deal as a young boy. My public school clinicians didn't cure me but they were sorely needed and I believe these experiences laid the foundation for my eventual success. Indeed, I'm certain that, without this early therapy background, my therapy as an adult would have been much more difficult. But most valuable of all was the gift of caring. They cared! I was made to feel some worth as a human being despite my stuttering. Because of this experience, stuttering did not destroy my self-concept the way it does in many young stutterers. The caring and warmth I received from my school clinicians helped me to stay together as a person.

Although I remain grateful to all the public school clinicians who helped me, I believe that much more can be done than they were able to do. Most importantly, they should have tried to reverse the progressive course of stuttering. Unfortunately, too many borderline and mild stutterers become severe, confirmed stutterers and we feel the public school clinician can prevent this. There seems to be at least two reasons why so many stutterers get worse during their school years. The first is that they get no professional help in the early stages of their stuttering, and second is that the clinician hasn't been trained to provide the necessary methods for preventing its abnormal growth. It is our belief that the key to the problem of stuttering is early intervention so that the progressive growth of the disorder can be reversed.

Theoretically, it seems possible that a child might get worse because he has been taken out of his room for speech. He may consider this as being an indication that he is inferior or abnormal. If then he tries harder to speak perfectly his disfluencies may increase and he may become frustrated and fearful. Although this seems logical we have never seen it happen in reality, never once! Perhaps if the clinician's attitude toward the child were negative or if she shows an aversion to stuttering when it occurs then the stuttering might get worse, but our experience has been that most clinicians are loving, gentle people who accept and understand the child's stuttering. Such attitudes will not make the stuttering worse. Also, we must remember that many people have already been critical of the child's stuttering. People often claim that the child is completely unaware of his stuttering, but they are usually wrong. In our first meeting he usually tells us he stutters. It may be something as innocent as this: "I know my mom doesn't like it because she looks down when I do it." Usually, when the child is taken out of class it isn't the first time that attention has been drawn to his stuttering.

Another thing that school clinicians worry about is doing something wrong during therapy that will cause the child to get worse. Certainly we all make mistakes, but this is no reason to avoid seeing the child. Because of their resiliency, children are rarely affected for very long. If the clinician is alert to changes in the client's behavior she can always adjust her therapy accordingly. With each client our goals can be reached not only by following different routes but also by moving at different speeds. So let us have confidence in our abilities. Any good clinician will make a mistake occasionally but she is quick to recognize it and make appropriate adjustments. It is also true a child in therapy may get worse for reasons that have nothing to do with you.

Now that you have read Dr. Dell's statement, know that you too can make a difference with kids who stutter. Realize that when a stuttering child does not make the changes you want him to make, it does not mean that you are not helping him. Sometimes, no matter how caring and competent you are as a clinician of stuttering, there are children who will not, and cannot, make the changes in the time frame everyone else wishes or thinks they should. As Professor Ramig sometimes says to his students, "It's the nature of the beast, it's the way it is." Both authors hope you will, with the guidance and the ideas written in this book, seek out and work with children and adolescents who stutter, knowing that you truly can make a difference.

As stated earlier, our motivation in writing this book stems from the fact that the vast majority of speech-language pathologists report that they are uncomfortable with their level of expertise in providing clear and easy-to-follow behavioral models that individuals who stutter may implement to modify their speech. Part I of this book provides useful information for caregivers and clinicians on stuttering etiology, assessment, and treatment; it also emphasizes the contributions of caregivers, teachers, and other facilitators to the rehabilitation process. Part II of this book contains hundreds of specific activities to use during therapy. These techniques and activities are pooled from numerous sources and are grouped on the basis of different therapeutic goals for easier reference. We hope that the sheer number of activities included will stimulate the clinician's interest and creativity in stuttering therapy, rather than being taken as a definitive, inflexible treatment model.

This text is written primarily for certified speech-language pathologists and learners working toward a master's degree in speech-language pathology, but it may also serve as a resource to help many parents or other primary caregivers of children or adolescents who stutter. It is our hope that readers will learn factual information about stuttering and, as a result, feel more comfortable and capable in their ability to support the stuttering child or adolescent as he commences on the road to recovery. Caregivers are advised, however, to consult a qualified speech-language pathologist—one experienced in treating stuttering—before attempting to implement any of the specific therapy techniques and strategies presented in this text. This book is not intended to be a recipe or step-by-step manual on how parents or other caregivers should intervene and conduct stuttering therapy independent of professional advice and guidance. Although caregivers are encouraged to participate in the rehabilitation process, they should do so under the auspices of a trained professional speech-language pathologist experienced in treating children and adolescents who stutter.

We have chosen terminology that can be understood by parents and other caregivers reading this text. For the sake of convenience and clarity, we use the terms *parent, caregiver,* and *other caregiver* interchangeably. In addition, we refer to the child or adolescent who stutters by the pronoun "he" while referring to the therapist or clinician as "she." Our use of the term *child* generally refers to school-aged clients, including children and adolescents. We may also use the term *child* to refer to those of preschool through high school age. Figure 1.1 demonstrates the relationship between the child, the parents, and the speech-language pathologist.

The certified speech-language clinician is the most qualified person to tailor a specific stuttering therapy plan to a child or adolescent who stutters. The therapy strategies and activities described in this text are well suited for most children and adolescents who stutter, but some will be more appropriate than others, depending on the individual child. Despite our intention to provide a complete and comprehensive guide, the ideas, goals, and activities should be applied discriminately—considering the child's personality, age, stuttering severity, language development, and

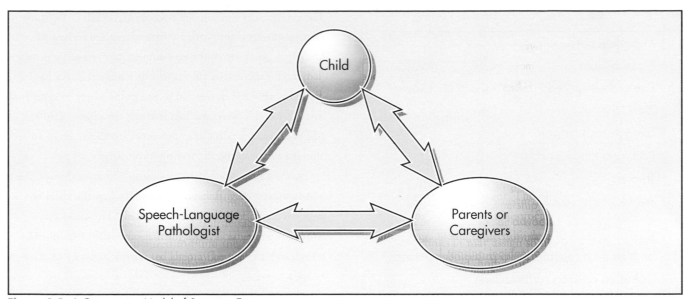

Figure 1.1　A Cooperative Model of Stuttering Treatment

emotional reaction to stuttering behaviors. The clinician must consider these important factors in crafting the best therapy plan. After she has worked with the child or adolescent for several sessions, she can better discriminate among the many therapy ideas presented in this text to help a specific client communicate in his everyday environment. As treatment progresses, she can implement more advanced strategies in response to the child's progress or other ongoing changes. During the course of treatment, parents should be encouraged to observe therapy sessions and ask questions before implementing changes at home. All activities suggested by the clinician should be understood by the parent and implemented with understanding, caring, and support. The young child or adolescent should never be made to feel guilty for stuttering or denigrated for failing to improve "if only he just put forth the effort and used his techniques." In our experience, children do not—with rare exception—consciously stutter for attention. Furthermore, we do not feel they can always and easily prevent stuttering in meaningful situations by implementing a single technique or activity that may have worked in the therapy room. Although substantial change and even complete recovery from stuttering is very possible with most children and adolescents, patience, openness, and understanding facilitate this process. Of the greatest benefit to a child or adolescent who stutters are a competent clinician and involved, caring parents.

What Is Stuttering?

Stuttering can be defined as an abnormally high frequency or duration of stoppages in the forward flow of speech affecting its continuity, rhythm, rate, and effortfulness (Guitar, 1998). Stuttering is characterized by an abnormally high number of dysfluencies, abnormally long dysfluencies, and physical tension that is often evident during speech. Chapter 3 includes a thorough description of stuttering for the purposes of diagnosis; however, Figure 1.2 lists a number of "warning signs" typically indicative of the onset and development of stuttering.

Some Possible Warning Signs of Stuttering

There are a number of possible warning signs for stuttering, listed in Figure 1.2 and discussed in more detail in the following section. These descriptions are adapted from *If your child stutters: A guide for parents* (Stuttering Foundation Publication No. 11).

Multiple Repetitions. Multiple repetitions mean repeating sounds of a word, such as "ta-ta-ta-ta-table," more than one or two times, faster than normal, or with irregular tempo. Although these have often been distinguished from whole-word repetitions, repetitions of short words such as "I-I-I" or "It-it-it" or "and-and-and" should be noted as well. These repetitions of short words may indicate an early attempt to

Figure 1.2 Some Possible Warning Signs of Stuttering

- Multiple repetitions
- Prolongations
- Use of the reduced "schwa" (i.e., "uh") vowel
- Blocking
- Struggle and tension
- Pitch and loudness rise
- Tremors
- Avoidance of speaking situations, words, or sounds
- Pauses, extraneous sounds, interjected words, and/or even repeated whole words or phrases
- Disturbed or irregular breathing
- Movement of other body parts
- Fear of speaking
- Additional behaviors

postpone or recoil from impending, anticipated feared words or sounds.

Prolongations. Abnormal prolongations occur when the child stretches out a sound at the beginning of or (particularly) within a word, such as "rrrrrrrrrabbit" or "raaaaaa—bit." It is important to distinguish these prolongations from easy stretches, which may be associated either with previous therapy or with a self-calming mechanism in response to tension or struggle.

Use of the Reduced "Schwa" (i.e., "uh") Vowel. Instead of saying "re-re-re-read," the child says "ruh-ruh-ruh-read," using the neutral schwa vowel. This behavior may indicate that the speech difficulty has become uncoupled from language and communication and is being felt as a performance struggle. It may also indicate that the child has lost a measure of awareness in response to the severity of the blocking experience.

Blocking. Blocking occurs when the speaker stops or gets stuck before or during the production of a sound or word. Blocks may occur at the respiratory, laryngeal, or articulatory level of speech production (Guitar, 1998). Blocking may be anticipated as the person approaches a word, or it may be used to close down the speech system to await a return of fluency or to minimize an overt display of stuttering.

Struggle and Tension. Struggle and tension may be seen in the nose, jaw, neck, cheeks, lips, forehead, and upper chest.

These behaviors can quickly become classically or instrumentally conditioned (identified with the original feeling of blockage), resulting in the recruitment of even more muscles. Increased muscular tension of the articulators accompanies stuttering that has developed to the point where intervention is indicated. To overcome this tension, the child recruits additional surrounding muscles and muscle groups in an attempt to overcome the feeling of blockage.

Pitch and Loudness Rise. A rise in pitch or loudness often occurs during prolongation of sounds, when the child is struggling to proceed to the next sound. The child may anticipate or feel that he is going to have difficulty on the sound and uses the pitch or loudness rise as a way to force his way forward.

Tremors. Quivering of the jaw, lips, and tongue as the person speaks (fluently or dysfluently) should be noted. These observations will assist in defining the loci of tension associated with stuttering. Tremors may be viewed as a more persistent reaction to stuttering blocks (Van Riper, 1982).

Avoidance of Speaking Situations, Words, or Sounds. The child's reluctance to engage in speaking activities may or may not indicate avoidance directly associated with stuttering. There may, however, be other cues that the child is attempting to avoid speaking challenges, such as continually wanting to change activities, wanting to stop an activity during which he is experiencing excessive dysfluencies, and postponing by acting out or creating distractions.

Pauses, Extraneous Sounds, Interjected Words, and/or Repeated Whole Words or Phrases. These may indicate an attempt to postpone speech to avoid stuttering or delay until the child feels that a word can be uttered fluently. More direct avoidance signs are word substitutions, silences, breaking off speech for another activity, or changing the topic.

Disturbed or Irregular Breathing. Upon anticipating stuttering, a child may hold his breath, take several breaths, or display other types of erratic or irregular breathing patterns such as rapidly uttering many words per breath group.

Movement of Other Body Parts. In response to stuttering, the child may jerk his head forward or back; move his arm, leg, or hand; close or blink his eyes; or attempt other unusual physical behaviors. These movements become conditioned to moments of stuttering, as they occasionally help the child escape from stuttering episodes (Van Riper, 1973; Guitar, 1998).

Fear of Speaking. One or more of the behaviors described in this section may indicate that the child is fearful of speaking. The clinician should attempt to distinguish between normal speech-related performance anxiety and fear associated with stuttering behaviors.

Additional Behaviors. Additional warning signs include aberrant voice quality (such as excessive vocal fry) and dysrhythmic phonation during prolonged sounds. Phonemic consistency of dysfluencies should also be noted; for example, the child may display a regular tendency to become blocked on one or more specific sounds (e.g., /s/, /f/, /b/, or /d/).

The Onset of Stuttering

One of the most useful pieces of information we have about the cause of stuttering is that it rarely begins from the child's first utterance (Yairi, 1997a). Children who go on to stutter do not seem to have difficulty with the earliest speech sounds, such as cooing and babbling. Additionally, most of them appear to build up a sizable vocabulary and demonstrate a good base of grammatical structure before ever exhibiting difficulty with disruptions of fluency (Watkins, Yairi, & Ambrose, 1999). There is general agreement that stuttering begins about the age of two years, with most cases being evident by the age of five (Andrews, 1983). However, a few children do not begin to stutter until as late as age seven or even later. Reports that children have stuttered "from the beginning" are generally unsubstantiated and may be the result of coloring provided by later parental memories (Lankford & Cooper, 1974). Some individuals may not begin stuttering until as late as the mid-teen years, but this is unusual and is more likely to be the result of physical brain trauma or an acute psychological reaction (Guitar, 1998). In our experience, initial reports by children or adolescents who began stuttering at the age of eight or nine are often revised by memories of relatively minor earlier fluency problems, which are refreshed once the stuttering begins to be resolved or early difficult speaking experiences are recalled.

There is no evidence to suggest that developmental stuttering is caused entirely by a physical or purely psychological trauma (Vabiro & Engelmayer, 1972). In our experience, case histories of individuals who stutter are usually devoid of such experiences. In fact, stuttering usually begins at a time when the child is integrating speech and language skills within a changing physical and neurological makeup during a dynamic expansion of communication demands, personal interactions, and situational experiences. As a result, stuttering is more accurately associated with an interaction between internal, physical characteristics and external, environmental factors (Starkweather, 1997; Guitar, 1998).

Some children begin stuttering as soon as they begin combining words, but most do not start until approximately one year later (i.e., $2^{1}/_{2}$ to 3 years of age; Andrews, 1983; Yairi, 1997a). About 90 percent of the children who stutter begin to do so before the age of six. Figure 1.3 illustrates the age of stuttering onset. Stuttering can begin either gradually or acutely, and its progression is often episodic, containing oscillations that range from no stuttering to mild to severe across communicative tasks and time. Repetitions of sounds or syllables occurring on initial words or utterances are the most frequent type of dysfluency noted in children who are beginning to stutter (Bloodstein, 1995). Other dysfluencies include stretching of the sound or syllable (i.e., prolongations) or momentary blocking during attempts to say a word.

Research indicates three-fourths or more of very young children who stutter are prone to recover without any form of treatment (Andrews & Harris, 1964; Glasner & Rosenthal, 1957; Johnson et al., 1959; Yairi & Ambrose, 1992; Yairi, Ambrose, & Niermann, 1993; Yairi, Ambrose, Paden, & Throneburg, 1996; Yairi & Ambrose, 1999), but it is important to note that such figures may omit many who will not recover their fluency. This high reported recovery rate may not apply to children over the age of five who have been stuttering for a year or more (Ramig, 1993). Although some indicators have been identified to help determine which children are more or less likely to recover from their stuttering, at this time we have no reliable and consistent protocol for doing so. As a result, most authorities on stuttering recommend positive, supportive early treatment in the belief that the eradication of stuttering is possible for those less likely to recover otherwise (Gregory & Hill, 1980; Starkweather, Gottwald, & Halfond, 1990; Starkweather, 1997).

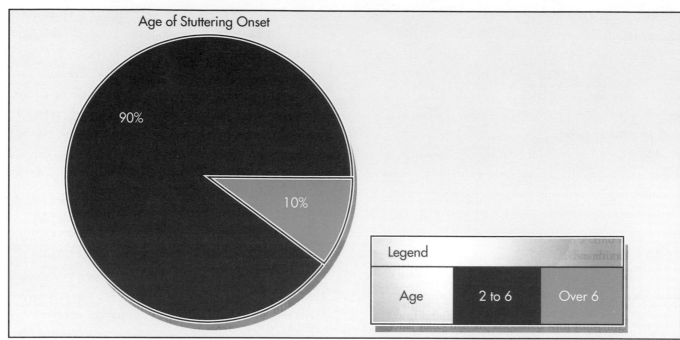

Figure 1.3 Age of Stuttering Onset

What Causes Stuttering?

One of the first questions that parents, people who stutter, clinicians, and observers ask is, "What causes stuttering?" Many theoreticians and researchers have tackled this problem, with only partial success. We perhaps know more about what does *not* cause stuttering, or about factors less related to its cause, than we do about the actual mechanism. As far as the development of stuttering is concerned, we have a considerable mass of observations, clinical experience, and personal anecdotes that, taken together, provide several possible paths of development, as well as a large body of information about the therapy and recovery process. Unfortunately, it is very difficult—some would say impossible—to quantify all this information in a manner that provides an indisputable, "objective," scientific base.

Persistent stuttering is a complex and multifaceted disorder (Zimmermann, Smith, & Hanley, 1981; Smith & Kelly, 1997). The specific cause(s) are not fully understood; however, significant gains in research in the past 10 years have contributed to our better understanding of its complexities. In the distant past, many theorists and clinicians—including speech-language pathologists, psychologists, psychiatrists, and physicians—targeted the parent as the most probable culprit

in the development of childhood stuttering (Johnson, 1942, 1955; Johnson et al., 1959). In sharp contrast, we want to emphasize that the vast majority of stuttering researchers and specialists currently do not believe parents or other caregivers directly cause children to stutter. Nor do experts believe that children "catch" stuttering from hearing a parent, relative, neighbor, or schoolmate who stutters (Yairi, 1997b; Guitar, 1998). There is no credible research to support these age-old theories placing blame on parents and other important persons in the life of the child. Understandably, we, as practicing specialists of stuttering, continue to see many caregivers who feel guilt, and even shame, fearing that they somehow are at fault for their child's inability to speak fluently. Fortunately, and in contravention of the old finger-pointing scenarios, recent research incorporating improved brain-scanning technologies and knowledge of genetics further supports what many of us now believe; that is, there is likely a neurological predisposition to stutter that is in many cases genetically transmitted (Felsenfeld, 1997; Ingham, 2001). Based on research, there appear to be differences in the neuromuscular and neurophysiological systems of persons who stutter (Zimmermann, 1980; Kent, 1984; Geschwind & Galaburda, 1985; Neilson & Neilson, 1987; Perkins, Kent, & Curlee; 1991; Wingate, 2002).

Therefore, it is increasingly clear that stuttering is not "in the ears of the parents," as Johnson claimed (1955). Indeed, parents and caregivers should be reassured that the underlying cause of their child's stuttering is unlikely to relate either to poor parenting skills or to anything they did in raising their child. That is, a child's predisposition to stutter is neurological, not parental, in origin.

Physical or Neurological Characteristics Associated with Stuttering

What physical or neurological characteristics may be associated with the start and development of stuttering? Unfortunately, that is very difficult to determine from the results of available research studies, which commonly use adults who stutter. As a result, it is very difficult to determine whether observable differences are indicative of the cause or the result of stuttering. The physical and functional differences measured by brain-scan research efforts suffer from the same uncertainties. Researchers at Tulane (Foundas, Bollich, & Corey, 2001) have measured statistically significant size and other physical differences in several areas associated with speech and language skills. Such results may indicate that a larger-than-normal fold in the brain area associated with voluntary speech planning and monitoring results in the creation of competing commands that interfere with fluent speech. However, an alternative interpretation argues that certain brain areas overdevelop in stutterers during early childhood due to the child's attempts to voluntarily control or monitor dysfluencies.

Likewise, statistically manipulated functional measurements using brain imaging equipment show that the left-hemisphere speech and auditory brain areas of people who stutter are significantly less active (and the right hemisphere more active) during stuttering than people who are fluent and the same stuttering subjects when they are speaking fluently (Wood, Stump, McKeehan, Sheldon, & Proctor, 1980; Pool, Devous, Freeman, Watson, & Finitzo, 1991; Wu et al., 1995; Fox, Ingham, Ingham et al., 1996; Ingham, Fox, Ingham, Zamarripa, Jerabek, & Cotton, 1996; Braun et al., 1997; Fox, Ingham, George, et al., 1997; De Nil, Kroll, Kapur, & Houle, 1998; Salmelin, Schnitzler, Schmitz, Jäncke, Witte, & Freund, 1998; De Nil, Kroll, Kapur, & Houle, 2000; Fox, Ingham, Ingham, Zamarripa, Xiong, & Lancaster, 2000; Ingham, Fox, Ingham, & Zamarripa, 2000; Salmelin, Schnitzler, Schmitz, & Freund, 2000; Ingham, 2001; Ingham, 2003; Stager, Jeffries, & Braun, 2003; Ingham, Fox, Ingham, Xiong, Zamarripa, Hardies, & Lancaster, 2004). One common interpretation of these results is that something is physically wrong with the observed, inactive brain areas that prevent them from functioning normally. However, an alternative interpretation holds that another part of the brain is disrupting the cortical areas that appear inactive during stuttering. The observed inactivity could thus be the consequence of stuttering, rather than its cause.

Another study of 15 people who stutter (Sommer, Koch, Paulus, Weiller, & Buechel, 2002) measured the diffusion characteristics of the neurons in the motor speech-language planning areas in the left hemisphere and found that the neurons were not aligned as well with the direction of transmission as the neurons in the brains of 14 people who were fluent. Again, this is an interesting and perhaps useful finding about the brains of people who stutter. But because diffusion and neuron myelination continue to develop throughout life, it may very well be that the disruption of speech-motor planning (or the attempt to control the planning process through inhibition) was partially responsible for the difference observed in people who stutter.

Does It Matter that the Precise Cause of Stuttering Is Not Known?

We know that there is a disruption of speech fluency associated with stuttering that is reflected by actual differences in the structure and function of the brain (Foundas, Bollich, & Corey, 2001; Ingham, 2001). Whether these neurological differences are the cause or the result of stuttering (or both) is less important than the fact that therapy techniques are available that can effectively alleviate these speech disruptions. In fact, other studies have reported increased normalization in speech-language brain function following stuttering therapy (De Nil et al., 2000). Although speech therapy would probably significantly improve if a precise cause of suffering were known, speech-language pathologists have demonstrated an ability to help clients to modify and reverse the development of stuttering through the use of many of the techniques described in this book. Also, the recovery process helps us infer quite a bit about the possible causes and dynamics of stuttering.

How Stuttering Develops

Once the child begins to experience disruptions in fluency, the progress and development of stuttering symptoms and behaviors can be surprisingly rapid (Yairi, 1997a; Guitar, 1998). Our theory of development involves the idea of the occurrence of original dysfluencies or events that cause the child's attention to his or her speech to become negatively stimulated. Contributors to the development of stuttering may be the negative aspect, the extent, or the intensity of this attention. Other contributions may be the child's unconscious and conscious attempts to cope with or correct dysfluencies (see Figure 1.4).

This process places initial speech dysfluencies in competition with a preexisting model of speech behaviors. Internally, this preexisting model of speech may include an innate or developed speech-motor or speech-monitoring "program" or

schema. Externally, it may represent the fluent speech patterns of others in the child's environment. Thus, the child may negatively compare early dysfluent episodes to previously developed internal and external references of fluency. In response to this negative emotional assessment, it appears that the child naturally attempts to cope with, control, or modify subsequent perturbations. For many or most children, this may involve pushing, tensing, and forcing of the speech articulators (e.g., vocal cords, tongue, lips, jaw) that introduce an inappropriate amount of energy into the speech-motor system, which precipitates further breakdowns.

At this point, this process is primarily internal to the child. It is for this reason that we and most other stuttering specialists believe that parents do not directly cause their child's stuttering. Stuttering begins with the child himself, and its initial appearance is related to one or more of the neurological factors discussed earlier. Even so, people in the child's environment can affect the development of stuttering and can positively or negatively influence the course of its development. For example, when others listen attentively and demonstrate acceptance during the child's dysfluencies,

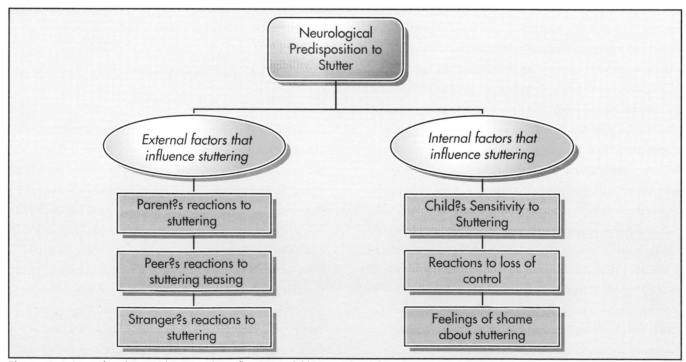

Figure 1.4 Internal and External Factors That Influence a Child's Neurological Predisposition to Stutter

negative external messages will less likely reinforce the child's negative internal reactions. One hopes that the child's internal reactions will diminish over time as they fail to resonate with external reactions from others. It is sometimes difficult, however, for listeners to totally mask emotional reactions when a child is experiencing problems, particularly if they care a great deal about the child. These reactions are natural and are not the fault of the parents or caregivers. In these instances, it can be helpful for others to verbally reassure the child of their support.

In our experience, several months after the onset of stuttering symptoms, the child's negative reactions to speech seem to become more difficult to reverse without direct intervention. Recent research suggests that children whose stuttering has persisted for more than 18 months without intervention are more likely to continue to stutter (Yairi et al., 1996). The central nervous system of a 3½ year-old child is developing rapidly and is highly susceptible to the creation of conditioned responses (automatic reactions to stimuli first described in the famous experiments by Pavlov). Negative experiences are more likely to have long-lasting effects on the implicit (unconscious) and explicit (conscious) memory systems of very young children. Because these early learning experiences strongly influence lifelong development of children, these memories are deeply ingrained and may indeed be permanent (LeDoux, 1996, 2001), creating long-lasting secondary responses that make stuttering worse and more difficult to overcome. This does not mean that stuttering therapy cannot be effective in increasing fluency, particularly in those who have a genetic predisposition for recovery (Kidd, 1984; Yairi et al., 1996). It does suggest, however, one reason why stuttering is so persistent and why a "cure" for chronic stuttering occurs only rarely.

Conture (1990) provides an excellent summary of the strengths and weaknesses of various theories of stuttering causation and development. For most purposes, it is enough to understand that a behavior as complex as developmental stuttering is not caused *exclusively* either by genetic or by environmental factors, but by an *interaction* of both factors. The therapy approach described in this book is designed to treat stuttering from an interactive and holistic perspective.

Parents Do Not Cause Stuttering, But They May Contribute to Its Development and Maintenance

As discussed earlier, evidence does not support the premise that parents are responsible for initially causing stuttering. It is nevertheless important to understand that once stuttering begins, they can and often do play a vital role in the child or adolescent's change and recovery (Sheehan, 1970, 1975; Van Riper, 1973; Starkweather, 1987; Bloodstein, 1995; Guitar, 1998). For example, a hectic, punitive, judgmental home environment—including parental pressures on the child to speak perfectly, to use complex vocabulary, or to continuously implement speech fluency techniques—may exacerbate his stuttering. Many of us believe the aforementioned examples fuel stuttering by reinforcing to the child that he can please his parents if he does not stutter. As a result, children naturally expend a great deal of physical and emotional energy attempting not to stutter. Some children may increase muscular tension to force through the stuttering; others may hesitate during speech and develop a vast array of avoidance strategies. These initial, internalized attempts to control or eliminate dysfluencies can produce a vicious cycle of stuttering that worsens over time (Figure 1.5).

In response to the fear of incipient stuttering, muscular tension levels often elevate and precipitate more stuttering. The additional dysfluencies amplify the child's fear of stuttering and his desire to avoid it in the future. Although these avoidance strategies may work temporarily for many, the long-term consequences of such behavior only produce more sophisticated and insidious avoidances as the old ones lose effectiveness (Sheehan, 1998). We call this the Vicious Cycle Syndrome: the more someone tries not to stutter, the worse the problem may become.

In contrast, a more relaxed, understanding, and accepting home environment may contribute to the reduction or

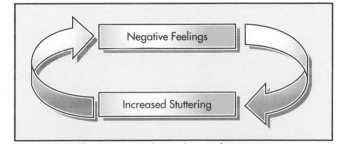

Figure 1.5 The Vicious Cycle Syndrome of Stuttering

eventual disappearance of stuttering in the young child. Once the problem manifests itself, the parents do play a significant role. Thus, parental involvement and responsibility become paramount. As explained earlier, caregivers do not explicitly cause stuttering, but a less-than-healthy home environment may contribute to its maintenance or exacerbation. The child, too, can be his own worst critic, possibly contributing unknowingly to his own difficulty. We have seen many children and adolescents who stutter who appear to combine perfectionistic tendencies with an increased sensitivity to environmental changes and activities. We know that stuttering is an observable disorder that parents and others can see, but for the child or adolescent it is also an internal process that appears to exhibit both conscious and unconscious elements. Because of the emotional impact stuttering can have, it is imperative for the caregiver and clinician to treat the child or adolescent with the utmost respect and understanding. Negative actions or words directed at the child or adolescent in response to stuttering are inappropriate and unacceptable.

Our View of Stuttering: Reaction to the Unpleasantness of Stuttering Often Creates Muscular Tension and Contributes to Increased Stuttering

Often, more stuttering is created as a result of pushing and forcing at one or more vocal tract locations during the articulation of speech. For example, when a /p/ sound is produced,

the lips come together to create a rapid, momentary buildup of air pressure behind delicately compressed lips. The lips then open, allowing a sudden release of air from the mouth, which creates the sound we perceive as a /p/. From start to finish, the speech mechanism produces individual sounds in milliseconds of time. For children and adolescents who stutter, however, the frustration of not being able to easily and freely generate fluent speech, as well as learned apprehension or fear they experience from feeling different, translate into an increase in muscular tension at the place of articulation and often throughout the speech mechanism and body. This increased muscular tension is part of the makeup of stuttering, and is in part largely responsible for an increase in the frequency and duration of stuttering. It is this buildup of tension that the child or adolescent produces in his attempts to force his way through the stuttering episode that often creates more stuttering. This response is a normal reaction to the unpleasant experience of feeling stuck, embarrassed, frustrated, and so on, but this normal reaction is counterproductive to the normal functioning of a very delicate and complex speech production system. In that regard, we strive to teach children or adolescents to react to anticipated stuttering without resorting to the gut reaction of fighting and forcing through it. Their innate reaction to apprehension, fear, and frustration only serves to interfere with the smooth operation of the complex, delicate system that is necessary for creating fluent speech. Although this frustration and tension is not viewed by most modern researchers as the cause of stuttering, there is little doubt that it is a contributing factor known to increase existing stuttering.

CHAPTER 2: Strategies for Counseling Parents of Children Who Stutter

Professional counseling of parents of children who stutter is one of the most important responsibilities we face as clinicians working in the area of fluency disorders. As described elsewhere in this text, parents naturally experience powerful emotions and develop genuine concern when faced with a child or adolescent who stutters. In our experience, the severity of stuttering exhibited by the child often influences the degree of parental concern. For example, most parents react with more concern if their child overtly struggles when speaking than if he exhibits occasional, less severe dysfluencies.

Why Parent Involvement Is Important

Articles and texts addressing parent involvement in the treatment of children who stutter reveal a wide range of expectations as to the role the primary caregivers are encouraged to take (e.g., Ramig, 1993; Ramig & Bennett, 1995; Rustin & Cook, 1995; Yairi, 1997a; Guitar, 1998; Zebrowski & Kelly, 2002; Hill, 2003; Onslow, Packman, & Harrison, 2003). Although most clinicians work directly with the child and counsel the parents during the intervention process, the Lidcombe Program of Early Stuttering Intervention described by Onslow, Packman, and Harrison (2003) trains the parent(s) to serve as the primary "clinician" from the beginning. Our approach has been one of cooperative collaboration between parents and clinicians who work in concert to facilitate the child's experiences with speech and communication (e.g., Ramig, 1993; Ramig & Bennett, 1997). Figure 2.1 illustrates what we consider to be a continuum of clinical expectations.

In our experience dealing with hundreds of parents and other primary caregivers of children whom we have evaluated, parents invariably express genuine concern about their child's stuttering. They want to understand what is happening to their child, why it is happening, and what they can do to help. In response, we answer their questions and provide encouragement and support. This support may be indirect to the child, as we work directly with parents to educate them in the best ways to help their child. In other cases, it may mean working directly with the child in therapy while providing general guidance and support to the parents. Whichever path the clinician chooses, parent involvement is highly encouraged.

It is natural for parents to attempt to help their child when he is having difficulty speaking. Before we are contacted for advice, many parents have already begun to intervene on their own: telling the child to "Slow down," to "Think about what you want to say," or to "Take a deep breath" in response to stuttering. Occasionally, parents respond in a negative, perhaps punitive manner when they interpret the stuttering as an attempt to get attention (Moncur, 1952; Kasprisin-Burrelli, Egolf, & Shames, 1972; Langlois, Hanrahan, & Inouye, 1986; Zebrowski & Conture, 1989; Yairi, 1997a, 1997b). Such negative reactions, though relatively uncommon, are particularly unhelpful (Conture, 1990).

Although the more common requests by parents to reduce speaking rate, or to breathe more easily, may seem logical, many clinicians of stuttering do not recommend that parents verbally correct their child in such a manner. As clinicians, we are concerned that these parental comments may cause the child to feel that he is doing something "bad" or "wrong" (Gildston, 1967; Yairi & Williams, 1971). After all, whenever the child speaks, his parents correct him! Because he learns through his parents' reactions that his speaking behavior is unacceptable, the child may begin trying harder to hide his stuttering, which often makes it worse (Van Riper, 1973;

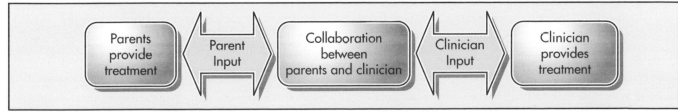

Figure 2.1 The Continuum of Clinical Expectations

Guitar, 1998). This may help explain how parents unintentionally exacerbate their child's stuttering (Starkweather, Gottwald, & Halfond, 1990; Starkweather, 1997). In other words, even if neither the parents' reactions nor the child's environment causes stuttering to begin with, their reactions may help or hinder the child's speech fluency.

In general, allow the child the time he needs to speak even if he is obviously stuttering (Gregory & Gregory, 1999). Patience is a virtue here. However, this does not mean a parent should ignore stuttering if the child verbally addresses his difficulty, or if he shows obvious signs of frustration or avoidance of speech (Logan & Caruso, 1997). For example, parents should be encouraged to address the child's reactions by casually commenting on signs of frustration:

- "Everyone has trouble talking sometimes. Mommy does, Daddy does. It's okay. Mommy will wait for you."

- "Yeah, that was a hard one. No problem, though, Daddy will always wait for you to finish."

- "Let's say that hard, bumpy word together so we can make it come out easier."

Completely ignoring the obvious by not addressing it when the child is reacting negatively can lead the child to believe that his stuttering is shameful and bad. He may begin to believe that his problem is so bad, not even Mommy or Daddy will talk about it. We believe this way of thinking is harmful to the child. As an alternative, it is important to emphasize that parents should respond to the child's reaction to his difficulty with comments that are casual and reassuring. We recommend this strategy because it is our intent to demonstrate, by our responses, that his "bobbles" are no big deal; as a result, it is our hope that he will be less likely to develop further fear and avoidance patterns.

Teaching strategies to change parental speaking style can be helpful in decreasing tension in the environment, and may be beneficial in slowing down the child's rate of speech (Starkweather, 1997). Such changes include slower rate, relaxed pauses, turn-taking, and other behaviors that are viewed as helpful. The logic here is that a more relaxed speech environment may help the child to be more fluent by allowing more time for coordinating the motor movements necessary to operate the highly complex and sophisticated

speech production system. However, as described earlier, the parent is discouraged from telling the child to speak in a different way. Instead, parents should be taught strategies such as pausing between sentences and before responding to others, that may eventually be learned by the child as a result of hearing this model from the parents (Van Riper, 1973). Figure 2.2 illustrates the beneficial effects of modeling in the home environment.

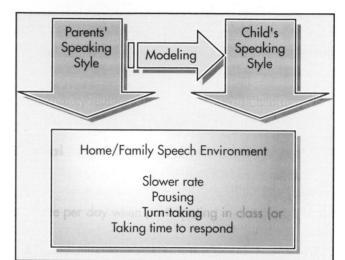

Figure 2.2 The Beneficial Effects of Modeling in the Home Environment

All knowledgeable and successful clinicians of stuttering have worked with some children who progress slowly in treatment and relapse periodically. Although this is a fairly common experience along the road to recovery, it can be frustrating to parents. For this reason, we include this topic of discussion as part of our parent interview during the evaluation process. We want parents to understand that this can happen and that it is not unusual (Gregory, 1991; Ramig & Bennett, 1995). In such cases, it is especially important that parents feel free to consult with us about their concerns, fears, and apprehensions. A concerned parent may need our support as much as, or more than, the child during periods of relapse. For information on counseling parents of children who stutter, the clinician is encouraged to view the Stuttering Foundation video, *Counseling: Listening to and Talking with Parents of Children Who Stutter* (2003). Accompanying this tape is a booklet that also contains important information for the professional speech-language clinician.

As described by Ramig (1993), parents should be encouraged to be active participants in the intervention process. Their involvement begins with their observation of several sessions. Next, they are encouraged to actively participate in a specified number of sessions. Specifically, they become part of the activities and practice the same strategies as their child. The clinician is the guide throughout all of the sessions involving direct parent involvement (Perkins, 1992). We have found this strategy to be helpful in ensuring that the parents become the positive role models we wish them to be, enhancing their ability to react and interact helpfully with the child outside of the formal treatment environment. Recall our mention of the Lidcombe program (Onslow et al., 2003), the underlying philosophy and approach of which encourage parents to be trained by the speech-language pathologist to become the primary "clinician." That is, the clinician's purpose is to train the parent to work directly with the child and to become the sole provider of what is, in most other stuttering treatment programs, the primary responsibility of the speech-language pathologist. Assuming that the clinician is properly trained in the Lidcombe approach, we feel this program is suitable for some young children who stutter and their parents, especially those cases in which parents want to play a dominant role in helping their child change. However, for other parents who are unable or unwilling to assume this responsibility, or if the clinician has not been trained to administer this type of treatment, this approach is not advised.

Much of what we have addressed thus far has dealt with changes that can be made through direct or indirect guided parent involvement. Pursuing the likelihood of parent influence on the problem of stuttering brings us to suggestions for helping parents identify and reduce possible disruptors of fluency that may exist in the home environment of the stuttering child (Botterill, Kelmaii, & Rustin, 1991; Kelly & Conture, 1991). Once the parents feel the caring and concern the clinician has for their child, and have a higher level of knowledge about stuttering, it is relatively easy to talk directly about environmental factors that could maintain or exacerbate the child's stuttering (Figure 2.3). These include, for example, parent(s) who speak rapidly or move quickly from task to task; dissension between family members; parents who schedule too many activities, have unrealistic

performance expectations, or are overly critical of the child's speech; or food products that can cause behavior changes in susceptible children (Ramig, 1993; Starkweather, 1997).

Figure 2.3 Possible Exacerbating Environmental Factors and Behaviors

- Speaking rapidly
- Moving quickly from task to task
- Creating tension in the home by dissension among family members
- Scheduling too many activities that could place stress on the child
- Having unrealistic performance expectations
- Reacting critically to the child's speech
- Eating foods that cause behavior changes in susceptible children

Similarly, siblings can have an undesired influence on the child who stutters if they tease him and/or dominate speaking interactions, causing him to become frustrated (Guitar, 1998). Creating a positive working partnership with parents is often as important as working directly with the child who is struggling with stuttering. When the parent interactions and home environment are in synchrony with factors that we believe facilitate fluency, the child's chances for recovery increase.

What Parents Need to Know about Helping Their Child Speak More Fluently

There are a number of things parents need to know that can be helpful in achieving greater fluency for their child. These are outlined in Figure 2.4 and discussed briefly in the following section.

Minimize Interruptions. Adults can set the example of waiting until the speaker is finished talking before they initiate speaking. Interrupting can create stress and possibly maintain or exacerbate stuttering.

Speak Slower. Slowing down the rate of speaking helps. This can be accomplished by pausing frequently between sentences and by slightly stretching out words within

Figure 2.4 What Parents Need to Know about Helping the Child Speak More Fluently

- Minimize interruptions
- Speak slower
- Respect silence
- Minimize rushing and hurrying
- Ask one question at a time
- Avoid "show and tell"
- Talk about meaningful topics
- Read to your child
- Talk about stuttering
- Lessen conversation when he is more dysfluent
- Insert short, easy, stutter-like mistakes in your speech
- Teach turn-taking
- Build self-confidence

sentences. This slower rate should be within the normal speaking and inflection range, but should be slow-normal. It should not sound mechanical or monotone.

Respect Silence. Silence is all right. Fostering and modeling normal periods of silence can help reduce the stress created from feeling pressure to speak.

Minimize Rushing and Hurrying. Starting off the day in a rushed or hurried manner can, for example, be significantly reduced by setting alarm clocks 10 minutes earlier during the workweek. Early-morning scurrying to eat breakfast, bathe, dress, and so on can create a stressful beginning to the child's day. Such experiences may create tension that can fuel stuttering.

Ask One Question at a Time. Asking multiple questions in succession is a common occurrence in even the most positive home environments. A way of reducing stress is to ask simple questions one at a time.

Avoid "Show and Tell." Parents often want their children to show family and friends how much they know. However, on days when the child is experiencing more stuttering, we recommend avoiding this possibly stressful performance situation.

Talk about Meaningful Topics. Talking about topics that interest the child is important. People, objects, activities, books, movies, and other items and areas of interest can be an enjoyable and positive speaking experience.

Read to Your Child. Using slightly exaggerated inflection, and a slow and relaxed rate, read books of interest to the child. Sitting on the parent's lap can be a positive and safe bonding experience for the child. Setting aside a consistent time to do this activity can be rewarding and fluency-enhancing for the child.

Talk about Stuttering. This is recommended only when the child shows signs of discomfort with his repeating, prolonging, or blocking of sounds. There is no need to fear addressing harder stuttering episodes to which the child is reacting. This is often a moment of discomfort, so support him by making nonchalant comments such as, "That's okay, Jimmie, everyone gets bumpy sometimes. Mommy does, Daddy does, everyone does sometimes. It's okay." This can be followed up with, "Mommy/Daddy will wait for you to finish." The speech-language clinician can offer other suggestions based on her knowledge of the child and his stuttering patterns.

Lessen Conversation when He Is More Dysfluent. Stuttering fluctuates. On days when the child is struggling more, we recommend asking fewer questions that require lengthy answers; instead, ask more questions that require one-word or two-word responses. Many children experience less stuttering when the complexity of the language is reduced through use of shorter, simpler utterances.

Insert Short, Easy, Stutter-Like Mistakes in Your Speech. Inserting normal-sounding "mistakes" in one's speech, such as frequent pausing, tension-free repeating, and occasional stretches of sounds, without any apparent reaction, can show the child that everyone makes mistakes when they talk. Instilling this concept through modeling can be helpful to children who are reacting to their stuttering.

Teach Turn-Taking. The dinner table is a place where turn-taking can be encouraged. Use an object the child likes as a way to signify whose turn it is to speak; this teaches others to wait while a family member is talking. The person speaks only when the object is passed to him. Upon completing his speaking, he passes the object to another family member who wishes to speak.

Build Self-Confidence. Promoting and supporting activities and experiences that help the child feel good about himself is another important goal. Persistent stuttering can erode a child's self-confidence, so it is crucial for parents to provide opportunities for him to succeed in whatever activities he enjoys.

Goals of the Assessment

This chapter is intended for the speech-language pathologist (SLP) who is tasked with the challenge of assessing the fluency of children and adolescents. An assessment of fluency disorders is not merely an "on-ramp" or an "off-ramp" for stuttering treatment. Although a primary goal of clinical assessment is to determine whether a problem exists that would require treatment, sometimes the severity of the problem and the prognosis regarding treatment cannot be determined from an initial assessment (Conture, 1997; Guitar, 1998). For one, the child may be having a good day and consequently not stuttering very much. Also, the child may effectively use postponement or avoidance strategies that, on the surface, hide any difficulties. In the case of aberrant or disorganized speech, it may be difficult for the clinician to differentiate between cluttering, stuttering, or a combination of the two. Although stuttering for attention is extremely rare, it remains a possibility. Also, the initial referral may be based on confusion between normal mistakes (disfluencies or normal nonfluencies) and stuttering.

Figure 3.1 illustrates the basic assessment procedure. The goal of the assessment should be to begin an investigation and exploration of speech behaviors that someone has identified as problematic. The strategies for the assessment should be selected to obtain information about the problem and create an environment conducive to allowing the child to demonstrate, reveal, and share feelings and thoughts about the problem in your presence. Only by keeping an open mind will the clinician be able to recognize the "problem" behavior for what it actually is. This does not mean that the clinician should leave her professional experience at the door. It does mean that this knowledge must be applied to objective, scientific inquiry. It can be too easy to jump to conclusions, for example, about the severity of stuttering behavior. Until all the evidence has been examined (including video and audio tapes made at the assessment or in the child's home environment), it is premature to make pronouncements of any kind.

Differential diagnosis (Figure 3.2) is an important element of fluency assessment (Ambrose & Yairi, 1999; Hill, 1999; Onslow & Packman, 2001). Differential diagnosis not only involves identifying the severity and impact of the problem displayed by the client, but also means discovering the behaviors that make up the individual's condition. In addition, it is important to document other concomitant and simultaneous speech and language problems, as well as environmental influences that may be causing, maintaining, or exacerbating the client's problem. Within the developmental stuttering population alone, there is an almost infinite variety of stuttering behaviors and severities, with an attendant infinite range of variations in the situations in which different severities of stuttering occur (Conture, 1997, 2001). There are other types of dysfluency as well that will have to be considered, including cluttering, neurogenic stuttering, and stuttering-like dysfluencies associated with language problems or delays.

Cluttering is a syndrome characterized by a speech delivery rate that is either abnormally fast, irregular, or both. In cluttered speech, the person's speech is affected by one or more of the following: (1) failure to maintain normally expected sound, syllable, phrase, and pausing patterns; (2) evidence of more frequent than expected incidents of disfluency, the majority of which are unlike those typical of people who stutter (St. Louis, Raphael, Myers, & Bakker, 2003). Neurogenic stuttering, in contrast, typically refers to the often-transient stuttering that results from a specific neurological insult or lesion. It is generally observed in adults who have suffered confirmed brain damage (ASHA, 2002).

Private Practice versus School-Based Fluency Assessments

Some important differences exist between the goals of assessments conducted in private practice and university settings and those associated with school-based special education services. The differences in resources and in availability of the primary caregivers must also be considered.

Advantages of the private practice-based or university-based assessment are that the clinician normally has more time to conduct the evaluation, one or more caregivers may be available for interviewing, and the child's dysfluencies have probably already been acknowledged as an appropriate

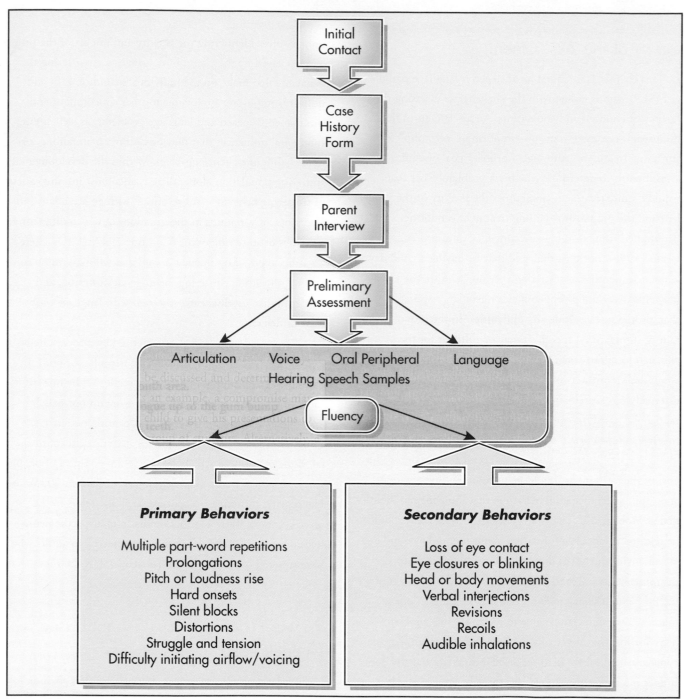

Figure 3.1 Basic Assessment Procedure

area for concern. The child's speech and language abilities may already have been evaluated by a school SLP or local diagnostic center and substantial language testing results may be available. Note that the presence of this information does not mean that the private practice or university clinician should not conduct a thorough independent evaluation. Many school clinicians have limited experience with stutter-

ing and may even be restricted by school policies or parental preference from working with dysfluent children, particularly stutterers in their adolescent and teen years. Disadvantages of private practice assessments are that the clinician may not have immediate access to other important people, such as teachers, in the child's communication sphere. Figure 3.3 highlights these relative strengths and weaknesses.

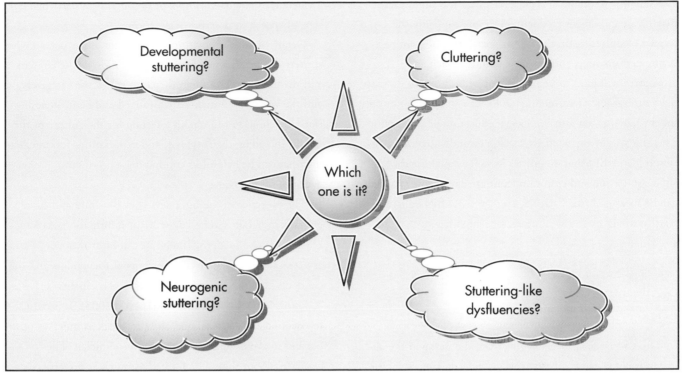

Figure 3.2 Differential Diagnosis

School-based clinicians may have several important advantages over those in private practice. For example, the school SLP may have access to the child at a time very early in stuttering development. There is also the opportunity to communicate directly with teachers who have observed the child interacting with his peers, and to observe the child in a classroom setting, where stuttering behaviors may be more severe. Disadvantages include the possibility that the school SLP will experience resistance to a stuttering assessment or its results from the parents or caregivers. Parents who bring their child to a private practitioner may already be committed to the idea of proceeding with treatment. If the goal of the

Private Practice and University Assessment	
Advantages	*Disadvantages*
Usually more time for evaluation Caregivers available for interview Dysfluencies are already identified as a concern Previous testing may be available	Teachers may be unavailable for interview

Figure 3.3 Relative Strengths and Weaknesses of Private Practice and University Assessments

assessment is to obtain special services for the child, there may be a requirement to document more explicitly the impact of stuttering on the child's social development, academic performance, and learning abilities. Such an assessment will have to be performed with an eye to developing a rationale for treatment, should it be indicated, not only for the parents, but also for special education administrators. The SLP will be expected to develop an individualized education plan (IEP) that quantifies as well as qualifies the child's stuttering and communication behavior in a way that can be measured (see Chapter 4). Figure 3.4 highlights the relative strengths and weaknesses of school-based assessments.

Strategies for Conducting the Background Interview

The assessment process begins from the moment the clinician is contacted by the person needing therapy or by his caregivers. During initial contact, the activities planned for the assessment should be explained in a manner that motivates the parents to participate in the assessment process. For example, a clinician should provide a rationale for requesting a videotaped language sample or for eliciting a particular type of speech in the assessment room.

Details about the environment and life of the person who stutters can be obtained by paying attention to the content and manner of questioning, the concerns of the caregivers, and the way appointments are arranged and kept. In addition, the clinician can obtain a feeling for the culture of the family, including their style of, and expectations for, interacting, that can be helpful in conducting a productive background interview.

The objective of the interview with the child and caregivers is to obtain several key types of information. As long as these are obtained, the interview can be as short or as long as necessary, focusing on the concerns of the parents and the child, and building rapport among the participants (Haynes & Pindzola, 1998; Conture, 2001; Hill, 2003). It is critical to encourage the parents and child to speak as much as possible and to avoid long discourses by the clinician. The clinician's input should be limited as much as possible to asking questions that elicit detailed and open responses and providing information about specific questions and concerns.

Beginning the interview with a few minutes of relevant light conversation, such as the child's ease or difficulty in

School-Based Assessment	
Advantages	*Disadvantages*
Early access to child	May encounter resistance
Teachers available for interview	Must document educational impact
Able to observe child in school environment with peers	

Figure 3.4 Relative Strengths and Weaknesses of School-Based Assessments

making it to the clinic or plans for the remainder of the day, is a good way of assessing the communication style of the parents and child. It may also provide information about the pace with which they would like the assessment conducted, and provide important cultural cues that can be used to guide the interview and assessment process. Interviewees who are anxious to "get down to business" may be easier to obtain information from, but they may also be more interested in completing the interview in a hurry. Excessive haste may result in the clinician not obtaining important facts.

Darley and Spriestersbach (1978) provide some general advice about interviewing style, such as avoiding yes/no questions, sequencing of questions according to the anxiety level of the information, building rapport by starting with more factual material, and maintaining a brisk pace to obtain more pertinent information. They also point out the importance of noting discrepancies in responses and returning to these later in the interview, rather than bluntly challenging the informant's honesty or consistency. Figure 3.5 provides some general categories of questions that a clinician may want to use when interviewing parents.

Figure 3.5 Parent Interview Question Categories

- Motivation
- Family background
- Characteristics of present stuttering
- Development course
- Communication abilities and style
- Degree of awareness, handicap, or adjustment
- Environmental influences
- Parent/child relationship
- Skills, interests, and locus of control

The clinician must always be prepared for, and be willing to welcome and learn from, expressions of emotion during fluency evaluations. Emotions that may be encountered or signaled by the behavior of interviewees include anger, frustration, anxiety, fear, sadness, grief, and even indifference. These expressions are not something to be downplayed, minimized, or "made better" during the interview. They provide critical information about the affects, personalities, and interactions of the caregivers and child. Feelings about stuttering can be extreme, particularly if the caregivers experience guilt about causing the dysfluencies. Terminating an interview to avoid or cut off emotional displays may send a message that the clinician believes that the feelings expressed are bad or unwanted. Therefore, expression of feelings should be encouraged, though the clinician must realize that attention may have to be tactfully redirected to fluency concerns if the information being provided ranges too far off topic.

Recommended Parent Interview Questions

Handout B: Recommended Parent Interview Questions, located in the Appendix, is a reproducible list of suggested questions for designing an interview session for a particular child. These questions are organized into categories of various kinds of information that you need to obtain to conduct a thorough evaluation. An alternative parent assessment form, developed by Westbrook, is available at the Stuttering Homepage Web site (http://stutteringhomepage.com). This excellent Web site also posts excerpts from the book *Spanish Phrasing for SLPs,* including a list of yes/no questions to ask parents during an assessment (Esckelson & Morales, 1998). These questions are also available on The Stuttering Homepage.

Recommended Interview Questions for Older Children

If the child is older and obviously aware to some extent of his speech problem, the clinician may want to ask some direct questions of the child regarding his awareness of, and reaction to, his stuttering problem. Handout B: Recommended Parent Interview Questions, located in the Appendix, contains a list of these questions for older children. This list may also be used to stimulate conversations about stuttering during therapy. It may be worthwhile to ask the questions again after the child has made some changes in his speech, or even at the end of the direct therapy process.

Preliminary Assessment of Stuttering Severity and Awareness to Determine Style of Evaluation

Even if characterized by prior discussions with the parents, the presenting severity of the child's stuttering and his awareness of his dysfluencies should be determined as soon as possible by eliciting some speech from, or interacting directly with, the child. This will help the clinician decide how direct or indirect the evaluation should be and make a final selection of activities for obtaining the speech samples. If the child is generally not aware of his stuttering, a more indirect approach—focusing on observation—should be used. If the child is aware of or obviously reacting to his dysfluency, this will provide the clinician with an opportunity to learn about the child's feelings about stuttering and (near the end of the assessment) to do some trial therapy or modeling of fluency techniques. This may also provide the child with some comfort and may assist the evaluation. Just a simple sympathetic comment, such as, "Yeah, getting stuck like that can really be tough," may elicit a flood of information that has been bottled up for months or years.

Feelings of Guilt Associated with Stuttering

The one area in which it may be appropriate to intervene during an emotional display is the expression by caregivers of guilt about causing the child's dysfluency. This should be handled factually, rather than by minimizing the expression of feelings. If the clinician senses or is told that feelings of guilt are involved, she should impart the factual information that research has shown that parental behaviors and inherited characteristics are not absolute predictors or causes of stuttering development or severity (see Chapter 1). Some parents may want to argue with this, based on their beliefs about the importance of parental influence on the child's behavior. This should be considered important information for the evaluation rather than a springboard for philosophical discussion or debate at this point.

Materials Required for an Assessment

The assessment process always begins at the first contact with the caregivers or the child. Considerable information can be obtained and imparted over the telephone or, at times, in e-mail communications. The notes made at this time should be saved for incorporation into the assessment. Building rapport and establishing good communication as early as possible—including understanding of cultural factors and family norms and expectations—can save time and increase the accuracy and usefulness of the assessment. Whenever possible, the clinician should send a background information form that can be filled out before the assessment (see Handout B in the Appendix). Permission should also be sought to obtain information from school clinicians and special education personnel, including copies of previous speech and language assessments, psychological assessments, and IEPs.

If possible, an audio or video tape recorded by the parents of the child's speech in the home should be obtained prior to the interview. Such a recording may provide important information about the child's interaction with parents and siblings within the home. Characteristics of speakers within the child's communicative environment, such as speaking rate, turn-taking, and other pragmatic issues, may more efficiently be assessed. This information is also helpful if the child is either shy or uncooperative during the formal assessment.

Equipment at the assessment should include an audiotape recorder, videotape recorder, and plenty of blank tapes (see Figure 3.6). A variety of reading and speech stimulus materials should also be at hand, including standardized tests and games or toys (suggested by the parents before the assessment) for use with young children. Such materials may also be useful to provide scenarios for observations of child and parental interaction. Whenever possible, the clinician should avoid making notes during the interview. Rather, shortly thereafter, she should consult the audio and video tapes made during the interview and make notes during her review.

In addition to the scoring sheets used in tests, such as the *Stuttering Severity Inventory-3 (SSI-3)* (Riley, 1994), the clinician may want to use a reproducible form, such as Handout D: Fluency Evaluation Results, which is provided in the Appendix. Such a form can help limit the writing that has to be done to document the primary and secondary stuttering symptoms observed during the assessment. It also helps make key diagnostic information more accessible.

Figure 3.6 Assessment Materials

- Videotape recorder
- Audiotape recorder
- Plenty of blank video and audio tapes
- Developmentally appropriate reading materials
- Language sample material
- Standardized tests
- *Stuttering Severity Inventory-3 (SSI-3)*
- Parental perception of self-rating forms
- Articulation/phonology tests
- Language tests
- Oral-peripheral test form

The Clinician's Speaking Style during the Assessment

A word of caution must be given here regarding the tendency of clinicians to adopt (consciously or unconsciously) a soothing speaking style that could be detrimental to the assessment process (Figure 3.7). Although speaking too abruptly may be stressful to the parents and the child and should be avoided, it is also undesirable to use too many fluency-enhancing behaviors when the child is present. The clinician may have a habit of using stretches, slow rate speech, or a phonation style that features continuous voicing when interacting with children. Such behaviors may provide the child being assessed with a fluent speech model that tem-

porarily reduces the severity of his stuttering. This is particularly important in the case of stuttering clinicians who may use fluency-enhancing behaviors as a normal part of their verbal interactions. Of course, the child's response to such modeling might be a valuable piece of information near the end of the assessment, when trial therapy or modification stimulus may be conducted.

Strategies for Obtaining Speech Samples

The assessor should vary speaking tasks to provide a broad sample of types of speech by the child. Questions, explanations, responses or answers, and other contextual and noncontextual speech tasks should be used in the assessment. Speech samples should be at least 200 to 300 words in length (Riley, 1994). Samples that reflect a number of communication modes and situations are more useful in diagnosing stuttering than single-task samples. In addition, rather than documenting a single "severity level" of stuttering, the conditions under which various types of dysfluencies were elicited should be carefully recorded and referenced in the assessment report. Discussing severity within a functional context may increase credibility for parents who may be skeptical of, or unduly anxious about, unitary severity results. Such an approach may help parents understand why they have not observed significant stuttering at home but have received reports of high dysfluency levels at day care, preschool, or school.

Contextual versus Noncontextual Speech

Research has indicated (Yaruss, 2001) that noncontextual speech is often associated with more dysfluency than contextual speech that references objects and situations in the immediate environment (or context) (see Figure 3.8). It is important for the assessor to monitor the type of speech commonly used by the child being evaluated and to vary the type of speech her stimuli may elicit. Contextual speech provides the child with visual aids that can be used to limit speaking demands. For this reason, asking the child to describe speech stimulus pictures may not result in satisfactory speech samples, because there may be excessive pointing or use of empty descriptive words such as "this" or "that." If the child tends to resort to such language, the SLP may want to ask questions requiring a more specific answer.

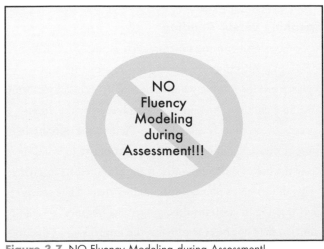

Figure 3.7 NO Fluency Modeling during Assessment!

Badgering or short question–answer exchanges (e.g., "What's this?" or "What's that?") should typically be avoided, though, because they may cause the child to withdraw. Borrowing from the Stocker Probe (Stocker, 1980), "easier" contextual speech situations come first and more difficult, abstract tasks come later.

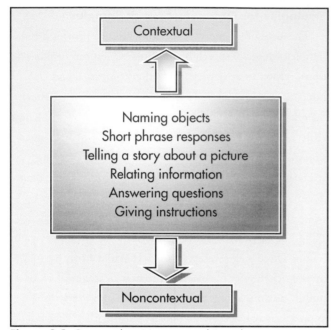

Figure 3.8 Contextual vs. Noncontextual Speech

Using Play or Games to Elicit Speech Samples

One way to obtain natural speech samples in very young children, particularly when the clinician wants to be indirect, is to engage in play with age-appropriate games or toys. Because these are sometimes used in therapy as well as assessment, it is important to avoid teaching or modeling fluency techniques. The assessment itself is a time for interacting and observing.

Most games and toys, such as train sets, farmyard sets, board games (e.g., *Candyland* or *Snail Race*), card games (e.g., *Rug Rats Uno*), and memory-matching games, feature different colors, characters, or objects that provide opportunities for eliciting speech. Games such as *Mr. Potato Head* or *Lego Creator* allow the clinician to set up a request format, in which the child gets to add to a construction pieces that he requests from the clinician. This format is particularly valuable for modifying the stress or time pressure associated with the speaking task.

Determining the Stutterer's Response to, and Feelings about, Stuttering

The clinician should perform some noticeable pseudo-stutters to elicit responses from the child being assessed that indicate his attitude toward or awareness of dysfluencies by others. These should be performed without announcement or drawing attention. Responses may range from early recognition and even criticism (e.g., "Hey, you stuttered! You're not supposed to do that!") to apparent or feigned indifference. At other times, the clinician may have to try many pseudo-stutters before the child appears to notice.

Simplifying Speech to Hide Stuttering

In our experience, children may lower their register (the level of linguistic sophistication used in speech) or simplify their speech to ease the pressure they feel during the assessment. This may simply be a consequence of the stress a child feels when he is expected to perform, but it may also help him hide his stuttering by reducing the complexity of thought and language or to avoid higher-stress speech demands, such as when he is expected to describe without pointing. The assessor should note if the register being used by the child seems inappropriate for his age. If the child's lower register is hindering the collection of more natural speech, the assessor may want to attempt to maintain her own register (assuming it is still age-appropriate for the child) rather than resort to "baby talk." The parents may be able to provide some insight regarding the child's usual speech style and responses under stress.

Speaking versus Reading

Some assessment instruments, such as the *SSI-3* (Riley, 1994), may substitute the description of a picture as a replacement for reading when collecting speech samples from preschool children. It is important to recognize the differences between these speaking tasks. Picture descriptions are more contextual and offer ample opportunities to avoid or delay the use of difficult words. If the child resorts to saying, "This thingy here's gonna crash," rather than, "The spacecraft is going to crash into the gingerbread house," the clinician may not be able to tell if the imprecision is due to avoidance, word-finding difficulties, or the child's expressive language style. However, reading offers no such opportunities, so avoidances or delays are much easier to spot, assuming that the level of the reading material is appropriate for the child's age and ability. In addition, reading and describing are two different tasks that may have different motor or emotional skill associations for the child and therefore may elicit different severities and types of stuttering.

Games during which a child is expected to produce a word or series of words on demand may be a better replacement for reading. Such games include memory-matching games, situation or sequence cards, or request games, where the child must ask for a specific game piece or object to complete, for example, a *Mr. Potato Head* or a *Lego* construction.

Analysis of Stuttering Behavior

The clinician should be able to differentially diagnose normal dysfluencies from the dysfluencies that have been identified as danger signs or warning signs indicating that the child may be at risk for developmental stuttering. Figure 3.9 lists these danger signs.

Figure 3.9 Analysis of Stuttering Behavior: Identification of Danger Signs

- Multiple part-word repetitions
- Prolongations
- Use of the schwa vowel ("uh")
- Struggle, tension, and speed
- Pitch or loudness rise
- Tremors
- Habitual eye closure, rolling, or glazing during dysfluencies
- Avoidance of speaking situations, words, or sounds
- An unusual number of pauses, interjected words, or extraneous sounds
- Fear of speaking

Multiple Part-Word Repetitions

The clinician should note repetitions of first sounds of a word, such as "tu-tu-tu-tu-table," more than one or two times, faster than normal, or with irregular tempo. Although

these have often been distinguished from whole-word repetitions, repetitions of short words such as "I" or "it" or "and" should be noted as well. These may be postponement behaviors to avoid anticipated or feared words or sounds later in an utterance.

Prolongations

Prolongations occur when the child stretches out a sound at the beginning of or (particularly) within a word, such as "r------rabbit" or "raaaaaa----bbit." It is important to distinguish easy stretches (which may be associated with previous therapy or—more unlikely—represent a self-calming mechanism) from prolongations associated with tension or struggle.

Use of the Schwa Vowel ("uh")

Instead of saying "re-re-re-re-read," the child says "ru-ru-ru-ru-read." This behavior indicates that the child is struggling to overcome a feeling of blockage or loss of control. It may also indicate that the child's articulators are in an inappropriate position for the required sound and that the child has lost a measure of awareness due to the impact of the blocking experience.

Struggle, Tension, and Speed

Increased muscular tension in the articulators and rapid movement transitions accompany stuttering that has developed to the point where intervention is needed. To overcome this tension, the child recruits additional surrounding muscles and muscle groups. These behaviors can quickly become conditioned (identified with the original feeling of blockage). This struggle and tension may be seen in the nose, jaw, neck, cheeks, lips, forehead, and upper chest.

Pitch or Loudness Rise

These phenomena may occur at the end of prolongations, when the child is struggling to break out of a block and proceed to the next sound. The child may anticipate or feel that he is going to have difficulty on the sound and the pitch or loudness rise results from the extra energy used to force his way through the block.

Tremors

Tonic quivering of the jaw, lips, and tongue and clonic tremors as the child speaks should be noted. These observations will assist in defining the loci of tension associated with the individual child's stuttering.

Habitual Eye Closure, Rolling, or Glazing during Dysfluencies

Eye involvement of this type may indicate that a pattern of unconscious "escape" behavior has emerged.

Avoidance of Speaking Situations, Words, or Sounds

The child's reluctance to engage in speaking activities may not always indicate avoidance associated with stuttering. There may, however, be other cues that the child is attempting to manage the situation to avoid speaking challenges. These can include continually wanting to change activities, wanting to stop an activity during which he is experiencing a lot of dysfluencies, and postponing by acting out or creating distractions.

Unusual Number of Pauses, Interjected Words, or Extraneous Sounds

An unusual number of pauses, interjected words, or extraneous sounds, and even repeated whole or partial words may indicate an attempt to postpone speech to avoid stuttering or delay until the child feels that a word can be uttered fluently. More direct avoidance signs are word substitutions, silences, breaking off speech for another activity, or changing the topic.

Fear of Speaking

One or more of the behaviors described previously may indicate that the child is aware of stuttering and may be fearful of speaking. The clinician should distinguish between simple speech and performance anxiety and actual stuttering.

Other behaviors that tend to be associated with these danger signs (but are not in themselves indicative of stuttering) include hard onsets of phonation, shallow or irregular breathing (gasping or gulping) during speech, aberrant voice quality (such as excessive vocal fry), and dysrhythmic phonation while prolonging sounds, and abnormally high speaking rates (more than 220 syllables per minute).

Phonemic consistency of dysfluencies should also be noted; for example, a tendency to become blocked on one or more specific sounds such as /s/, /f/, /b/, or /d/, or on vowels, voiced sounds, or unvoiced sounds exclusively.

The evaluator should try not to express conclusions that the child is at risk for chronic stuttering based on the presence of one or a few of these danger signs during the assessment. Interrupting an interview or play session to make an announcement of a diagnosis can be unsettling for the parents and child and may make the evaluator appear arbitrary, impulsive, or insensitive.

Molecular Evaluation of Speech Samples

The clinician should thoroughly evaluate the video and audio speech samples to identify the individual behaviors that together characterize the child's stuttering. This will provide a baseline to help identify progress and stuttering development, and will also assist in the development of a treatment plan. The *loci of stuttering* will describe the parts of the speech apparatus that exhibit tension, tremors, and other disordered movements. An inventory of *core* and *accessory behaviors* will identify the observable speech behaviors that result from the disordered movements. Note that "core" does not refer to underlying or internal causes, but rather to behaviors that are actual speech movements, as opposed to those that involve other physical movements (e.g., hand or eye movements).

Loci of Stuttering

Comments about the loci of stuttering should include a physiological description of what happens when the person stutters. For example, this section of a diagnostic report could read:

> *When saying the /s/ sound, child grits teeth and hunches his shoulders. Forcing to produce the sound includes excessive audible airflow through the mouth area and teeth, and sudden snap-like opening of lower jaw and eye blinking during transition to the subsequent sound. Subsequent vowel often exhibits vocal fry, indicating laryngeal tension or possible pathology.*

Sometimes the primary locus of tension can be identified. The three primary loci include the upper chest and torso, the laryngeal area, and articulators in mouth and facial area, particularly the jaw. Occasionally only one characteristic type of tension (such as teeth clenching) must be described. This may be helpful for later stuttering identification and desensitization or deconditioning activities.

Inventory of Stuttering Events

The following core and accessory stuttering behaviors should be inventoried for the speech sample. The inventory should include the number of events and the approximate percentage of occurrence of each event relative to the overall number.

Core Behaviors

- Sound/syllable repetitions (with or without schwa vowel)
- Whole-word repetitions
- Phrase or sentence repetition
- Sound prolongations (with or without pitch or loudness rise)
- Inaudible prolongations or blocks

Accessory Behaviors

- Verbal interjections
- Eyebrow raising
- Eye blinking, rolling, closure, or enlargement
- Head or jaw jerking
- Hand, arm, or other movements of extremities
- High speaking rate

Considering Stuttering-Like Dysfluencies

Yairi and Ambrose (1992) developed the concept of "Stuttering-Like Dysfluencies" (SLDs) as a way of considering and including behaviors other than "within-word dysfluencies" in fluency assessments. We discuss the SLD concept here mainly because of its fairly wide use in the field. The SLD concept acknowledges that children who do not stutter also are dysfluent. It provides a way to factor into clinical observations the idea that the dysfluencies of children who stutter are qualitatively different. The SLDs include sound/syllable repetitions, monosyllabic repetitions, tense pauses, and dysrhythmic phonations (i.e., ones that disrupt

or distort the flow of speech). It should be noted, however, that this definition of SLDs has been critiqued as imprecise and, in fact, invalid (Conture, 2001; Wingate, 2001). For example, using Yairi and Ambrose's SLD measure, a child whose dysfluencies were comprised of 34 percent SLDs would not be considered to be stuttering, whereas a child who stutters would have an SLD percentage of 72 percent. However, such numbers are statistical means for large populations of children who stutter and cannot be reliably used in a differential fluency assessment without considering other factors. The value of SLDs lies primarily in determining the characteristic types of dysfluencies of an individual child. For example, if an individual child stuttered on 40 percent of his syllables, but only 25 percent of these dysfluencies were SLDs, he would still be exhibiting 10 percent SLDs and would be considered to be a child who could benefit from fluency therapy (Conture, 2001).

An important caution when considering SLDs is that the clinician may miss important clues (for various reasons, including the child's actions) that indicate that the child is experiencing or avoiding a real stuttering disruption. For example, whole-word repetitions such as "I-I-I-I" or "The-The-The-The" may result from an expectation of an actual stuttering dysfluency on a subsequent sound. It is not possible to read the mind of a child who stutters through his gestures alone. Also young children cannot be expected to be able to describe their internal experiences.

Length of Dysfluencies

Assessment instruments (such as the *SSI-3*) commonly have a provision for factoring in the length of time that speech is disrupted by stuttering blocks. Even when not using such a formal assessment, the clinician should measure and note the longest disruption and the average disruption associated with each type of dysfluency.

The length of the stuttering disruption can have a far more important effect on the perception of stuttering severity—for the child and for observers—than the sheer number of stuttering events. Accordingly, the clinician will want to qualify judgments regarding stuttering severity based on frequency with observations of length. Disruptions that last for two or more seconds can have a far more damaging effect on the child's psyche and self-image. In addition, such long durations may indicate development of considerable secondary or accessory behaviors that come to be strongly associated—through conditioning—with the stuttering block. These accessory behaviors can include postponements, interjections, struggle and tremor, inappropriate movements of the trunk or limbs, restarts, and loss of awareness. Fleeting dysfluencies or those that are less than half a second in length are usually less of a concern, if only because of their minor impact on the child's communication effectiveness. However, that does not mean that their impact is always commensurate with their length, particularly if they are frequent and involve violent tension-releasing behaviors, such as jaw snaps.

Teen Assessments

An important difference in older teenaged child assessments is that parents may not be present. This may limit the collection of early childhood information and may result in inaccuracies of such information as the age at which stuttering began and details of previous stuttering or other treatment. The attitudes of the parents toward stuttering will also be difficult to determine from the child's description. However, questionnaires collecting information on the child's feelings and attitudes toward stuttering and communication may be more insightful for this age group (see Johnson, W., et. al., 1952, 1980; Woolf, G., 1967).

Formal Assessment Instruments

Most formal assessment instruments are more useful for examining contributory language and developmental characteristics than the stuttering itself. The school-based clinician may have more formal testing instruments at her disposal than a clinician in private practice. However, the language element that is most critical to test—the relationship between expressive and receptive language abilities—can be determined with either of two pairs of tests that are relatively easy to administer and score: the *Expressive One-Word Picture Vocabulary Test* (*EOWPVT*) (Gardner, 2000a) and the *Receptive One-Word Picture Vocabulary Test* (*ROWPVT*) (Gardner, 2000b), as well as the *Peabody Picture Vocabulary*

Test-III (*PPVT-III*) (Dunn & Dunn, 1997) and *Expressive Vocabulary Test* (*EVT*) (Williams, 1997). These tests, when used together, can help the clinician determine if the child's receptive language skills are somewhat ahead of his expressive language skills. Such an imbalance can result in the child attempting to reproduce complex utterances that he has heard from various sources in a manner that is beyond his present ability to coordinate all the elements of speech motor movements.

Articulation and phonology disorders are the highest co-occurring disorders for children who stutter (Blood, Ridenour, & Qualls, 2003). Also, although additional factors are necessary for reliable prediction, poor phonological ability during incipient stuttering appears to be a contributing factor to the differentiation of persistence and recovery (Paden & Yairi, 1996). Articulation tests such as the *Goldman-Fristoe Test of Articulation-2* (*GFTA-2*) (Goldman & Fristoe, 2000) should also be conducted, particularly if obvious articulation inaccuracies or delays are present. The presence of phonological processes may indicate underlying oral peripheral anomalies. These may be cause for concern and referral to an ear, nose, and throat (ENT) specialist and should be factored into the overall plan of intervention.

Oral Peripheral Assessments

Whenever possible, it is desirable to perform a full oral peripheral examination, using props such as peanut butter (if appropriate for the child) or a sucker, if required. The child's oral-motor coordination skills are of particular interest in the fluency evaluation. These can have a bearing on the techniques the clinician may use for therapy, as well as providing an indication of potential triggers for some stuttering behavior. Improvement in oral motor coordination may facilitate reduction of stuttering (Riley & Riley, 1986). The child may have issues about how his speech sounds or feels that could affect his confidence in himself as a speaker. If so, these issues will have to be taken into account.

With some children, it will be difficult to perform a hands-on examination of the oral peripheral region during the initial assessment. The clinician should carefully observe key characteristics of the region, however, and should make note of voice quality and resonance, hypo- or hypernasality, excessive or restricted movement of the articulators, tongue thrusting, and other features of the child's speech. These can be addressed in more detail at a later date. If possible, the clinician should at a minimum elicit some diadochokinetic "puh-tuh-kuh's" from the child, noting regularity, speed, and the presence, absence, or resolution of dysfluencies.

Areas of particular concern are hypernasality and poor voice quality (including raspiness, hoarseness, or excessive vocal fry). Hypernasality may be due to oral surgery (removal of adenoids), a visible or submucous cleft, velopharyngeal weakness, or some other organic anomaly. It is critical to obtain a definitive diagnosis from a physician should a problem be discovered or suspected. It may be even more important to make a referral if there is no apparent reason for a case of noticeable hypernasality. The child's awareness of resonance problems could cause him to be excessively concerned about his speech.

Excessive tension or force while speaking can result in voice quality that is raspy or hoarse. However, this could also be a sign of laryngeal pathology, such as vocal fold nodules, cancer, or other pathology. Caregivers may be able to provide information about the child's speaking style (i.e., whether the child yells or screams a lot, habitually talks loudly, or commonly imitates loud machine or animal sounds) that may be a source of laryngeal overuse or irritation. The consistency of poor voice quality should also be noted. It may resolve when the child speaks more easily or more slowly. If the clinician is concerned about voice quality, she should consult a physician to provide the appropriate diagnosis. A form for conducting the *ASHA Oral Mechanism Examination for Children & Adults* is included in Appendix C.

Strategies for Deciding Who Needs Therapy

Emphasis is placed on the fact that stuttering involves more than just observable behaviors. Specifically, the speaker's experience of stuttering can involve negative affective, behavioral, and cognitive reactions (both from the speaker and the environment), as well as significant limitations in the speaker's ability to participate in daily activities and a negative impact on the speaker's overall quality of life. There is also a range of possible approaches to referral for

child stuttering therapy, from discouraging therapy for most children to accepting everyone. The former is the approach used by some professionals, who unfortunately use a "too soon, too soon, too late" strategy for handling their uncertainties about stuttering. With this strategy, children are considered most likely to "grow out of" stuttering, until it is clear they are not going to do that. It may then be too late to help them take advantage of the window of time during early childhood when remediation appears to be most effective for many.

For teens and adults, it is sometimes possible to determine whether therapy is indicated by determining the amount of handicap the person is experiencing due to dysfluencies. When the impairment of stuttering disables the person and creates handicaps, the severity of the person's stuttering may be secondary to its effect. The definitions of *impairment, disability,* and *handicap* were developed by the World Health Organization (WHO, 1980, 1992, 1993) and still form the basis for framing the impact of disorders in the health field. They are also featured in a tool called the *Overall Assessment of the Speaker's Experience of Stuttering* (*OASES*) developed by Yaruss and Quesal (in press; see also Yaruss 1998; Yaruss & Quesal, 2004).

Under the OASES definitions, an *impairment* is the actual physical issue that affects the functioning of the individual. For stuttering, this impairment is evidenced in the brain scans of people who stutter, which show that the brain regions involved in speech language functioning are dramatically hypo (or less) active compared with these regions in people who are fluent. The *disability* caused by or associated with this impairment is the actual inability to speak in a normal, fluent manner. The *handicap* associated with this disability is of particular concern when it comes to deciding whether children and adolescents can benefit from therapy. When the impairment (i.e., temporary disruptions of fluency) creates a disability (i.e., perceived speech breakdowns that disable the person from communicating in some situations), and this handicaps the person by hindering him from seeking the job he wants, meeting people, establishing relationships, using the telephone, or going to the store, then the severity of the person's stuttering is secondary to its effect.

In reality, there are few teens and adults who stutter who are not handicapped to some extent by their impairment. At this point, the benefit of stuttering treatment must be weighed, balancing the potential improvements in communication ability, on the one hand, with the person's ability or willingness to invest in therapy, the availability of time, and commitment to engage in a change process that may take an extended period of time, on the other hand.

We believe that all stuttering is a disability. However, the question of handicap is complex and this complexity must be considered if handicap is used as one criterion for therapy. The primary issue is the person's perception of handicap, relative to the actual handicap or the "handicapping" of the person by others. For example, a certain person may not feel that he is disabled by his stuttering and can easily perform a job that is, in actuality, entirely within his capabilities to perform (i.e., he is not handicapped). At the same time, a teacher or employer may handicap the person by assuming that he would not be able to perform the job or would not reflect well on the company or would disrupt a classroom (a judgment, of course, that involves perceptions of societal acceptance of stuttering). For another person, with another teacher or employer, this situation could be entirely reversed.

The situation is different with young children, many of whom may not even be aware of their stuttering and who, therefore, are not (or not yet) severely handicapped by stuttering. As a result, the risk of stuttering development must be strongly considered in the therapy decision. Because there is always a risk that even mild or infrequent childhood stuttering may develop and grow to be chronic, or that the environment may change, this is a difficult decision.

If the assessment has been thorough, several measures will be useful for determining the risk of continued or developing stuttering. Each of these measures should be used only as a guide to whether the child is "more likely" or "less likely" to require treatment, as none have been shown to be precise predictors. These measures are outlined in Figure 3.10.

Total Frequency of Stuttering or Dysfluencies

A frequency of more than 10 percent syllables stuttered is commonly thought of as a threshold for stuttering that will be more likely to need intervention. Frequencies of less than 6 percent are thought to indicate a problem that may not require treatment to abate. However, other factors, such as the severity of stuttering episodes and the length of time the

Figure 3.10 Deciding Who Can Benefit from Therapy

- Total frequency of stuttering or dysfluencies
- Sound prolongation percentage relative to total number of within-word dysfluencies
- Score on *Stuttering Severity Instrument-3*
- Score on *Stuttering Prediction Instrument*
- Length of time the child has been stuttering
- Severity and number of observed secondary stuttering behaviors
- Imbalance of receptive and expressive language abilities
- Inventory of temperamental risk factors
- Inventory of environmental risk factors
- Sex of child
- Family history of stuttering
- Concomitant problems
- Age

child has been stuttering, have to be considered as well. If the frequency is less than 3 percent and the type of dysfluency is not among those in the list of risk indicators, treatment may not be indicated for a child.

Sound Prolongation Percentage

Sound prolongation percentage relative to the total number of within-word dysfluencies is a useful measure in evaluating the severity of stuttering events. Sound prolongations within words—particularly when accompanied by pitch or loudness changes—are considered to be indicators of more severe stuttering. If such events constitute more than 30 percent of the total number of dysfluencies, at least 30 percent of the child's stuttering events are severe. If such events characterize the child's stuttering, and the total frequency of stuttering is 10 percent, therapy is definitely indicated based on severity alone.

Score on *Stuttering Severity Instrument-3*

The *SSI-3* (Riley, 1994) includes measures of the frequency of stuttering, the duration of severe stuttering events, and a measure of stuttering severity based on the visual appearance of the stuttering and accessory behaviors.

Recommendations for interpreting the results are provided in the test manual. Because it is probably the most widely used evaluation instrument, this chapter was written partly to help clinicians interpret the results of the *SSI-3*.

Score on Stuttering Prediction Instrument (Riley, 1981)

The *Stuttering Prediction Instrument (SPI)* is not a totally reliable test because it has not been sufficiently normed with outcomes, but it does provide a quantitative measure of risk factors that have been correlated with a low number of subjects. In general, a score of 10 on this test may indicate that a child is more in need of stuttering treatment. Scores of more than 16 would certainly provide sufficient rationale for therapy, if only because of the frequency and type of dysfluency that such a score indicates. Yaruss and Conture (1993) have used the *SPI* to evaluate the degree of chronicity of a child's stuttering.

Length of Time Child Has Been Stuttering

This measure is based on clinical evidence (Yairi, Ambrose, Paden, & Thromeburg, 1996) that children who stutter for more than 18 months prior to intervention are more at risk for continued chronic stuttering behavior. However, this does not imply that an individual child who has been stuttering for less than 18 months should not be treated or that a particular child who has stuttered more than 18 months will not recover. The duration of stuttering should not be considered in isolation from the child and his needs.

Severity and Number of Observed Secondary Stuttering Behaviors

Accessory or secondary stuttering behaviors fall into two general categories:

1. Spontaneous behaviors that the child uses to express the difficulty he is experiencing (such as grabbing the mouth area to "pull" words out or foot-stamping to express frustration)
2. Conditioned or stereotypical behaviors that are used habitually to "help" the child break out of, time, or delay the stuttering disruption

During the assessment, these behaviors should be noted and categorized. The presence of the first kind of accessory behavior exclusively may indicate an earlier form of stuttering. The presence of the second type of accessory behavior indicates that the stuttering has developed in a way that places the child at greater risk for continued chronic stuttering, if only because he may be prone to creating behaviors that make the stuttering more inaccessible.

Supporting Assessment Information

Additional information that supports a fluency evaluation may be obtained from various other test instruments and observations. Some of these are discussed in this section.

Imbalance of Receptive and Expressive Language Abilities

There is clinical evidence of a bimodal population of stuttering children. One mode consists of children whose expressive language abilities are generally low. The other includes children who are skilled in language acquisition, have high receptive language skills, and may have language and speech environments that are very highly stimulating. It could be theorized that the abilities of such children to comprehend and remember long and complex utterances (indicative of high receptive language skills) may outpace the child's more slowly developing expressive language capabilities. Children at risk for stress in this manner may be identified by considering the parent's speaking style, together with their hopes for, or comments about, their child's language or intellectual development. A score on the *EVT* that is significantly lower than the child's *PPVT* score indicates an increased likelihood that such a dynamic is present. In the presence of some stuttering during descriptive, noncontextual speech tasks, such a dynamic may be sufficient to recommend treatment, if only to help the child cope with his rapidly developing speech and language skills.

Inventory of Temperamental Risk Factors

One or more of the following temperamental factors, in conjunction with some stuttering or dysfluency, usually indicates a need for treatment:

- Extreme inhibition
- Extreme extroversion
- Extreme reactivity to stimuli
- Difficulty attending or focusing
- Speed-directed behaviors or impatience

Inventory of Environmental Risk Factors

One or more of the following risk factors, in conjunction with moderate to severe stuttering, usually indicates a need for treatment:

- Parental speaking rate greater than 250 syllables per minute
- Parent observed to interrupt or speak over child
- Divorce or separation of parents
- Frequent moves or moves during child's social expansion years (ages 6 to10)
- Differential analysis—other disorders

Cognitive Abilities

Although a cognitive assessment is usually beyond the scope of a fluency evaluation, formal information on the child's cognitive skills should be obtained, if possible. The clinician will also want to assess the child's participation in conversation and play to roughly determine his developmental stage. Overall cognitive skills may be more important for designing a therapy regimen for older children, whose recovery will be enhanced by their ability to understand the purpose and limitations of therapy procedures and techniques. For younger children, the clinician will want to determine what kind of activities are most appropriate when therapy begins.

A thorough assessment is an important precursor to designing a tailored treatment program for the child and his family. The information learned provides knowledge pertaining not only to core and accessory behaviors, but also to the child's total receptive and expressive abilities. In addition, important information on family dynamics and possible behaviors that maintain and exacerbate the problem can also be learned.

Note on Cluttering

Assessment and diagnosis of cluttering is discussed in Chapter 12. If the child's speech is rapid or uneven, unintelligible, disorganized, or exhibits abnormal pauses or breathing, cluttering should be considered.

Within the education environment, individualized education programs (IEPs) are required for all children who are evaluated or treated under the federally mandated Individuals with Disabilities Education Act (IDEA) program. For the IEP team that determines that a child should be eligible for treatment under a school program, care and accuracy in documenting a determination of eligibility are critical. A narrow (and therefore prejudicial) interpretation of the guidelines for inclusion in special education services will, unfortunately, focus on grade performance alone. Such a perspective may lower the probability that a child who stutters will receive services, because average or slightly above average grades are not unusual even for children whose other school activities are severely hampered by their stuttering disability (Schulz, 1977; Cox, Seider, & Kidd, 1984). It is possible that some children who stutter have been denied treatment in the public schools because they had been determined ineligible for benefits on narrow academic grounds, even though they exhibited severe stuttering. Incidentally, children who clutter may be more likely to receive services than those who stutter, because cluttering is often associated with learning disabilities and may receive intervention as a related service under existing IEPs (Tiger, Irvine, & Reis, 1980; Daly, 1992).

For most individuals who stutter, however, an accurate determination for services necessitates a broader interpretation of the inclusion criteria—an interpretation that is clearly supported by the language in IEP documents. Obviously, grade performance alone is merely one measure of the student's progress in preparing for a productive life in society. Successful preparation also includes the development of social interaction and personal presentation skills, active involvement in learning, and opportunities for appropriate continued education or training following graduation from high school. A child or adolescent who may avoid academic opportunities and ultimately a college education because of stuttering should be identified and appropriately supported by the school's special education programs.

Impact of School Participation on Children Who Stutter

Stuttering is unique among the various disabilities because its severity may actually be aggravated and its negative effects increased *as a result* of participation in school. We have seen cases in which the effects of school participation have been the leading environmental factor driving the development of chronic stuttering. This is not to say that schools should be blamed in some way. Rather, the school setting—the child's first, significant participation within organized social activity—is the crucible in which his genetic predisposition to stutter is combined with environmental stressors to aggravate chronic stuttering behavior.

There is an important implication here that will be touched on several times in this chapter: namely, that because confirmed stuttering is developmental in nature and usually worsens over time (Van Riper, 1973), school experience may be a key ingredient in the development of severe stuttering. If a particular special education department tends to focus on treating very young children, and assumes that milder or less significant problems will continue to decrease in importance as a student progresses in school, the stuttering children whose symptoms are worsening may fail to receive adequate attention.

Defining the Child's Performance and Education Needs

Typically, "Present Levels of Performance" are defined on a separate page of the IEP form, on which the following instructions are provided (taken from a Denver-area IEP).

> Describe how the student's suspected or identified educational disability affects the student's involvement and progress in the general curriculum. For preschool children, reflect how the child's disability affects participation in appropriate activities. If appropriate, consider the results of the child's performance on any general state or district-wide assessment programs. Address any lack of progress toward annual goals when the term "reasonable education benefit" is narrowly interpreted. [Identify if] a stuttering child is performing one or two grades below the level predicted by testing (or is receiving Cs or Bs when testing or earlier academic achievements would predict As), and consider the most recent evaluation results and information provided by the parents.

During a determination of eligibility, "involvement and progress in the general curriculum" should not be constrained to a narrow, academic interpretation of performance. Instead, a more appropriate conceptualization of "involvement" would include class participation, ability to make required presentations in class, engagement or interest in school academic activities, and ability to interact with peers in class study or activity groups. Teachers are well positioned to provide much of this information.

Focusing on the information provided by the parents will be particularly helpful in identifying factors that may affect performance. Parents may be aware of attitudes, changes in performance, and emotional factors. They may be acutely aware of an older child's reluctance to go to college because of stuttering or tendency to select a career path dictated by fear of speaking.

Determination of Eligibility Form

Discussion of the "Determination of Eligibility" form is based on the current version of IDEA as of the date of publication. Although this law may be revised after the publication of this book, the basic strategies have been designed to be flexible enough so that they can be applied to future permutations of the law.

The eligibility form essentially consists of a yes/no gating system, in which an answer of "yes" to any question passes the student on to the next criterion determining eligibility, but a "no" answer to any question essentially excludes the child from eligibility. These gates are discussed in the following quotation (from the same IEP form as previously quoted) in terms of children who may be exhibiting either cluttering or stuttering behavior.

> *Have sufficient assessments been completed, documented, and considered to determine eligibility and to determine the student's educational needs? Based on current levels of functioning, achievement, and performance?*

In this paragraph, the concepts of "functioning," "achievement," and "performance" are critical to establishing a baseline assessment. For a stuttering child, *functioning* may include the

actual speech impairment. It is critical to document the observable primary symptoms of stuttering as well as the secondary ones, which may in fact have more impact on the child's performance in school. These include word avoidance, lack of participation in class and academic speech activities, and accessory physical behaviors that may make a child look peculiar to classmates and teachers, such as struggle behaviors involving the body, limbs, head, or face (including lack of eye contact).

Inclusion of secondary symptoms has an important implication for school SLPs. As children enter their teens, it is more likely that such symptoms will be degrading the stuttering student's academic achievement, because social stigmatization has a greater effect on the student's overall performance. Key evidence of such effects includes a student who is underperforming based on the expectations of earlier assessments of intelligence, language abilities, and actual grade performance. Simply labeling a student who stutters as an "underachiever," without treating the stuttering, is problematic.

Under this criterion, the SLP would need to have a documented record proving that the child is exhibiting dysfluent speech that can be classified as stuttering or cluttering. This record should include the results of a detailed fluency evaluation using an accepted stuttering assessment protocol such as the *SSI-3*.

> *Can the student receive reasonable educational benefit from general education alone?*

Because the effects of stuttering are in no way alleviated by "general education," the answer to this question should be "no" if the SLP views stuttering as having a negative impact on the child's education. However, this is the criterion used to exclude many people who stutter from special education services. If "general education" (i.e., existing class activities) has not helped, this is a clear indication that fluency therapy may be beneficial.

> *Does the student have a disability as defined in the State rules for the Administration of the Exceptional Children's Education Act?*

The disability or disabilities must then be identified from a list, as seen in the following box. The disabilities often associated with stuttering or cluttering *are highlighted in italics* and discussed in detail hereafter.

This disability is:

- Significant limited intellectual capacity
- *Significant identifiable emotional disability*
- *Perceptual or communicative disability*
- Hearing disability
- Vision disability
- *Speech-language disability*
- *Preschool with a disability*
- Physical disability
- Traumatic brain injury
- Autism
- *Other physical disability*
- *Multiple disabilities*
- Deaf-Blind
- *Multiple disabilities with cognitive impairment*

Significant Identifiable Emotional Disability

A child who does not "fit in," or who is often in conflict with peers, is easier to identify with regard to emotional disability than one who is liked by other students and has a lot of friends. Nevertheless, it is sometimes the latter who is most disabled by emotional factors associated with stuttering and other dysfluencies. Some children who stutter may overcompensate for their speech difficulties by trying too hard to please other children. This can lead to excessive showing off, clowning in class, or doing things that "look cool" at the expense of activities that are educationally efficient or productive. All of these may be indicators that the child has chronic low self-esteem.

Perceptual or Communicative Disability

The inability of children to say specific words required to communicate their thoughts is a clear instance of a disability. It could be argued that many children who stutter manage to communicate fairly well in spite of their dysfluencies (and this is clearly so in many instances), but the quality and even the content of this communication is changed in subtle ways by the strategies used to overcome the speech impairment. For example, it is very unlikely that a fluent child would purposefully modify a statement of fact, making it less precise and thereby risking that the communication will be misunderstood. However, children who stutter consciously and unconsciously make such modifications on a regular basis in an attempt to make their speech acceptable to listeners. In addition, the presence of stuttering behavior communicates emotions that distort the child's intent and modify his or her personality and image. Some children may project fear, anxiety, or nervousness because of their stuttering when called upon to speak. Such appearances distort communication and may cause listeners to devalue the child's thoughts and opinions or even to turn away from him.

In addition, stuttering may involve several important changes in sensory perception. These have been corroborated by brain scans that compare the brain function of stuttering and nonstuttering speakers, including hypo-function of the left temporal brain areas involved in hearing and word recognition. These changes are difficult to quantify, but their presence is indicated by the inability of some children to hear their own dysfluencies. Attention may also be severely affected by stuttering. A child who is extremely fearful or anxious of an anticipated in-class speaking task will not be as likely to attend to class activities before and after the feared task.

Speech-Language Disability

It should be obvious that stuttering is a speech-language disability, but there is no strictly definitive legal ruling that this is so under the Americans with Disabilities Act (ADA), which is often cited as defining legal disabilities in the United States. One reason for this is that individual court cases cannot define disability for a disorder with as many degrees of severity and handicap as stuttering. The definitions of *impairment*, *disability*, and *handicap* provided in a new assessment tool, called the "Overall Assessment of the Speaker's Experience of Stuttering" (OASES) developed by Yaruss and Quesal (in press) may provide some guidance in this regard. The OASES questionnaire is based on the definitions formerly used by the World Health Organization

(WHO, 1980, 1992, 1993), which are the basis for framing the impact of disorders in the health field.

Under the OASES definitions, an *impairment* is the actual physical issue that affects the functioning of the individual. For stuttering, this impairment is evidenced in the brain scans of people who stutter, which show that the brain activity involved in speech-language functioning are dramatically different compared with these regions in people who are fluent. The *disability* caused by or associated with this impairment is the actual inability to speak in a normal, fluent manner. The *handicaps* associated with this disability include problems in communicating, emotional distress, and the various difficulties in functioning in school and other settings discussed elsewhere in this chapter.

There is a tendency, in evaluations of function by children who stutter, to confuse disability with handicap. This seems to be the source of many people's reluctance to acknowledge that children who stutter have a disability. Perhaps many children who stutter are not handicapped by their stuttering in a major way within the confines of the classroom, but that does not mean that they are never handicapped by stuttering. Such problems with language and complexities in the effect of impairments are treated in the new WHO classification, documented in the framework titled *International Classification of Functioning, Disability and Health* (WHO, 2001).

The revised WHO classification scheme can also provide guidance in the definition of effects of stuttering on the individual (WHO, 2001). Indeed, the new guidelines provide specific examples of difficulties in education experienced by children with impairments. The new guidelines discuss various domains in terms of the *performance* and *capacity* of the person to participate. "Resulting difficulties with activities and participation are then discussed as *limitations* in activity or *restrictions* in participation, rather than as disabilities or handicaps" (Yaruss & Quesal, in press).

Other Physical Disability

It may be obvious that even a minor stuttering problem that exists in association with a physical disability could result in performance or adjustment problems. A disfigurement in conjunction with stuttering may also result in a greater risk of teasing, ridicule, and (unfortunately) even physical abuse by other children.

Multiple Disabilities with Cognitive Impairment

The category of multiple disabilities would apply to children who were cluttering, with associated stuttering behaviors, and who also had learning or attention disorders. (When children are cluttering, it is very rare that absolutely no stuttering symptoms will be present.) It would also apply to children who evidence autistic spectrum disorders in addition to stuttering. In any cases where stuttering is present with other disorders, it is vital to address the stuttering as well, because of its corrosive impact on emotional health.

Determination of Academic Impacts

For several reasons, including its focus on test performance and the lack of verifiable baselines, the literature is very unhelpful regarding the impact of stuttering on academic achievement. However, because cluttering often co-occurs with learning disabilities, children who are cluttering may be easier to qualify for in-school services. Although some impact of stuttering on school grades and learning has always been suspected, the effects are subtle and difficult to measure because each child is an individual with unique potentials. Because stuttering is a speech performance disorder rather than a language disorder, the stuttering child without concomitant disorders has ways of compensating for his disability within the academic system. He may, for example, focus on writing as a means of expression, thereby demonstrating increased academic competence relative to peers. Many (perhaps most) children who stutter have less difficulty maintaining fluency when they read aloud or recite a prepared script.

Because of his ability to compensate academically, a major negative effect on the child's performance in school may be the lack of creation of social bonds (with teachers as well as with peers), which are often considered to be outside the realm of academic performance. This effect can be manifested in subtle ways, such as a relative inability of the child to discuss problems or concerns, or to create positive bonds, with teachers. Ironically, it may also result in the creation of parent-child–type relationships with teachers, causing the child to be viewed negatively by peers.

Fluency Goals

A review of many IEPs for children who stutter will reveal treatment or achievement goals such as: "will speak with 95 percent fluency" or even "with 100 percent fluency." In some cases this may be supplemented with specifications for various speaking situations. In all cases, such narrow goals are counterproductive and should be avoided.

Progress in therapy is very situation-dependent, mirroring the situation with stuttering frequency itself. Furthermore, once children are in the school years (i.e., older than five years), progress rarely achieves a total cessation of stuttering. The school SLP is then placed in the role of a support person who is helping the child to manage fluency and facilitate recovery as he or she progresses through school. However, it is important not to view this in the negative light of case management. The gradual recovery of children out of stuttering has been documented in many cases. This can occur as a continuous or (in some cases) stepwise progression throughout the school years. Given this scenario of gradual recovery, it is crucial for the school SLP to set reasonable goals for the child who stutters. A goal of complete fluency in all situations will not be met in most cases. If the child and SLP "fail" to achieve this goal, then all parties concerned (child, parent, teacher, and SLP) may find themselves backed into a corner of their own making—and it is the child who will be most damaged by the notion that he has failed, because therapy and fluency management may be eliminated as an option. If speech therapy is dropped for lack of cost-effectiveness, then all parties have lost.

The loss of contact with older stutterers in junior and senior high school settings can lead to another bifurcated problem that has not really been recognized: the possibility of relapse and recovery later in the teen years. Children whose stuttering has been largely reduced in many situations may find that the added speaking and social stresses of later teen life cause a resumption of situational dysfluencies; that is, stuttering can increase in formerly fluent speaking situations. If stuttering is associated with failure and shame, such teens may be reluctant to seek out therapy and may respond instead by withdrawing or becoming more covert stutterers. On the other end of the spectrum, a teen may experience a natural reduction in stuttering that is related to the self-esteem issues that are so fragile in this age group. If the SLP has maintained contact with the child, even in a very casual fashion, this increase in fluency may be nurtured and reinforced. Without such contact, the increased fluency may be undermined by environmental factors and an opportunity may be lost.

Setting Realistic IEP Goals and Objectives for Children Who Stutter

IEP goals and objectives for any child must be developed in a way that recognizes what the child can realistically achieve. For children who stutter, this means that goals or objectives should not anticipate or expect huge improvements in fluency, ability to use modification techniques, increases in self-awareness or self-monitoring ability, or transformations in self-concept. For some children, merely maintaining the *status quo* may be an achievement at some points in their development. The suggestions in this section should be used with this overall guidance in mind.

Short-Term Instructional Objective

"Short-term instructional objective" is an official term with which an SLP writing an IEP would be familiar. For the child who stutters, short-term instructional objectives can include the following (see Figure 4.1 for an example of short-term objectives in a sample IEP goal):

- Use of fluency-enhancing behaviors such as continuous voicing or gentle onsets in specified situations
- Use of stuttering modification techniques such as initial sound stretches, pullouts, and cancellations in specified situations
- Reduced frequency of use of a secondary stuttering behavior
- Reduced use of a stuttering avoidance technique, such as interjections, word avoidance, pretending not to know an answer, or avoiding speech
- Measured stuttering severity in a therapy setting
- Class participation, such as asking questions and volunteering to answer questions posed by the teacher

- Participation in groups and extracurricular activities that require various speaking skills, such as music groups, choirs, sports, crafts, chess clubs, writing clubs, stage set preparation, and management groups

- Participation in activities that require speech, such as debating clubs or drama groups

Methods of Measurement

It may be very difficult to obtain an objective measure of stuttering frequency that indicates progress or regression in a nontherapy setting. In all cases, however, measurement will require the participation of teachers who have been trained by the SLP to observe stuttering behavior, as well as therapy techniques or so-called fluency controls.

Special Considerations for Classroom Settings

By their very nature, many of the objectives set for children who stutter have a potential to elicit reactions from other students. These must be anticipated and managed by the teacher and SLP for the objectives of therapy to be achieved in the school setting. This may require some degree of class preparation and education about stuttering.

For example, an objective calls for the student to speak with a pronounced slow bouncing behavior on nonfeared words—but such behavior may precipitate negative comments or teasing by other children in the classroom. Also, a requirement to participate more in class may cause the student to speak more openly, and therefore stutter more, in class, possibly leading to reactions by other students.

Sample IEP Goal

Sample Short-Term Objective
Will increase use of noticeable prolonged onsets to at least three per day when participating in class (or another situation, such as a reading group).

Method of Measurement
Teacher observation of general behavior; SLP observation and report; student report.

Schedule for Achieving Objective
Beginning date: January 12th
Target completion date: May 25th

Levels of Progress and Date
In this case, care must be taken to eliminate online verbal prompts or cues that may interfere with communication and undermine the child's willingness to perform the speech modifications. The danger here is that classmates may pick up on these verbal commands and use them to ridicule or try to gain control over the child when he is stuttering outside the classroom. Instead, prompts and cues can consist of offline reminders made by the teacher or by the SLP. In some cases, the student and teacher or SLP may want to develop a discreet nonverbal signaling system.

Objective Will Be Completed or Continued
By setting stepwise, achievable objectives, the IEP can provide the child and SLP with a way of measuring progress through recovery. The recovery path for stuttering is different and in many cases somewhat slower than for other challenges and this must be acknowledged. Continuing an objective for several semesters would not be unusual for stuttering therapy transfer and this should not be seen as negative or a failure.

Figure 4.1 Short-Term Objective in a Sample IEP Goal

Conversely, if students are made aware that the student is expected to perform a certain fluency modification behavior, there is a possibility that they will call for the stuttering child to perform that behavior to alleviate her stuttering—certainly a negative experience for the stuttering child, and one that is not conducive to successful therapy. Because of these possibilities, the teacher, student, and SLP need to work together to make the classroom safe for transfer activities.

Future Revisions of IEP Rules

IEP rules are now under revision and will change from the existing form. However, the principles provided in this chapter should provide sufficient guidance to handle virtually any future revision. The key points for children who stutter are to (1) focus on goals that involve speech modification, improved communication, and continued participation in school activities rather than mere fluency measures; and (2) consider the school environment as an arena for the development of the child's active and productive communication with and participation in society, and any hindrance to that development as qualifying the child for stuttering therapy, counseling and management services.

Teachers of children who stutter may serve key roles in diagnostic, therapy, and transfer processes (Gottwald, Goldbach, & Isack, 1985; Pindzola, 1985; Swan, 1993; Ramig & Bennett, 1995; Lees, 1999). Because she sees the child in numerous interactions with peers, under stress, and in performance situations, the teacher not only serves as a source of information about the child, but also can potentially provide an atmosphere that is conducive to open speaking and communication. In addition to Handout F: To the Teacher of a Nonfluent Child (in the Appendix), a checklist of fluency behaviors for teachers to complete during the assessment process, is available at the Stuttering Homepage Web site (www.stutteringhomepage.com).

An SLP's interaction with the teacher can take a variety of forms, from meetings at school or a private practice clinic to regular e-mails or phone calls. Whatever form this communication takes, the clinician should emphasize the importance of the teacher's role in the stuttering child's development and recovery (Lees, 1999). Teachers are key representatives of the world outside the family—a world in which the child will learn to participate during the school years. In our experience, a child who is encouraged to be open about stuttering within the school environment is more likely to develop a more positive long-term attitude toward communication.

Preparing for a Visit to a Private Practice

Inviting teachers to participate with the child in a private practice therapy session can provide benefits for everyone concerned. The teacher's presence may legitimize the therapy regimen for the child, emphasizing that therapy is important and that the child is not alone during the therapy process. The teacher will also learn more about the transfer process, including gaining a better appreciation of the difficulty of transfer itself. The teacher and parents will have another place to interact and discuss the child's therapy and transfer activities. Finally, the SLP can consult simultaneously with the parents, teacher, and child, providing an opportunity to share important information and to reach consensus.

Although a teacher visit to the therapy room might seem to be an uncomfortable experience for the child, in our experience it may be less stressful than activities involving the child's

peers. The teacher's direct participation within the therapy room can help reduce stress during the performance of later transfer activities in the classroom. Also, it can help the teacher understand how important it is to provide an environment free of teasing or bullying in which transfer activities can take place (Pindzola, 1985; Mooney & Smith, 1995).

Visiting the Classroom

Visits by the clinician to the classroom should respect the child's sensitivity to the possible reaction. The degree of direct class involvement, which may range from unobtrusive observation to open discussion of stuttering, should be in accordance with the parents' and child's degree of comfort. Although a great deal can be learned from such visits, their value can be undermined if the child does not want the clinician in the classroom. Furthermore, given the fact that IEPs are legal, confidential documents outlining intervention for identified disabilities, the SLP is advised to gain the consensus of IEP team members—including the student—before implementing overt classroom visits.

Counseling Teachers

Because of higher caseloads, it is increasingly likely that a school SLP will be expected to serve primarily as a consultant to teachers, rather than as the chief provider of direct speech therapy services for children who stutter. Although this service mode may be appropriate for academic activities such as reading, writing, and math, we do not see consultation alone as sufficient in the absence of other speech services. Children who continue to stutter in elementary school are usually past the age at which they can recover without direct intervention (Yairi, 1997a). Stuttering intervention, to the extent and degree described in this book, requires a sound basis in one-on-one activities with a knowledgeable speech-language professional. That said, there is still an important role for classroom teachers in the child's recovery from, or management of, stuttering (Dell, 2000).

Managing the Classroom Environment

Teachers play a key role in managing the environment to support the child who stutters (Hall, Oyer, & Haas, 2001).

By far the most important long-term role of the teacher may be to assist in helping the child transfer new speech behaviors outside the clinic. The classroom provides an excellent environment for the child who stutters to implement new behaviors and experiment with speech techniques. However, if the child is afraid of being teased or ridiculed for stuttering, or for using speech techniques such as stretches, slow bounces, pullouts, and cancellations, the transfer process will probably be jeopardized.

Another consideration is balancing the child's academic, social, emotional, and communication needs with his sensitivity to the more difficult aspects of transfer, such as classroom presentations. For example, the child may have extreme difficulty maintaining fluency during presentations and may request to be excused from them. Honoring this request may be important, but it is also a concern that the child be provided with the experience of presenting information in an oral mode. The solution to these issues is always individualized and should be discussed and determined by the IEP team members. As an example, a compromise may be struck that permits the child to give his presentations to the teacher or to a smaller group of students. Alternatively, a hierarchy of audiences (from comfortable to more difficult) can be devised and implemented to gradually prepare the student for regular classroom presentations.

Handling Teasing

Teasing of young stutterers by their peers may indicate that an undiagnosed child is having communication difficulties. It also often provides a clue as to why an identified child is having difficulty with transfer of new speech behaviors (Pindzola, 1995; Mooney & Smith, 1995). Although teasing that involves direct references to, or imitation of, dysfluencies is relatively easy to identify, teasing may be based on perceived differences in affect, such as shyness, a reluctance to participate in play activities, or reticence in defending oneself from verbal attacks.

It is true that the most effective way of protecting children from teasing may be to "bully-proof" them through counseling, teaching self-defense communication responses, and developing a positive (and more realistic) self image. However, the teacher also needs to counsel the teasers or bul-

lies. At times, this may require direct intervention and public admonishment. Today, teachers and school administrators are much more aware of the academic and social consequences of bullying, and it has been treated more seriously than previously (Parker & Asher, 1987; Sharpe, 1995; Hodges & Perry, 1996). Children who receive special education services may be at greater risk for experiencing teasing (Whitney, Smith & Thompson, 1994).

The teacher's role in the prevention of teasing and bullying is paramount. Stuttering intervention will be more successful when teasing and bullying become unacceptable to the peers of the perpetrators. Bullies often operate under the illusion that they are enforcing group mores or conventions, and they expect to receive positive recognition from other children. This reinforcement disappears when it becomes socially unacceptable within the classroom to tease a child who is stuttering or who is attempting to use stuttering modification behaviors. The development of this acceptance is one of the objectives of the classroom presentation on stuttering discussed later in this chapter.

Informal Teacher-Parent-SLP Team Meetings

Throughout treatment, the SLP should arrange informal, collaborative interactions with the teacher and parents of the child who stutters. These meetings are separate from the formal team meetings associated with the development of individualized education plans. Informal meetings involve practical matters related to the implementation of the IEP, such as discussions of upcoming classroom presentations or current problems, or addressing episodes of teasing. These meetings are particularly recommended when the child is being treated by a private practice clinician and does not have an IEP.

Teacher Participation in Transfer

Teachers sometimes ask if they can help the child's transfer activities by providing cues or requesting in class that the child "use" fluency techniques when he or she is having difficulties with speech. This may be helpful, but only if the teacher has a good understanding of some important considerations. In our experience, it is more important for the teacher to understand the role and intended effect of so-called fluency techniques. Though these techniques can indeed help in increasing fluency, they should not be considered magic tricks that make stuttering disappear. Openly demanding or requesting that a stuttering child use a technique can lead to humiliation when it does not work; such requests may also single out the child for special negative or critical attention by classmates. Instead, therapy techniques are intended to help the child demonstrate to himself that he can modify his speech in a way that can change stuttering and reduce its automatic and reactive nature. These changes may help the child feel better about speech, enjoy communication more, and experience a reduction in fearful anticipation.

Presentation on Stuttering

The most therapeutic classroom is one in which it is acceptable to stutter. Creation of a "stutter-friendly" environment may be greatly facilitated by providing information about stuttering to all students (Lees, 1999; Chmela & Reardon, 2001). Of course, the child who stutters should be comfortable with his level of involvement in providing such information. However, acknowledgement that the information is being provided because a stuttering child is in the class should not be a requirement, if the child is uneasy about this.

By far the most effective way of conveying information to the class is a presentation involving the child or children who stutter. It is helpful to provide the teacher with information and involve her in the planning of the presentation, so that she is comfortable with the topic before discussing it in class. This will help the teacher convey to the students that stuttering is neither a curiosity nor something to be feared. For example, if a child asks if other people can "catch" stuttering, the teacher will be able to provide definite and reassuring information that this cannot happen. Although the SLP leads the planning and preparation phase, participation by her during the presentation itself is not necessary, but will be influenced by feedback from the teacher and child who stutters.

Several stuttering organizations provide information and suggestions on class presentations about stuttering, including the Stuttering Foundation, the National Stuttering Association, and the Friends National Association of Young People Who Stutter. Table 5.1 provides an outline of a possible 30-minute classroom presentation on stuttering.

The teacher, child, and SLP may plan the presentation together. The child's actual role may vary considerably, depending on the child's stage in therapy and sensitivity. It can range from virtually no participation to the child leading the presentation or an activity, such as a quiz on stuttering or a presentation about famous historical figures who stuttered or well-known people who stutter. Indeed, some children who stutter are highly active communicators and may wish to do the bulk of the presentation themselves. This role should also be monitored by the SLP to modify the child's participation accordingly to help ensure that the experience is positive.

Participation by additional adults is encouraged because it provides support and demonstrates to the child who stutters

TABLE 5.1 Outline of a 30-Minute Classroom Presentation on Stuttering

Length	Person	Activity
2 minutes	Teacher	Introductions
5 minutes	SLP	What is stuttering?
5 minutes	Child	Famous people who stutter—Quiz
10 minutes	SLP	Video clip
5 minutes	Child	Stuttering—Quiz
3 minutes	Teacher	What did we learn today?
	SLP	Provides handouts to class

that numerous adults care about his well-being. The SLP may consider inviting the leader of a local adult support group to speak about stuttering. To this end, consult the National Stuttering Association (www.westutter.org) or one of the online discussion forums about stuttering. The SLP should meet with the person before the presentation to ensure that the information to be shared is consistent with that presented in therapy.

To help young people who stutter with ideas for class presentations, John Ahlbach, a high school teacher who stutters, has written the *FRIENDS Stuttering Presentation Guide*, which is available on the Friends Who Stutter Web site (www.friendswhostutter.org) as a downloadable PDF file.

Frequently Asked Questions about Stuttering

The following section presents some questions teachers frequently ask about stuttering in their students.

Q. **If a child is having extreme difficulties with his speech fluency, should I stop calling on him in class?**

A. This area requires your attention, but the way it is addressed should take the child's individual situation into account. The SLP can recommend some strategies for encouraging the child's participation while reducing the stress involved. One way of doing this may be to set up smaller reading or speaking groups, something that may actually benefit all of the children in the class. A meeting with the teacher, SLP, and student may also be beneficial in developing a strategy for increasing the student's participation and incorporating activities into the SLP's therapy program. This may even be helpful if the child is not on the SLP's caseload.

Q. **If stuttering is such a big handicap, why do many of the children who stutter seem to do well in school?**

A. The impact of stuttering on academic performance has not been accurately determined, because of the difficulty in establishing control populations for comparison (Bloodstein, 1995). However, it is clear from clinical experience and population studies that many children who stutter are extremely facile with language in modal-

ities other than speech (Guitar, 1998). Reading silently, writing, or working with computers may even be an expressive language outlet for many children who stutter, providing a compensation for their impairment. However, it is important to view school as a training ground for success later in life. By this measure, academic performance is not an adequate indication of the impact of stuttering on a child. If a child emerges from school with good grades but is afraid or reluctant to select a college or career path because of stuttering, the school has missed an opportunity to educate the child. However, this negative effect will not be factored into the school's performance, of course.

Q. **I hardly ever have children who stutter in my classes. If the prevalence of stuttering is 1–2 percent of the population, where are all the stutterers?**

A. There is a wide range of stuttering severity (Van Riper, 1973; Guitar, 1998). Many stuttering children and adolescents stutter so mildly that they can successfully hide their problem from others through the use of coping mechanisms such as situation avoidance, word substitutions, and self-distraction techniques. Unfortunately, cultural stereotypes of people who stutter are overwhelmingly negative, despite the many stutterers who have made positive contributions to society. This is probably because these people (e.g., James Earl Jones, Winston Churchill, John Updike, and others) are not known to be stutterers or are thought to be people who have been "cured" of stuttering or have outgrown it.

Q. **Why does progress with stuttering often seem to change during the teen years?**

A. This question has long been of great concern to clinicians and parents. For most teens, one reason is the influence of peer pressure and the fear of looking or feeling different. This perception can affect not only stuttering itself, but also the acceptability of speech therapy to the teenager. Because any previous therapy has not resulted in a complete cessation of stuttering, the teenager may interpret remaining dysfluencies as evidence of failure. For these reasons, he may then increase attempts to hide or minimize the residual or continued dysfluencies, which can worsen as a result.

Teachers can help reverse these trends by encouraging a teen to join a stuttering peer group. For many teens who stutter, who can largely hide their dysfluencies behind a façade of "coolness," detachment, aggression, and even academic excellence, any association with therapy or with other teens who experience difficulties may seem like an admission of weakness or failure. In our experience, despite any initial reservations, most students who stutter find the opportunity to talk with others who stutter beneficial, for it emphasizes that they are not alone.

Q. **My student rarely stutters. Should I tell him that his stuttering is not as important as he thinks it is?**

A. It might seem that it would be helpful to encourage a child who stutters by reassuring him that his stuttering is not as noticeable or as important to others as he may fear—but this message may backfire. The observed behaviors of stuttering are often only the tip of a very large iceberg of impairment, fear, and emotional pain. The child may be successful in hiding this from others, but still must deal, every minute of every day, with a problem that seems much bigger to him than it appears to you. Minimizing the problem may also make the child feel that he is being discounted or ignored. This may not seem logical, but it is a big part of the dilemma of childhood stuttering and underlies the reluctance of many children, adolescents, and young adults to seek or accept help and therapy. The attempt to hide stuttering is also a part of its development. By saying that the child is "okay" because he does not stutter very much, the teacher is actually reinforcing the child's continual attempt to hide or minimize his dysfluency, which can make the problem worse over time (Van Riper, 1973).

Q. **Would it help the student if I encouraged him to take charge of or take responsibility for his stuttering?**

A. Probably not, if this advice is not accompanied by an acknowledgement of the powerlessness stutterers often experience when they lose control of their speech. Many teens who stutter are consumed by their speech difficulties. It may seem like an insensitive put-down to be told to take ownership of an impairment with which they must struggle every day, and which can make it difficult to go to school each day (requiring a huge amount of emotional energy and even courage). The understanding that the stutterer can have a huge impact on the way he speaks and thinks about his stuttering involves a series of insights and usually requires a series of successes during the therapy process.

Q. **If the teenaged student does not want to discuss stuttering, should the teacher just ignore it and not say anything about it to the student or his parents?**

A. The teacher should discuss the student's stuttering openly with him and with his parents. Because many teens may have more or less difficulty with their speech at home, parents need to hear about how the student is either coping or not coping with stuttering in the academic environment.

Q. **How can a teacher be encouraging to a child who is stuttering when the child does not want to discuss stuttering or becomes embarrassed when the subject is mentioned?**

A. The teacher can provide support to the child or teen who stutters by rewarding participation and communication—regardless of level of fluency—and by acknowledging the extra effort the individual must make to do things that others may take for granted. For many dysfluent teens, some activities (such as oral book reports) may involve not only extra preparation but significant feelings of fear that can potentially lessen the teen's desire to participate in other school activities.

Basic Principles Underlying Treatment of Stuttering in Children

Children and adolescents can be conflicted by the concept of stuttering therapy. On the one hand, it may be important for children to learn to stutter more openly; on the other hand, they may believe that involvement in therapy for stuttering implies that it is bad to stutter. Children cannot help that they stutter, and many older children are unable to become normal speakers; it is our goal to help them become more accepting of their dysfluency as they learn that they can speak or stutter in easier ways that are less forceful, tense, avoidant, and debilitating. When children stutter, let us help them to increase their tolerance as we work together to do everything we can to increase their comfort level. It stands to reason that they will be more accepting of their own stuttering when others in the environment model acceptance, too. In addition, we encourage children and adolescents who stutter to talk openly and freely while working on reducing stuttering severity and demonstrate to themselves the possibility of eventual reduction or elimination of dysfluencies. These thoughts guide the definition of basic principles for the treatment of stuttering in children:

We work at developing an open child-clinician relationship as an important component for building trust, confidence, and understanding.

For children who react negatively to their dysfluencies, it is important to help them express and understand their feelings about stuttering. We encourage the clinician to share other children's experiences and validate embarrassment, pain, and frustration with caring, understanding, and support. We also try to reflect in our words what the child or adolescent may have difficulty expressing. Figure 6.1 reiterates the basic principles underlying the treatment of stuttering in children.

We base treatment on a continuum, as stuttering can be a progressive disorder compounded by cyclical variability (Ramig, Stewart, Ogrodnick, Bennett, Dodge, & Lamy, 1988; Ramig & Bennett, 1995). Treatment plans for many children have to be flexible and designed to meet each child's

Figure 6.1 Basic Principles Underlying Treatment of Stuttering in Children

- Develop an open client-clinician relationship.
- Help the child express and understand his feelings about stuttering.
- Individualize treatment plans to meet each child's changing needs.
- Make therapy enjoyable and rewarding.
- To build self-confidence, structure therapy activities on a level at which the child can experience success.
- In therapy and in the home environment, use a slowed speaking rate with increased pause and response time and maintain appropriate eye contact.
- Help teachers understand how to positively react and interact with a child who stutters.
- Avoid punitive attitudes or intervention measures in or out of the therapy room.
- Conduct sessions outside of the clinic or therapy room to allow the child to experience increased fluency in meaningful environments.

changing needs. Some children and adolescents may not overtly demonstrate an intrinsic motivation to change their speech; therefore, it is important to make therapy enjoyable and rewarding.

Building self-confidence is important and is targeted throughout treatment by providing the child with successful speaking activities. Success with fluency and easier speech is paramount. As a result, therapy activities should be structured on a level at which the child is able to experience success. Single-word and phrase-level tasks may be continued long after the child achieves fluency at that level.

During therapy and in the home environment, we recommend using a slowed speaking rate with increased pause and response time, and maintenance of appropriate eye contact during both fluent and stuttering episodes (see Figure 6.2). In addition, clinicians and clinician-trained caregivers are encouraged to use and model other techniques and strategies

Figure 6.2 How to Speak to a Child Who Stutters

- Use a slowed speaking rate.
- Increase pause and response time.
- Maintain appropriate eye contact during both fluent and stuttering episodes.
- Model techniques and strategies such as easy onsets, easy stuttering, and smooth and easy transitions between sounds.
- Pseudo-stutter to model acceptance.

such as easy onsets, occasional easy stuttering, and smooth and easy transitions between sounds.

Teacher understanding of how to positively react and interact with a child who stutters is very important; thus, teacher education is crucial in meeting our desired goals. The child should never be exposed to punitive attitudes or intervention measures in or out of the therapy room.

Though success in the therapy room lays the foundation for permanent change, long-term changes almost always require the child to successfully experience his increased fluency and use of therapy strategies in everyday speaking situations. Consequently, conducting sessions outside of the clinic or therapy room, when possible, is highly encouraged. When planning stuttering therapy activities, the beginning therapist may be confronted by a dilemma: Am I demonstrating fluency-shaping or stuttering modification techniques or using these therapy activities in a way that will really benefit the children? If we are using commercial games during therapy with children—as this book supports doing for many children—are we sure that they are actually helping improve the child's speech, or are we just making ourselves feel that we are doing something positive? Over the years, we have learned some basic skills of planning, executing, and evaluating therapy sessions that can help us ensure that we are providing real benefits.

Modeling Speech Modification Techniques

The therapist needs to be completely comfortable with all of the speech modification techniques used in stuttering

therapy, including: (1) fluency-enhancing techniques (easy onset of phonation, continuous voicing, easy stretching, light/soft contacts, etc.); (2) stuttering modification techniques (slow bounces, pullouts, cancellations, and exaggerated articulatory movements); and (3) fake or pseudo-stuttering, including hard or tense contacts, repetitions, initial and midword prolongations, and hard or silent blocks.

Methods for teaching (and demonstrating) these techniques are addressed in Chapter 8 of this text. Without continuous, rigorously accurate modeling by his clinician, the child will have difficulty learning the techniques and will lack the motivation to use them. If parents are modeling the techniques at home, they need to perform them properly, with smooth movements and minimal tension, so they will have to be taught by the clinician as well. To make absolutely sure that the client is getting a strong and accurate model, clinicians may observe each other or may wish to watch themselves performing easy onsets, easy stretches, pullouts, and other techniques in a mirror or (even better) in a close-up video recording. Refer to the article by Ramig (1993), "Parent-Clinician-Child Partnership in the Therapeutic Process of the Preschool- and Elementary-aged Child Who Stutters," for more suggestions on involving and training parents to become effective partners in the intervention process.

Therapy Activities

Some clinicians are determined not to play games with their child clients, preferring to use conversation or drill activities to provide a context for learning and practicing the use of speech changes. Other clinicians may prefer to develop game-like activities of their own to help structure therapy sessions. Still others may want to use standard or prepackaged games because children are excited by them or have a special interest in the characters (e.g., Pokémon, DragonBall Z, or Yu-Gi-Oh).

This section focuses on generic types of activities that can be used to structure therapy, with reference to available games that exemplify them. When the clinician becomes adept at using commercially available games, these guidelines can be modified to create activities that provide the specific characteristics needed to enhance therapy for individual children. Of course, some clinicians may prefer to design their own structured games or to modify the commercial games to meet the specific needs of a client. This may be particularly useful with some younger children for whom complex games are too difficult. It is important to remember that games are not therapy; rather, therapy lies in the speech and communication that happen while games are being played. The clinician needs to guard against becoming complacent and allowing the successful use of a game to become the objective of a therapy session. The actual speech activities occurring during the game should be continually reassessed for efficacy.

Why We Use Structured Speech Activities

It is important to have a rational explanation of the therapeutic value of every treatment activity. This is particularly important for games that look like they may be "too much fun" for the child to derive any benefit from them. The benefits of structured speech activities using games include the following.

Games Stimulate Interest in Therapy

Games also have a standard form and series of responses, providing greater ease of comparison within the clinical course for a child as well as across children to help define areas of relative strength and weakness. Create a realistic distraction that can provide practice in attending to the production of speech changes in the real world outside the clinic.

Games Serve as Home Therapy Transfer Activities

Playing games is an important part of childhood, and games used in therapy can serve as home therapy transfer activities. Many children who stutter may be limiting their participation in games—and thus limiting their interaction with other children—because of the speech challenges that the games present. Such children, upon learning that they can be more fluent while playing games, will have an easier time overcoming fears and anxieties.

Types of Games

Some of the different types of games that can be used in therapy are listed in Figure 6.3 and discussed in the following subsections.

Memory-Matching Games

Memory-matching games can address *language complexity at the word level and carrier phrase level.* Memory-matching

Figure 6.3 Types of Games

- Memory-matching games
- Blocks and Legos
- Toy trains; role-playing with story sets and figurines
- Card games
- Board games
- Question games
- Simple dice games
- Complex dice games

games typically involve matching pairs of cards or chips that are shuffled and placed face down on a table. Players draw one card and then try to find its match. Speech activities can involve announcing the content of the cards in one or more words ("flower; bee") or using a carrier phrase; ("I found a flower; I found a bee.") Fluency activities could include stretches or slow and easy bounces on the words ("flo-flo-flower; bbbbbbbee") or on specified components of the carrier phrase ("IIIIIII found a ffffffflower"). Stuttering modification activities could include a combination of stretches and pullouts ("IIIIIIII found a b-b-b-bbbbbbee"), slow bounces and cancellations ("III-III-III found a b-b-b-ce/bbbbbecee /bee") or whatever is appropriate for the child.

Variations or commercially available games include:

- *Go Fish*
- *I Spy* (Briarpatch)
- *Pie Face* (Hassenfeld Brothers)
- *Battleship* (Milton Bradley)

Blocks

Games using blocks can address *language complexity at the word level, the carrier phrase level, and the conversation level.* Building blocks can be used together with drill activities as rewards. For example, a child can be awarded a building block for each successful production of a target activity (easy onsets, stretches, slow bounces, pullouts, etc.) They can be used in request activities, employing carrier phrases (such as "IIIII want a yyyyyyyellow block") or they can be used in free-form play, with the therapist and child interacting and conversing as they build a house or other structure. During the latter, the clinician can allow a talkative child to converse, or can elicit speech by asking leading questions ("How do you think we can make this part of the garage higher?").

Toy Trains and Role-Playing with Sets and Figurines

Many very young children (ages two to four) respond best to play with toys rather than games involving verbal stimuli. The clinician's challenge is to turn nonverbal play into a stimulating speech-language activity without intruding on the child's creativity. If the child is used to playing in silence, the first step is for the clinician to begin actively vocalizing in ways that reinforce or mirror his play, without being intrusive. Such vocalization should reflect the level of cooperative play the child is accustomed to engaging in. If he desires or is used to parallel play, the clinician can matter-of-factly make statements about what she is doing and what the child is doing. After a while, this may stimulate the child to begin mirroring his own activities with vocalizations. The goal is to encourage cooperative play, which is age-appropriate for most children who are beginning to stutter. Of course, the ultimate goal is to encourage open speaking, open stuttering, and open modification of stuttering behaviors.

One child we worked with never tired of a game involving a plastic flying dinosaur (the child's stuttering) and a Batman action figure (the child as self-therapist). During the game the child (in the role of Batman) would first use "hard" speech (fluent speech with hard onsets of phonation) and imitations of "pushing" behavior, which would cause the dinosaur (controlled by the clinician) to take off and start destroying a block city. If Batman continued to address the dinosaur using hard speech, the destructive activities would simply increase. However, if Batman used a gentle speaking style employing "easy" speech (stretches and slow bounces), the dinosaur would calm down and eventually go to sleep. With the dinosaur close at hand, the clinician could monitor the child's productions during the remainder of the therapy session. If his speech began to get hard or be rushed, the dinosaur might come back to life, requiring a return of Batman and his easy speech to save the day once more.

This play activity reinforced a behavioral change that is crucial for the success of stuttering therapy for young children: replacing a strategy of forcing, tension, and pushing with one of ease, relaxation, and compliance. It also places the child in a position of power and control with regard to his stuttering, giving him a greater feeling of comfort.

Card Games

Card games used in therapy can address *language at the word level and carrier phrase level.* Some clinicians have said that all they need to conduct stuttering therapy is a child and a deck of *UNO* cards. Though this might be an exaggeration, much can be done with a simple card game.

The main difference in playing a card game for stuttering therapy is that all moves and activities are announced openly in speech, using a fluency or modification technique. For example, in *UNO*, rather than just playing a card, each player uses a carrier phrase to announce: "IIIII have a green ssssssiiix," "IIIII have to dra—dra—dra—draw," "I pppp-paass," and so on. The pace of the game is such that dozens of repetitions of these techniques and others can be accumulated in a very short period of time.

The limitation of simple card games like *UNO* is that, with their limited word set and language complexity, they may quickly become too easy for some children to benefit. However, they can still be used as warm-ups or to practice newly introduced techniques.

Board Games

Board games can be used in therapy to address *language at the word level and carrier phrase level, reading, and complex utterance.* Board games come in a large range of type and complexity, from word-level games to games involving carrier phrases, complex reading skills, and conversation. They offer the advantage of engaging the clinician and child in a cooperative activity where speech can be open (yet structured) and modifications can be modeled by the clinician and performed by the child in a nonthreatening environment. Basic categories of games, including commercially available examples, are listed here; however, some of these games are more enduring than others.

1. Question games
   - *Battleship* (Milton Bradley)
   - *Guess Who?* (Milton Bradley)

- *Mystery Garden* (Ravensburger)
- *Outburst* (Hasbro)

2. Simple dice games
- *Candyland* (Milton Bradley)
- *Blue's Clues Game* (University Games)
- *Dora the Explorer Game* (Mattel)
- *Monopoly Junior* (Parker Brothers)
- *Yahtzee* (Milton Bradley)
- *PayDay* (Parker Brothers)
- *Yu-Gi-Oh* (Vintage Sports Cards)

3. Complex dice games
- *Pokémon Master Trainer* (Vintage Sports Cards)
- *Clue* (Parker Brothers)
- *Monopoly* (Parker Brothers)
- *The Game of Life* (Milton Bradley)
- *Risk* (Parker Brothers)
- *Lego Creator* (Lego)

Which Game to Use?

A hierarchical approach should be used when selecting games for use in therapy. Early in the intervention process, it is important to use very simple games with which the child can achieve success in increasing fluency without continual reminders from the therapist. The definition of *simple* will vary from child to child, but most memory games, *UNO*, and games that can be played with rote responses involving numbers, letters, or colors (such as *Battleship*) will qualify. If excessive cueing is required, this may be an indication that the game is too complex for the child to manage while simultaneously working on fluency-shaping or stuttering modification techniques. The focus should always be on speech activities, rather than the games that are coincidently used to provide the speech stimulus.

In *Battleship*, for example, each player may simply announce the location of the square he wants to hit, using an easy prolongation, stretch, or pseudo-stutter. Alternatively, a simple phrase such as "I hit E six," or "I shoot C nine" can be used, with an easy prolongation on the "I" and the number. Similar use can be made of memory games, in which the

child turns over two tiles at a time, seeking a match. He can either identify the object on the tile ("antelope") or be encouraged to use a short carrier phrase ("IIII found an aaaantelope.").

Once the child has mastered easy games and his therapy moves on to longer carrier phrases and sentences, the more complex types of games listed earlier can be used. Expressive language and reading speech modalities can be explored by selecting question-response games (such as *Mystery Garden* or *Guess Who*, in which players seek to identify a tile or card held by the opponent) or games such as *Twenty Questions* or *Pay Day*, which use cards that must be read aloud. *Outburst Jr.*, which uses both of these modalities and employs short questions and one- or two-word answers, is a good intermediate game.

Using Structured or Programmed Fluency Therapy Programs

Some clinicians may desire the confidence derived from using a preprepared fluency therapy package, such as *Easy Does It-2,* to provide structure and easy-to-use activities for therapy sessions. Other clinicians may even be required by their school districts or other jurisdictions to use these programs. If this is the case, there is certainly nothing wrong with doing so. In addition, some of these programs provide speech modification, games, drill activities, role-playing scenarios, and counseling activities that can be readily adapted to the integrated approach advocated in this book.

Using Delayed Auditory Feedback Devices in Therapy

The use of delayed auditory feedback (DAF) devices for short, therapeutic periods, is advocated for older children in several places throughout this resource manual, with the focus on several different therapy goals. These include:

- Slowing the child's speaking rate (cluttering and stuttering)
- Providing the child with a model of more fluent speech
- Helping the child feel the movements, tactile feelings, and proprioceptive aspects of fluent speech

Based on our experience with using DAF technology for many years, and on findings provided in recent research (e.g., Kalinowski, Armson, Roland-Meiskowski, Stuart, & Gracco, 1993; Kalinowski, Noble, Armson, & Stuart, 1994; Kalinowski, Armson, & Stuart, 1995; Kalinowski, Dayalu, Stuart, Rastatter, & Rami, 2000; Kalinowski & Dayalu, 2002), we do not believe that delayed auditory feedback helps generate more fluent speech in people who stutter simply because it slows speech rate. Stuttering is also reduced when normal or even faster-than-normal rates are used in the presence of DAF. People who stutter commonly report a feeling that they are less vulnerable to stuttering at fast as well as slow speech rates. Accordingly, we use DAF at a number of target speaking rates for different purposes. Because the slowest speaking rate involves a very slow (70 to 90 syllables per minute), highly exaggerated, and blended style of speech that can seem very unnatural, the clinician will need to learn to model this for the child. It is valuable for the clinician to experience the difficulty some children may have in maintaining the slow rate for more than a minute or two, as well as resisting the tendency to gloss over syllables that should be pronounced slowly.

The faster speech rates are used to beat the delay imposed by DAF and help children focus more on the feeling of speech movements. Most speakers will have to ignore the *sound* of their voices as much as possible and monitor the tactile and proprioceptive feeling of speech gestures very strongly to maintain their fluency and not get tripped up by the delay.

Therapy with Portable Electronic Fluency Devices

Recently, improvements in miniaturized electronic circuitry have enabled the development and use of highly portable altered auditory feedback (AAF) devices that may incorporate DAF and/or frequency altered feedback (FAF) technology. Such devices may inhibit stuttering to a significant extent with continuous, long-term usage. Although the inhibitory effect has been shown by preliminary studies to be maintained for an extended period for many users, there is little or no carryover effect for most. That is, when the person stops using the device, he is likely to resume stuttering much the same as he did before. Fluency devices are normally provided by a certified clinician trained in their application by

the company that distributes the device. The authors have dispensed such devices for teen and adult stuttering clients who have requested them and who have been shown to benefit from them in trial usage, but we generally do not recommend extended use of these devices by younger children and adolescents younger than 12 or 13 years of age. There are several reasons for this:

- The devices may be complicated to wear, requiring extreme care in use, cleaning, and maintenance that may be difficult for some younger people.

- The continued benefits of traditional therapy may not yet have been realized by young children. The devices are most effective when the user has received traditional therapy and continues to employ fluency-enhancing techniques used in such therapy.

- There may be interference with normal hearing caused by the altered feedback, which could be detrimental in classroom learning and some conversational situations for some children.

Because of the increasing use of such devices, clinicians may be confronted with the need to assist a child who is having difficulty maintaining fluency or who seeks to increase his fluency with a successful device. In our experience, traditional fluency-shaping and stuttering modification techniques (particularly initial sound stretches and cancellations employing easy initial-sound prolongations) are beneficial to device users. However, if continued use of the device is desired, it is important that the child actually be wearing the device while receiving supplementary therapy in the clinic. It is also our experience that lack of success with these devices may be partly associated with a previous lack of desensitization to stuttering or to increased attempts to avoid stuttering in the presence of listener expectations of fluency. Because we feel that counseling and working with attitudes about stuttering are integral parts of the therapy process, such emotional work would have to be undertaken with the child if he is to be successful with his fluency device.

Rewards, Classical and Otherwise

Until most children are nine or ten years old, they will initiate change activities or respond better to directive or potentially unpleasant activities if they are provided with tangible rewards. This is as true in stuttering therapy as it is in any other type of activity. The choice of reinforcement should be determined by observing the child's response to various types of rewards. Some children only need the recognition of how much work they have done (counters), along with verbal encouragement and praise. Others need the pleasure of acquiring a valuable commodity (such as a trading card) or a favorite food item. Still others need a combination of these approaches, with counters representing discrete work accomplishments (easy onsets, stretches, bounces, pseudo-stutters, or cancellations) that are translated into trading cards, pieces of fruit, or small candies. The clinician should, of course, take her cue from the parents regarding what is acceptable to them.

It is important, however, to keep a flow of praise going to the child for all accomplishments, no matter how slight, and to avoid letting tangible or concrete rewards take the place of social ones. Eventually, the clinician will look for the child to leave tangible reinforcements behind and respond to the internal rewards of feeling more fluent speech and being able to express his feelings and needs to friends, family, and teachers. Without a generous flow of verbal reinforcement, it may take longer for this transformation to occur.

A very useful approach is to treat more enjoyable therapy activities as rewards. The therapy sessions can begin with drill, with the promise that good effort in the drill activity will result in being able to play the child's favorite board game. When the activity itself is rewarding, the child moves closer to the time when tangible rewards can be left behind. Success is much more likely if the child enjoys therapy, rather than experiencing it as a temporary hardship that results in a consolation prize.

Counters

Counters can be controlled by the clinician or used to provide the child with a measure of control over himself or the therapy activity. They also strengthen cognitive awareness during therapy sessions, on the part of both the clinician and the child. Positive and negative behaviors can be counted, with the emphasis on the former. However, sometimes it can be better to simply count negative behaviors or missed opportunities rather than orally reminding the child, because this is less intrusive. The child will then realize that the therapist is counting something that he has just missed and will have to self-monitor to discover what he didn't do.

Counters can be used in conjunction with rewards at first. When the child is weaned from classical rewards, just the behavior count can serve as a measure of his success and accomplishment.

Trading Cards and Other Collectibles

The child should perceive any rewards as having value. That means the clinician will need to listen to the child's preferences and place them above her preconceived notions of what a child should want. The clinician will want to maintain an ongoing awareness of the latest fads and trends in the various media outlets of interest to children. That does not mean that we need to spend Saturday mornings watching cartoon shows. It does suggest that the clinician should develop the habit of asking the child what he is interested in at the moment and encouraging him to bring play activities to the clinic.

Food and Candy

All reinforcements should receive the approval of parents, but this is even more essential when candy and food rewards are contemplated. Of course, nuts and foods like peanuts should typically be avoided because of the possibility of allergies. High-calorie candy bars are not recommended because they may interfere with normal meals and nutrition, and the child may too strongly anticipate them as a reward in the future. Smaller hard or chewy candies may be used, however, to reward speech changes. Counters should be used to quantify the rewards, rather than handling the candies while therapy is going on, to minimize health risks, reduce distractions, and prepare the child for the day when tangible rewards will be replaced by verbal praise.

Although it is essential to maintain a positive tone during therapy and to acknowledge the difficulty of the child's tasks, the possibility of not getting a reward or receiving a lesser one should be maintained. Some children may not respond well to the punishment of withheld rewards, but many children will be motivated to do better next time if they receive a reward that reflects poor performance.

Transfer Activities

One of the best ways of creating synergy between in-clinic and outside speech activities is to present transfer activities such as visiting stores, ice cream shops, and other enjoyable venues as rewards for work in the clinic. Additional information on handling these activities and making them relevant to therapy is provided in Chapter 11. As with all activities, it is important that the clinician performs all of the activities asked of the child. Some children may not be able to perform these activities without assurance that nothing bad will happen, and the clinician can demonstrate this through modeling.

Summary

We have provided detail regarding basic principles in working with children, as well as information on the use of a variety of games and other pertinent therapy-room ideas and activities. Although we recommend and support the use of these activities in working with children and some adolescents, we must emphasize that behavior change is more likely to occur when the clinician's focus is the elicitation of as many target responses per session as possible in the context of high quality comunication. Incorporating games and other fun activities with children helps ensure the child's continued interest in the intervention process, but it is ultimately the number of responses per session that changes behavior. In that regard, it is important that the fun activities be pre-planned and organized so the session moves along at a steady pace.

Those who provide therapy for both preschool and school-age children realize that preschool children are very different from older children. Preschool children stutter differently, react to therapy differently, recover their fluency differently, and require slightly (and sometimes radically) different therapy techniques (Van Riper, 1973; Bloodstein, 1995; Conture, 1997; Guitar, 1998; Dell, 2000). These differences have always been the reason for the existence of two different approaches for treating children in this age group: direct and indirect. Within each of these approaches, there are techniques that can be classified as active or passive. Until the 1980s, indirect therapy, involving environmental modification in the home, was the most popular therapy approach. However, beginning with techniques employed by Carl Dell (2000) and others, direct treatment, employing fluency-shaping and even stuttering modification techniques, was employed for those children who were found to benefit. Recently, an indirect method, in which the parents are taught to praise fluent speech and ignore stuttered speech, was developed by Onslow, Packman, and Harrison (2003) at the Lidcombe Institute in Sydney, Australia.

Indirect Therapy

Indirect therapy is provided by parents, with consultation by the SLP. It can also be used as a supplement for direct therapy by the SLP. The techniques for implementing this therapy approach vary considerably in style and intensity, including:

- Simply making changes in the child's communication environment

- Interacting with the child in ways that are intended to facilitate greater fluency

- Making changes in speech to provide the child with various types of models for change

- Praising use of the models provided by parents and the SLP

- Parental conduct of a structured indirect therapy program employing modeling, contingent praise of fluent speech or speech modifications, and parental reporting of progress to the SLP, including recording of speech samples

News that preschool children may recover their fluency just by being praised for their fluent speech and being "punished" (actually, ignored) when they are dysfluent has been a source of controversy over the last few years. Increased Northern Hemisphere experience with the Lidcombe Programme developed in Australia (Onslow, Packman, and Harrison, 2003) has indicated that parent-administered praise and punishment actually do have a positive effect on the fluency of children who are less than five years of age. We currently do not advise the use of this program with older children, given the lack of supporting research with older children at this time.

It is important to realize that an indirect approach such as Lidcombe requires a strong commitment by the clinician to train the child's parents and hand over the therapy process to them. Clinicians who want to try this approach will need to attend a special training program, administered by a person with experience in the Lidcombe Programme. Experimenting with a personal or modified approach to this program is not encouraged by the developers (Onslow et al., 2003).

For other clinicians, a degree of indirect therapy is always an integral part of a more traditional fluency-shaping/stuttering modification regimen for preschool children. Modeling of modified speech by other speakers and modification of the speech environment within the home will help to reinforce direct therapy by making fluency—slower, easier speech—seem more natural to the child. Praise for the conscious or unconscious use of fluency-enhancing speech behaviors will help increase the child's confidence. Although merely simplifying the parent's language complexity or reducing speech rate have not been found to be effective in increasing the child's fluency (Miles & Ratner, 2001), the real benefit of such changes may be to help and encourage the child to transfer his more fluent behaviors across environments.

We feel strongly that it is inappropriate to treat the use of fluency-shaping or stuttering modification techniques as a "performance" that should be executed at the command or request of others. Such expectations are unhelpful for school-age children and should be specifically avoided for preschool children.

Direct Therapy

Direct therapy means any therapy approach that is conducted primarily by the SLP. Although a direct therapy regimen may (and should) include some indirect therapy by the parents and other caregivers, the SLP's role is preeminent. Direct therapy by the SLP may include the full range of intervention approaches, including play and play-drill therapy, modeling, fluency shaping, and stuttering modification, using the variety of techniques discussed in this resource guide.

Awareness of Stuttering

The clinician's biggest challenge when working with some children may be figuring out how to discuss stuttering when the child is not aware of (or is not acknowledging) his own speech dysfluencies. Such a child may perform many repetitions, but may not be aware of the relationship of speech to the feeling that he is "stuck" or that "something" is holding him back. It is important to acknowledge this distinction. Although the child may not perceive his speech productions as distorted words, he is aware of a difficulty in speaking; specifically of *feeling* stuck.

To help such children develop a new understanding of their speech, it is helpful for the clinician to demonstrate the relationship between the sensation of getting stuck and the resulting speech productions. The act of "putting stuttering in our own mouths" (Van Riper, 1973) helps to illustrate this difference and to make the child more aware of what he is doing. In the example in Figure 7.1, the clinician could explain: "Sometimes I get stuck when I talk. That sounds like this: 'He-he-he-he-he-he-he-help.' But my speech feels better when I say it like this: 'He-hhhheeelp.'"

Another strategy for creating positive awareness, and building the child's sense of self-efficacy and confidence, is commonly referred to as playing "Speech Patrol." In this activity, the child identifies times when the clinician is getting stuck on words. This helps the child see instances when it would be appropriate to modify speech so that it feels better. If the child recoils in horror upon hearing the clinician, she may reduce the severity or frequency of the imitated stutters until the child can tolerate them. Incidentally, the emphasis on feeling here is intentional. The powerless feeling that results from a loss of control often concerns children more than the actual speech dysfluencies. Once the child learns how to be a "speech cop," the clinician can introduce the idea of helping each other to get unstuck from stuttering. Success with this activity will result as the child feels more in control by learning to modify his stuttering behaviors.

In our experience, it is probably best to model a type of dysfluency that is not very distorted (i.e., that does not involve use of the schwa vowel). Also, if the child commonly stutters on a particular word, such as "I" or "he," it is good to select another common word so the child does not feel that the clinician is teasing or ridiculing him. Otherwise, it is appropriate to imitate the child's stuttering, so that he may be able to generalize your behavior to his more easily. However, we have found it important to reassure the child that such imitation by the clinician is meant to help rather than to mock or tease.

At some point, the child may verbalize the concept that he gets stuck, too. Sometimes such a realization will not be volunteered, so the clinician will have to break the ice. The child may then deny that he gets stuck, particularly if he feels a lot of shame about it. In some cases, it may be effective to play a recording of the child to create self-awareness of dysfluencies. Great sensitivity, of course, is required when doing this, so that the child will be less likely to feel shame or disgrace that someone has "found him out."

Which Word Is the Stuttered Word?

It can sometimes be important to determine on which sound the child feels blocked when stuttering. When the child is repeating the word "I" in the utterance "I-I-I-I th-th-think

> **Child:** "He-he-he-he-he-he-he-he-he-help me to open this."
>
> **Clinician:** "OK, I'll he-he-hhhheeelp you with that" (modeling a modified dysfluency).
>
> **Child:** "Whatt's he-he-hhhheeelp?" (not recognizing the word).

Figure 7.1 Clinician Modeling Modified Dysfluency

the bear is tired," it could be that the child is anticipating difficulty on the "th" rather than stuttering on the "I" itself. Nevertheless, even if the anticipated difficulty on the "th" sound is the source of the "I" repetitions, it is still beneficial to help the child to make the "I" easier, less tense, and less forceful. The feeling of an easier "I" may help extinguish the expectation that the subsequent sound will be difficult. When starter or postponement repetitions are habitually said in a less forceful way, the habit may generalize to other sounds and help to extinguish the development of tense speaking patterns. This will set the child up to initiate the feared or anticipated stuttering sound in a less forceful way as well.

Fluency-Enhancing Activities

The clinician's primary job in working with the preschool child is to create an environment conducive to communication activities that facilitate more fluent speech. Unless specific types of stuttering modification or desensitization activities are being conducted, the clinician's speech during therapy should be slow, tension-free, and characterized by gentle onsets of phonation and continuous voicing. Rhythmic speech activities and even singing may be used to further enhance the child's feeling of fluency.

Easier and more relaxed speech can help break the cycle of building tension that can contribute to dysfluencies. Stuttering is not a habit, but the behaviors that support its development may become habitual, and the strategies the child uses to avoid, escape, push, or force himself through dysfluent moments may perniciously increase the severity of stuttering. It is important to break this cycle as much as possible.

Stuttering Modification Activities

For preschool children, stuttering modification activities are not as specific or as precise as those for older children and teenagers. They involve making hard stuttering moments easier and "repairing" stuttering after it has occurred to demonstrate control. Once again, these types of modifications should be modeled by the clinician as much as possible during all therapy. An example of a modeling interchange between the clinician and child is provided in Figure 7.2. Note that the clinician should not expect any particular type of response from the child.

> **Clinician:** I have been getting stuck when I try to say some words today. Would you help me by telling me when I get stuck so I can get unstuck?
>
> **Child:** [may respond in some way.]
>
> **Clinician:** When I get stuck, it sounds like this: "Th-th-th-the boy is walking his dog."

Figure 7.2 Example of Modeling Interchange

Throughout these activities, it is important to emphasize that stuttering is always acceptable. We are helping the child to produce an easier form of stuttering that will help him make his speech feel better and help him feel more confident about his communication abilities.

Activities are always aimed at increasing the child's participation in the therapy process. Because it is actually the child who must make the speech changes, it is vital that the child's active role be rewarded, through either concrete means or actual improvements in speech. To reinforce the effect of speech changes, the clinician should be extravagant and unconditional with her praise, as long as the child is making some effort. It is likely that an apparently small or insignificant effort on the child's part is the result of a great deal of effort of which the observer is not aware. Just as stuttering may be likened to an iceberg, with only a small part evident to the observer, (Sheehan, 1970), so may be speech modifications.

Changing Form of Stuttering

One of the most disconcerting (and interesting) aspects of direct work with preschool children is that their stuttering behaviors and reactive strategies may change from session to session. This requires the clinician to be extremely flexible in the development of speech activities or targets. Failure to address a new behavior rapidly may result in lost time. This is not critical for the child, whose speech is too fluid at this point to be permanently damaged by a few days of delay, but it is important for the efficiency of the therapy process.

Primary behaviors such as prolongations and repetitions may appear, disappear, and reappear, depending on the child's mood and the stressors he is experiencing. Some secondary behaviors that the clinician thought had been extinguished may suddenly reappear, requiring retrenching or a return to an earlier phase of therapy.

Examples of common preschool behaviors that may crop up without warning are forcing and pushing, tensing and holding, changes in the number or speed of repetitions, whispering, and introduction of starter words (Figure 7.3). It is important to develop a good rapport and constant information exchange with the parents to provide news of new behaviors or the reappearance of old ones. Whatever the new behaviors are, it is key to address the primary event(s) to which the child is reacting by modeling changes and modifications, developing negative-practice games, or selecting other activities. It may be possible to address some secondary behaviors (such as inserting starter words) directly, but this should not be pressed if the child is not receptive or able to engage in a nonthreatening, entertaining extinguishment activity (which should always involve making a therapeutic modification—such as an easy stretch—to address the feeling that is causing the reactivity).

Figure 7.3 Common Secondary Behaviors of the Preschool Stutterer

- Forcing and pushing
- Teasing and holding
- Changing either the number or speed of repetitions
- Whispering
- Introducing starter words

Being Less Directive

On some days, virtually nothing can be done in terms of active direct therapy, because of either the child's mood or his physical condition. That is a part of working with this age group. The therapist just needs to stay relaxed, modeling easier forms of speech, and go with the flow. There may be other days when the child's dysfluencies are very severe and he is under considerable stress for one reason or another.

These are good times for performing nonspeech activities such as drawing, playing with a train set or tea set, or smashing toy cars together. There are always ways to praise and build the confidence of children.

Often, the therapist may be able to accomplish her objectives by adapting them to the child's preferences. This type of flexibility may be uncomfortable for some therapists, but it can pay dividends for the child. For example, if the child refuses to play a board game the clinician was hoping to use for a drill-play activity, the blocks or play set that the child prefers on that day may provide opportunities for similar work. Or the child may be encouraged to speak while drawing.

How Do Preschool Children Recover Fluency?

Evidence shows that up to 75 percent of preschool children who stutter will recover their fluency naturally; this may indicate that very young children do recover differently than older ones. It is as if many preschool children have an innate ability to work things out that older children lack or have lost. This may also be evidence for the important role of neurological conditioning in stuttering development. Recent clinical evidence (Yairi & Ambrose, 2004) indicates that the types and severity of stuttering behaviors exhibited by children are not valid predictors of success in therapy or recovery, at least when early intervention is accomplished. This may indicate that children who have not been conditioned for extended periods can more easily learn or use imitated or alternative adaptive techniques to overcome or inhibit the reactions that seem to accompany stuttering behavior. Perhaps it is largely by interfering with the development of stuttering and changing the overall dynamics of reactivity to stuttering that therapy helps preschoolers recover their lost fluency. These are questions that we hope will be answered soon, so that more effective treatments that will help all stuttering preschool children recover their fluency can be developed.

Unfortunately, not all children recover their fluent childhood behaviors—even with treatment—before they enter kindergarten. That does not mean that recovery will be impossible, just that it will be more difficult and may not be accompanied by complete fluency. With increased awareness and consciousness may come increased reactions to the feeling of dysfluency. However, greater cognitive abilities also allow the use of more active direct therapy techniques by the clinician.

Sample Activities

Preschool children require special accommodations and types of activities. By following the child's lead, the clinician may learn activities (some very simple in nature) that will enable her to structure speech productions during therapy.

Commercial Games

Commercial board or matching games may be difficult to use conventionally with preschool children under four years of age, who may be overly competitive (and who therefore may find it painful or stressful to lose) or who may not know how to share or follow rules. Such games may be used in nonconventional ways to provide speech opportunities. One simple example is using the special tiles in *Candyland* as tokens for prizes (when the object is named with an easy

stretch) rather than requiring the child to lose his position on the board.

Speech Patrol

In "Speech Patrol," the clinician asks the child to stop her when she repeats a syllable multiple times. The clinician can also ask the child to remind her to use easy speech when she repeats a syllable multiple times. This activity can be conducted while playing with puppets or toy sets. If the child seems squeamish about hearing the clinician repeat sounds, puppets can be used to role-play. One puppet can play the role of speaker and the other the role of helper. (It is helpful to use puppets with mouths that open wide.)

Request Games

A modified request game has the clinician ask for items held by the child. As long as the clinician repeats or pushes or struggles on the first syllable of the word without modification, the child withholds the item. When the clinician turns the repetition into a stretch, the child agrees to offer the item. The clinician and child should alternate these roles.

Before identifying stuttering behaviors, it is vital to engage the child in exploring his fluent speech (Dell, 1993; Nelson, 1998; Ramig, 1998b). This involves the child in a process of inquiry and exploration, provides a useful working vocabulary (for example, voiced and unvoiced sounds) to facilitate communication during therapy, and forms a basis for later speech modification work. There is also considerable desensitization value for some children who may consider their vocal anatomy an adversary or—at least—an uncooperative partner (Healey, 2004). It makes sense that if we are hoping to assist the child in producing more fluent speech, we first explore the fluent speech that is available. It is also useful for the child to discover that his physical speech apparatus and mental capacities for speech are essentially normal, in that all the elements needed to produce fluent speech can be made to work properly, albeit inconsistently at present.

Emotional Aspects

Sometimes exploring the speech process can be an emotional and embarrassing experience for children and adolescents (Zebrowski & Kelly, 2002). Some children may consider themselves to be physically flawed or imperfect in the area of speech. We have seen children tear up or begin to weep when confronted with a line drawing of the speech anatomy. When this happens, it may be best to take a short break to validate the child's feelings with words acknowledging his reaction: "Yeah, it's a little strange talking about this stuff, isn't it?" or "Stuttering isn't very much fun, is it?" The best antidote, when the child is ready, is to make the process of exploring normal speech interesting and fun. This is all part of the process of being scrupulously open about speech and stuttering. As the process unfolds, the child will probably begin to experience a profound feeling of relief.

Becoming an expert on speech can be a positive reinforcement for the child. Speech is taken for granted by most people and by schools, so most people never learn about the mechanics of speech. This can be an area of special knowledge for the child who stutters. To help him develop a sense of expertise, consider teaching him the following concepts:

- Voiced and unvoiced sounds
- Articulatory movements
- Role of breathing in speech
- Speech anatomy
- Resonance
- Gentle or easy onsets of phonation
- Continuous voicing
- Speed and rate of speech
- Co-articulation (slow and fast)
- Conscious and unconscious aspects of speech
- Relationship between letters and sounds

Sample Activities

Working together to explore the child's fluent speech offers a chance to establish rapport and clinical rituals that provide structure and a feeling of safety for the child. Rewards for success also can make speech therapy into something positive that will be looked forward to instead of dreaded or feared. A list of sample activities is provided in Figure 8.1. A more detailed description of some key activities is provided in the following subsections.

Teach Anatomy of Speech Production Using a "Speech Person" Model

Depending on the child's age, a drawing or a cardboard cutout model can be used to help him locate the various "speech helpers" involved in producing speech sounds (Ramig, 1998b). If this aid is realistic rather than schematic, it will be important to have several drawings of boys, girls, adults, and people of different racial backgrounds. The components should include the diaphragm; lungs; windpipe, (trachea); voice box (larynx), oral and nasal cavities; and the articulators, such as the jaw, lips, tongue, teeth, and the "gum bump" (alveolar ridge) that is used to create many sounds.

If the child is developing a speech notebook, a drawing of the speech person or a copy of the SLP's picture can be one of the first things he puts into it.

Figure 8.1 Natural Speech Production Activities

- Teach anatomy of speech production using "speech person" model
- Use picture word cards to teach syllable components
- Use *My First Phonics Book* to demonstrate co-articulation
- Demonstrate the function of breathing in speech with long and short "ahs"
- Feel voice-box vibration to distinguish voiced and unvoiced sounds
- Use voiced and unvoiced pairs to teach the differences between sounds
- Use a mirror to demonstrate normal mouth opening
- Discuss and demonstrate gentle onsets of phonation
- Teach fluent stretching of consonants
- Teach stretches to children with articulatory delays

Use Picture Word Cards to Teach Syllable Components

Cards published by School Zone Publishing Company have two sides that feature single-syllable words appropriate for two age groups. The clinician can also make such cards. The first side has a picture with the associated word (e.g., "book") that is appropriate for children under less than six or seven years of age. The second side has a simple list of one-syllable words that rhyme, such as

- Book
- Took
- Look
- Cook

This side is useful for talking about the constituents of syllables, practicing consonants, and teaching gentle onsets of phonation. Such cards can also be developed by the clinician or even by the child with the clinician's input.

Use *My First Phonics Book* to Demonstrate Co-Articulation

My First Phonics Book (Dorling Kindersley Publishing, 1999)—and other similar products—features language sam- ples with highlighted phonemes in various positions: initial, medial, and final. These can be used to illustrate the differences between the articulation and voicing of sounds when they are at the beginning of words and when they follow and are blended with various other sounds.

Demonstrate the Function of Breathing in Speech

For this activity it is useful to have a stopwatch (with a sweep second hand, if you can find one). Have the child sit still (if possible!) with his hand resting lightly on his stomach. Ask him to relax for a minute and then say, "Say 'ah'." Ask if the child felt his stomach expand when he said "ah." If he did not or could not remember, ask him to make his stomach move outward the next time you ask him to speak. Repeat the process a few times if necessary. Once he reports that his stomach is moving just before he speaks, have him say "ah" as long as he can. Let him start when he is ready. (The clinician can also model this for the child.) The point here is to note how much more air is needed and how much tension is present in the upper chest area as the child tries to squeeze out the last little bit of air.

Feel Voice-Box Vibration to Distinguish Voiced and Unvoiced Sounds

Voicing is an important concept and activity to teach to stuttering children. It is the basis of teaching the gentle or easy onset. "Turning on" the voice is often the point in the utterance where the most stuttering occurs. Most young children (and even many adults) have never been exposed to the concept of voicing and are interested in learning about the mysterious voice box that vibrates in their throats when they speak.

Use Voiced and Unvoiced Pairs to Teach the Differences between Sounds

One of the easiest ways to teach the difference between voiced and unvoiced sounds is to have the child demonstrate to himself the difference between voiced and unvoiced pairs such as /d/ and /t/, /b/ and /p/, /k/ and /g/, /s/ and /z/, /f/ and /v/, and so on. The clinician should focus on the fact that these sounds are created using exactly the same articulatory movements. The only difference is in the activation of vibration and sound in the voice box on the voiced component of the pairs. Once the concept is learned, testing the child's knowledge gives him an opportunity to demonstrate competence. By asking which sounds are voiced and which are unvoiced, the clinician can give the child an opportunity to demonstrate knowledge and competence in speech—an area where incompetence may formerly have been assumed by the child.

Use a Mirror to Demonstrate Normal Mouth Opening

Production of vowels can be easier to demonstrate if the clinician points to her mouth opening during vowel-sound production and then invites the child to observe his own mouth in a mirror. Because smooth, tension-free mouth opening and jaw movement can help ease tension in the laryngeal area, this demonstration can be repeated during later work on fluency-enhancing skills. The vital point here is that mouth opening is an element of normal speech.

Mouth opening can be a way to begin the discussion of how the vowel sounds are centered in different parts of the oral cavity. Low vowels ("uh" and "ah") can allow more normal mouth opening than higher vowels like /e/. Explanation of this can teach normal expectations for mouth opening, lessening the chance that the child will add tension to vocalizations by opening his mouth too wide.

It is important to mirror the child's findings throughout these exercises. Figure 8.2 illustrates this interaction.

Fluency-Enhancing Techniques

The teaching of fluency-enhancing techniques (*fluency shaping*) is performed in our therapy in a way that distinguishes them from stuttering modification techniques. There are several reasons for this, including their logical association with normal speech, the ease of teaching them, and the desirability of increasing the child's confidence and giving him a feeling of success early in the treatment regimen.

Gentle Onsets of Phonation

Though not all fluent speakers use gentle onsets in their speech, such onsets are considered an important part of normal speaking. Therefore, teaching the child or adolescent how to reliably produce gentle onsets on vowel sounds is an

Clinician:	Let's try an "e" sound now.
Child and clinician:	"eeeeee"
Clinician:	that sounded like an "e," didn't it? Now how about if we try it with our mouths open as wide as it was on that "a" sound?
Child and clinician:	"aaaaaaaaa"
Clinician:	What did you notice about that?
Child:	I guess it sounded more like an "a" than an "e."
Clinician:	How about that! I guess that we need to keep our mouths closed a bit when we say an "e."

Figure 8.2 Mirroring

excellent way to begin the self-demonstration of normal and natural speech.

One of the pitfalls of teaching gentle onsets is that the child (and the clinician) can get caught up in trying too hard to do them exactly "right." It is important for later modification work to achieve a high degree of skill and accuracy in intentionally performing gentle onsets; nevertheless, the clinician needs to demonstrate that she does not always do them correctly and that this is acceptable. The point that hard onsets are not the cause of stuttering can be reinforced by having the child observe the speech of fluent speakers, many of whom do not always perform gentle onsets. For older children, however, it may also be worthwhile to discuss the way hard onsets can trigger stuttering because they make us feel less fluent or have become connected (through classical conditioning) with stuttering events. The discussion of what causes hard onsets in the first place should be left until the exploration of stuttered speech, where the gentle onsets taught here will provide a way of illustrating the differences.

The concept of gentle onsets may be introduced in several ways, depending on the child's age and intellectual level. For older children who have been introduced to graphs in school, a graph such as the one in Figure 8.3 may be useful. This shows two hypothetical speech onsets, plotted with voice

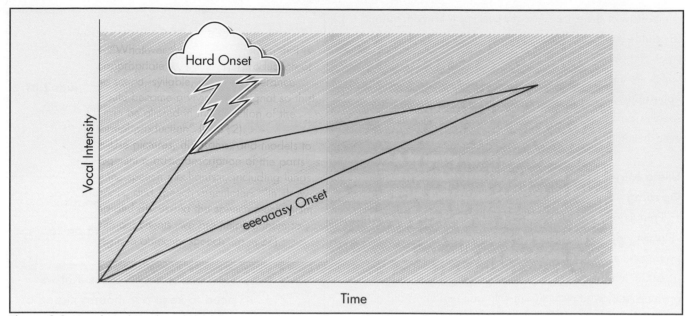

Figure 8.3 Hypothetical Gentle and Hard Onsets. Vocal intensity (voice volume) is on the Y axis and time is on the X axis.

volume on the Y axis and time on the X axis. The hard onset obviously involves a large increase in volume or loudness in a very short amount of time (less than 0.2 second). The gentle or easy onset illustrates a gradual increase over a period of one to two seconds. The clinician should model the two examples so that the child can clearly relate the graph to actual speech.

The concept of stretching a sound out should be taught first. Merely doing this will help to elongate the onset, distributing the force of the attack and helping to make the onset a bit easier. Such long durations will probably be difficult enough for the child at first, and it is important not to overwhelm him with too much. Two seconds is a good duration for practicing vowel sounds. A sweep second hand is much easier to use as an aid than a digital clock, because it helps illustrate how long a second actually is. Children often think that a second is a very small duration and will be amazed at how much can happen within a single second. (This concept can also be thought of as one of the first attempts to address the stuttering child's sense of time passage and time pressure.)

Younger (i.e., three- to five-year-old) children may not have to be trained beyond the two-second prolongation and a strong model of easy onsets by the clinician. In our experience, their onsets often become very gentle, perhaps because

hard onsets have not been reinforced or repeated often enough to become automatic. Older children and teens will probably require additional training. Once the older child has mastered prolonging several vowel sounds for two seconds, the clinician should encourage him to imitate gentle onsets modeled by the clinician and illustrated in the graph. Rather than doing one of these at a time, the child should try at least four or five in succession, separated with long (two- to four-second) relaxed pauses. This will encourage experimentation, increase carryover learning and improvement from production to production, and take the performance pressure off of each attempt. To begin to encourage the child to focus on the feeling of speech, rather than the sound, the clinician could ask him which one felt the best.

For children who have difficulty creating gentle onsets, some clinicians have advocated adding an /h/ sound to the beginning of an utterance to set up an initial flow of air. We have found, however, that this can become an unneeded crutch if it is maintained beyond the initial difficulties. It can even become a hindrance to communication; for example, changing the word "eight" to "hate" or "I" to "hi." The /h/ becomes very problematic if it is inserted in the midst of words, such as in the transition between an unvoiced consonant and a vowel (as in "Sssssss-hhhue" for "Sue"). Finally, a habit of forcing relatively large volumes of air through the vocal folds may even lead to excessive dryness or irritation of the delicate epidermal layer.

There is at least one electronic device that can aid clinicians in teaching gentle onsets. The "Desktop" version of the delayed auditory feedback device marketed by Casafutura Technologies includes a biofeedback device with internal programming similar to the voice monitor used in some intensive fluency-shaping programs.

Continuous Voicing and Reduced Rate

We work on the concepts of continuous voicing and reduced rate together because they are mutually supportive. However, they are fluency enhancing only if the proper use of reduced rate is recognized. Continuous voicing involves maintaining phonation (vocal-cord vibration) as much as possible between sounds and syllables of speech. Phonation cannot be truly continuous, of course, because there must be at least a slight pause of phonation on unvoiced consonants and when breaths are taken. However, maximizing the blending of sounds will help to produce the feeling that the voice is always "on."

Continuous voicing can be supported in several ways. The most important is probably by requesting (and modeling) a slightly more exaggerated movement and opening of the mouth. Such movement is required to bridge over the gaps between sounds and facilitates closing the gaps surrounding unvoiced consonants. The second major supportive target is the feeling of the continuous buzzing of the vocal folds. This can be reinforced by having the child feel his voice box with his hand or fingers, to verify that it is vibrating virtually continuously. Yet another method is by requesting (and modeling) the prolongation of the ends of sounds and syllables. We do this to avoid the tendency to set up for upcoming sounds by "turning the voice off" for a few milliseconds. (This can be associated with a slight tightening of the vocal folds, which may be a conditioned stuttering behavior.)

The role of reduced rate is integral (or natural) to continuous voicing. If we just reduce the number of syllables per minute without slowing and blending the transitions between sounds and syllables or increasing mouth movement, there is a risk of producing stilted, halting, on–off

words or syllables with sizable gaps between them that can result in blocking.

The reason that continuous voicing and reduced rate are so fluency enhancing is probably that they are so dissimilar to the speech patterns associated with stuttering. The attention required to increase articulatory movement and monitor the vocal-fold vibrations may also provide a distraction. However, such distractions should not be confused with those provided by accessory or secondary stuttering behaviors (such as arm waving and foot stomping). Continuous voicing and reduced rate actually provide high-stimulus versions of the sensations and tactile feedback that are a natural part of fluent speech. Thus, they are adaptive rather than maladaptive.

These techniques do not by themselves constitute all that is needed to permanently increase fluency for most children who stutter. In particular, they are not reliable methods of modifying stuttering moments, either inside or outside the clinic; in fact, they provide excellent examples of "clinic fluency." Their value is in providing a model of more fluent speech and, with constant clinical use, giving the child greater confidence in his ability to be more fluent. Some children will catch on very rapidly and will experience the joy of sailing smoothly through sounds with which they almost always have difficulty. Because these techniques cannot be used to modify stuttering reactions, though, they simply do not hold up when used in isolation. That said, these techniques may be useful ways of reinforcing and stabilizing the feeling of fluent speech for many children after they have achieved greater fluency through therapy.

Teaching Fluent Stretching of Consonants

Work on consonants will draw considerably from the practicing of voiced and unvoiced sounds and particularly the pairs of sounds that were worked on previously.

Unvoiced Consonants

The fluent stretching of consonants is a vital skill for all stuttering children and is the building block for fluency-shaping and stuttering modification techniques such as the pseudo-stutter, pullout, and cancellation.

Unvoiced plosives or *poppers* can be particularly difficult for some children and adults to hold or stretch because they involve speech movements and sounds that will seem relatively unnatural. Sounds such as the /t/, /p/, and /k/ may be especially difficult. These will require a lot of modeling by the clinician. With these sounds it is essential to emphasize to the child that he will not be expected to use extremely exaggerated stretches in normal conversation. Rather, what we are aiming for is a reduction of tension and force in the shorter stretches that the child may manage to actually use in normal communicative speech. Each of the plosives has a characteristic sound that is generated by constriction of the airflow by properly set articulators. For the /p/ sound, this is like air escaping from a balloon, which when contracted in time becomes a more normal /p/.

Fluent stretches of each of these sounds may be taught by having the child "set" his articulators in the proper position first, without any sound. For example, for the /t/ sound, this can be done in a step-by-step way:

---

1. Relax your entire mouth area.
2. Lift the tip of the tongue up to the gum bump behind the top front teeth.
3. Relax the tongue there.
4. Take a deep, relaxed breath.
5. Let some air out through the mouth, feeling it flow through a tiny space between the tip of the tongue and the gum bump.

Getting the appropriate /t/ sound quality will be achieved by modeling this for the child and having him compare what he is doing with what you are doing. Ask him if it sounds right, rather than judging his efforts. To help in achieving this quality, the clinician may model and have the child imitate two similar sounds made with roughly the same articulator position. For example, alternate between the unvoiced /s/ and /t/ (and, for that matter, the voiced /z/ and /d/) to demonstrate the subtle differences in the position and tensioning of the tip of the tongue used to create the qualities of those sounds.

Unvoiced consonants should be taught and practiced in combination with subsequent vowels to reinforce the gentle onset practice and prepare the child for voiced consonants.

Voiced Consonants

Voiced consonants, of course, require a combination of stretched articulatory sounds and gentle onsets. For this reason, some stuttering children may be particular sensitive to them. Also, because the sound volumes created when generating them can be higher, they may sound stranger than unvoiced sounds, particularly plosives. The stretched /d/ sound, for example, has a distinctive /z/ quality to it that, when subjected to time contraction, acquires a more normal quality.

Nonetheless, because these sounds seem to have more substance to them, stretches of these sounds are quite often easier to elicit. Most have considerable vibratory characteristics that provide the child with a lot of feedback. The clinician can call these sounds *buzzers* to distinguish them from poppers or sliders.

Guiding the child in producing these sounds requires changing step 5 in the previous section from letting air pass through the mouth to "gently 'turn on' the voice." It should be demonstrated that less air flows out of our mouths on voiced consonants than on unvoiced ones. This concept can be taught by having the child hold his hand in front of his mouth when producing a loud /f/ and then a loud /v/. The difference in airflow (much less on the /v/) will be immediately obvious. This concept can be taught by showing the child how holding one's nose during the production of a /m/ or /n/ indicates that a small amount of air is actually moving through the nose during these sounds. Again, however, as with unvoiced sounds, the sounds should be demonstrated by first asking the child to place his articulators in the appropriate set position, relaxing in that position, and then proceeding with easy-onset voicing.

For both voiced and unvoiced consonants, the clinician can construct or use games that require many productions of these sounds. For example, in *UNO* and some other card games, the players must use the /p/ very often when they have to "pass" because they have no playable card.

Teaching Stretches to Children with Articulatory Delays

Early childhood stuttering is often accompanied by co-occurring articulatory delays. When the sounds affected by these delays are also associated with stuttering, the clinician may face a dilemma: Should easy talk or easy stretches be modeled using the proper or the delayed form of the sound? We do not advocate reinforcing or modeling articulatory errors, but it is important to avoid stressing the child if he seems to be aware that he is having difficulty with the sound.

This awareness may be due to listener comments or even, in some cases, parental cueing. Such cueing, when identified, should probably be suspended at once. However, if the child keeps pronouncing the sound (for example, "lellow" instead of "yellow") in the delayed manner in response to the clinician's "yyyyellow" prompt, but manages to do so in an easier, less tense way ("llllellow), by all means continue this prompting, with appropriate praise for the easier form of speaking. If the child seems to react to the disparity between the clinician's production and his own, then it may be best to suspend work on that particular sound for a while until he is ready to begin articulation therapy cycles.

CHAPTER 9: *Strategies for Desensitization and Teaching Stuttered Speech Production*

It will often not be desirable to jump right in to work on the child's own stuttered speech productions. It may be best to begin speaking about "getting stuck" or "having bumpy speech" in a general way, exploring various possible ways in which people may stutter. From this, the older child or adolescent may be able to focus—with the clinician's help—on some of the ways that best characterize his particular brand or range of stuttering. Younger children, particularly preschoolers, will require a more indirect or passive approach. It will be helpful to build on the previous work on nonstuttered speech, using some of the same aids or demonstration devices. It is important to link the various types of stuttering with specific areas of tension in the vocal apparatus, at first with a drawing of a "Mr. Speech Man" or "Miss Speech Woman" model and then of the child's own speech organs.

Concepts to Teach

Primary stuttering symptoms include repetitions, prolongations, and silent blocks (Van Riper, 1973; Guitar, 1998). Although each child will have his own particular way of stuttering, and may exhibit one or two forms of primary stuttering more than the others, the characteristics of each type are fairly similar across stutterers. When beginning to describe each behavior and teaching the child how to reproduce or pseudo-stutter in each way, it is important to remember that these behaviors are a product of responses or reactions to an internal experience. Each behavior (see Figure 9.1) involves and requires a buildup of excessive tension or force in the laryngeal area and the speech articulators. These are not the actual core of stuttering, although (when conditioned) excessive tension and force can trigger stuttering events (Van Riper, 1973; Guitar, 1998).

It is also important to remember that fear, whether conscious or unconscious, is often associated with stuttering events, and that the child may not be able to verbalize his feelings of fear. At its most automatic, fear is a physiological reaction to a threat of some kind (Kagan, 1994; Gray, 1987; LeDoux, 1996, 2001). This reaction may be mild or severe. If the child is not fully aware of fear, the reaction may not be

1. Classic primary (core) stuttering symptoms
   - Repetitions
   - Prolongations
   - Blocks
2. Areas of tension associated with each core symptom
   - Articulators
   - Larynx
   - Upper chest/neck
3. Other or secondary behaviors
   - Vocal fry
   - Rapid speaking rate
   - Running out of air
   - Interjections
   - Avoidances
   - Anticipation
   - Extraneous body movements
   - Loss of eye contact
   - Loss of awareness

Figure 9.1 Concepts to teach

manifested in overt behaviors. Nevertheless, the presence of tension, forcing, and other inappropriate behaviors to facilitate speech indicate that some aspect of the child is attempting to overcome an anticipated or perceived disruption of speech. As this experience is repeated and begins to attract the attention of listeners, the fear will become more and more overt until it becomes the primary emotion associated with stuttering. Because of this association, stuttering behaviors become strongly fear-conditioned, and the child will become highly sensitized to this (Van Riper, 1973; Guitar, 1998). He will not want to perceive and feel the stuttering behaviors, and he definitely will not want to consciously assess them, analyze them, and perform them intentionally—yet these activities are one of the more certain routes to desensitizing him to his stuttering, and thus to being able to modify and gradually to extinguish them.

Areas of Tension

Though this is an oversimplification, it is useful to characterize the types of tension associated with stuttering blocks into two major loci: laryngeal and articulatory. Silent blocks, vocal fry, abrupt or hard onsets of phonation, and other voice-related behaviors are associated with laryngeal tension. Repetitions, tremors, and prolongations are primarily associated with tension in the articulators: the tongue, the lips, the jaw, and facial and orofacial muscles. Of course, tension primarily originating in one area can easily be transmitted to or associated with tension in other areas through the complex muscular connections in the neck and facial area.

Higher-Level Behaviors

Tension in the laryngeal and articulatory areas can be reflected in complex, high-level behaviors that are used to attempt to avoid, postpone, or break out of core stuttering behaviors. These include fast speaking rate, running out of air, interjections, avoidances and postponements, anticipation of stuttering, and others. Other secondary symptoms include extraneous limb, head, neck, and torso movements; arm and even leg and foot movements; loss of eye contact; lack of awareness (young and older children) and loss of awareness (older children).

Perhaps the most misunderstood concomitant or secondary behavior is loss of awareness or consciousness. Van Riper used the term "la petite mort" (the little death) to describe extreme manifestations of this loss (Van Riper, 1973). Based on our experience and a recent survey (Heite, 2000), a range of consciousness loss may occur, from a simple inability to detect the presence of primary stuttering behaviors (repetitions, prolongations, or blocks), to a feeling of being disassociated from the self, to a virtually total—albeit brief—loss of consciousness.

Evidence of such behavior may range from testimony by the child that he did not notice a rather obvious stuttering event to an appearance of glazing in the child's eyes, to actual rolling back of the eyes and a fleeting loss of facial muscle tone. Because this is a real unconscious event that is not intentionally perpetrated by the child, the clinician needs to be careful about blaming his inability to catch stutters on denial or lack of effort. This would be simply frustrating or alienating to the child. Like other concomitant behaviors, some children seem to be more susceptible to them than others.

It is usually not necessary to have the child purposefully work on stopping these higher-level behaviors, though awareness of them (if possible) can be important in some cases. Drawing attention to such behaviors should always be done carefully, in a way that is sensitive to the child's anxieties and fears and that focuses on the positive. Admissions of awareness should be rewarded extravagantly, as triumphs or victories, not regarded negatively as "I told you so" events. Loss of awareness or consciousness, as described earlier, may be a reaction to the severity of stuttering blocks. When the severity diminishes, we usually see these episodes diminish in intensity as well. All of our modification activities are designed to help increase awareness of speech movements. It is this movement awareness that later helps the child come out of his thrall during moments of stuttering.

Sample Activities

The following sections discuss some sample activities, including:

- The child as SLP
- Hard-easy contrasts
- Modeling stuttered speech for the older child
- Massed reading with pseudo-stutters
- Modifying speech outside the clinic

Child as SLP

Allowing the child to catch your bumpy speech (voluntary or real) can provide a younger child with a nonthreatening way of exploring the various types of stuttering. It may also be easier for the child to see stuttering behaviors in other people than to recognize them in his own speech. Stuttering may be perceived as a feeling, rather than as a behavior, with associated movements.

Like many other activities, this may be done in many contexts: while playing a game, while discussing something, or while playing together with blocks, toy trains, or puzzles.

Hard-Easy Contrasts

Here we are actually discussing stuttering-fluent contrasts, but it is useful to emphasize that the manner of speaking can be something the stutterer does in response to the expectation or the experience of speech disruption. It is the pushing and forcing that over time (and sometimes a very short time) turns the speech disruption into observable stuttering behaviors.

Here, as in every activity, the clinician must be an equal participant. This gives the child the experience of doing something (showing a speech stimulus) that causes another person to stutter. It provides an example for the child to imitate, and it provides an opportunity for the child to critique the clinician, giving him a chance to feel some power.

Practicing hard-easy contrasts is an important first step before pseudo-stuttering is attempted by older children, and is a useful awareness activity for all children. There are at least two major techniques: (1) producing separate productions of the same sound, first in a tense, hard manner and then in a soft, easy manner; and (2) starting with a hard, forcing production and then gradually making it easier, softer, or less tense. If the clinician has done good groundwork by helping the child explore how the various sounds are made, it will be relatively easy for him to figure out what to make tense for the various sounds (lips for /m/, jaw and tongue for /s/, etc.). Various types of feedback can be used to assist the child in discriminating between hard and soft: looking in a mirror, feeling his face with his hand or fingers, viewing a videotape or monitor.

The objective, as in other elements of our therapy, is to increase the child's ability to *feel* what he is doing when he speaks, and to give him an experience of success and mastery in changing or modifying the way he speaks.

It is quite possible that just performing hard contacts will result in stuttering blocks, as a result of conditioning. The clinician should welcome this as an opportunity to work with real stuttering in the clinic. It will be important to acknowledge what is happening and to realize that this experience may be scary for some children. It can also be an exciting experience of discovery, as the child learns that something over which he has control (at least at some times) is causing stuttering and can (at least at some times) be changed to cause less stuttering.

Modeling Stuttered Speech for the Older Child

With older children, it will be possible to model various types of stuttering directly, inviting them to imitate your examples or to tell you where they observed tension or blockage when you performed an example of stuttering behavior. This initial exploration will eventually result in the child learning to produce fake or pseudo-stutters that mimic or approximate his own stuttering behaviors (see Goal 4).

If the clinician is a stutterer, it will be possible to provide the child with some real examples of observed stuttering. If not, and the clinician does not have experience with voluntary stuttering, it will be necessary for her to learn how to produce stutters of various types that look and sound real. Repetitions and silent blocks are fairly easy to learn, but prolongations, or "sticky" speech, may be more difficult. Such blocks occur in the middle, rather than the beginning, of words, and are occasioned by an upcoming disrupted sound, such as the /b/ in "mayyy_ be," where the "y" sound is accompanied by struggle and tension as the speaker tries to form a /b/, but finds it impossible to do so for a while. This type of block is very characteristic of the chronic adolescent stutterer. It is easy for them to feel, though they may not want to acknowledge its presence. Sticky prolongations become mysterious and difficult to treat as long as the child does not realize that the feared word is actually the one after the prolongation.

Massed Reading with Pseudo-Stutters

When the child is having a difficult time generating realistic stuttered speech, the lack of success may be caused by performance anxiety. Getting a stutter "just right" can be just as difficult as speaking fluently. Therefore, having the child do many massed pseudo-stutters, where the onus is off any one particular production, may result in greater success.

Preparing a text for pseudo-stuttering practice can be as easy as underlining about one word per line on which the child is to stutter. Try to select a variety of different sounds, so that the child can have the experience of reading fluently a sound on which he has just pseudo-stuttered.

Modifying Speech Outside the Clinic

As soon as practical, and assuming that this has the approval of parents, the private practice clinician should begin conducting some activities outside the clinic to demonstrate how speech modification techniques can be used in the child's life. Of course, the school clinician has a variety of situations within the school to do this.

A stuttering situation hierarchy can be used as a guide to control the difficulty of performing speech modifications and pseudo-stuttering in other settings. The clinician should also use her knowledge of the child to ensure that demands are reasonable and that success is likely. Here is a possible progression of transfer activities:

1. The clinician and child play a card game after eating ice cream in a restaurant, during which they use speech modifications.
2. The clinician performs several obvious stretches or slow bounces when ordering ice cream in a store.
3. The child performs one or two stretches on nonfeared words while ordering ice cream.

4. The clinician performs a pseudo-stutter and then a pseudo-stutter and cancellation while ordering in a restaurant.
5. The child performs a cancellation on a pseudo-stutter in a restaurant.
6. The clinician and child go to a book or toy store and use speech modification techniques when talking to each other.
7. The child asks a store clerk a complex question about a toy or book he is interested in.
8. The clinician models asking a complex question while performing some speech modification techniques.
9. The child uses stretches, slow bounces, and finally pseudo-stutters with cancellations while discussing a toy with a store clerk.

Of course, these activities should be tailored for the child and planned to take advantage of local facilities. Transfer activities in the classroom are discussed in Chapter 11. Many additional activities are provided in Part II.

Modification Techniques versus Fluency Tricks

Though none of the techniques discussed in this book should be considered panaceas, that is especially true of the stuttering modification techniques discussed here. These techniques are not magic, and the clinician, child, and parents should not consider their use to be guarantees of more fluent speech. When performed in a therapeutic manner, pullouts and cancellations can be effective in helping the child to change his stuttering to an easier and—if this is a goal—more acceptable form. However, if they are thought of and used as tricks to avoid dysfluency, they will be no more therapeutically effective than the stutterer's secondary stuttering behaviors.

Some clinicians do not employ the techniques described here because of the tendency to use them as fluency tricks. We find the techniques to be effective because they help the child self-enforce important principles of therapy by providing a learnable technique. This also helps maintain clinical communications in environments where clinicians must be changed or rotated for various reasons. The clinician will need to continually monitor her child clients to ensure that the techniques are not being misused. This will require listening very closely to the language the child employs to describe use of the techniques in transfer activities.

Pullouts or In-Block Corrections

The pullout can be taught as a combination of a pseudo-stutter and an easy stretch. Because it is so difficult for people who stutter to produce real pullouts on command, it is often more productive to produce fake ones first. Of course, because a pullout is designed as a modification activity for real stuttering, the pullouts performed in the clinic may not necessarily look or sound like those produced in real speaking situations. It is therefore essential that the child progress to "real" pullouts in the clinic at some point. Without this experience, he will have a very difficult time transferring the technique to speaking situations outside the clinic.

Hard-easy contrast drills are the key preparation for pullouts. These are required to teach the *feeling* of relaxing the articulators.

The *pullout*, or *in-block correction* as it is sometimes called, is nothing more than an intentional freezing of the sound repeated in a stuttering repetition, followed by a relaxation of tension in the articulators producing the sound. This will result in an easy stretching out of the sound and a blend into the subsequent sound in the syllable. It is essential to freeze on the first sound of the word or syllable, rather than on the second or third sound in a blend or on the vowel in a normal onset-rime pair. For example, a pullout on the word "three" freezes the unvoiced /th/ sound rather than the /r/ sound. Going back to the first sound ensures that struggle or tension produced on that sound to force the speaker's way through the word will not be positively reinforced. It also ensures that the tension in the sound that was originally the culprit will be treated. In addition, it is easier for the listener to understand if the sound is significantly prolonged before relaxation can be achieved, as can sometimes happen.

On the word "thanks," a pullout from a repetition could be represented thus:

Thu—thu—ttttthhhhaanks

Note that the repetition is halted as soon as possible, on the second or third production, before the freezing and relaxing of the sound. The remainder of the word, after a slightly prolonged and relaxed second sound, is said at relatively normal rate. Catching the repetition as quickly as possible in practice is vital because the clinical representations of pullouts are usually much more precise than their manifestation in the real world. The longer the repetition and tremor lasts, the more difficult it may be for the child to freeze it, and the greater the possibility that a loss of attention or consciousness will plunge him into a longer stuttering episode.

If the child commonly prolongs sounds when he stutters, the pullout should be from a hard fricative sound on the /th/: TTTHHHHHHtttttthhhhhaanks.

An excellent bridge between fake pullouts and real ones—and one that involves a cooperative activity between the child and the clinician—is taking turns catching the other person just as she or he starts to stutter. Cue the speaker to freeze the sound using a tightly closed fist, held up where it is visible. As the cuer's fist gradually opens, the person doing the pullout gradually relaxes the articulators and relaxes out of the freeze.

As in all other areas of speech modification, the *feeling* of the modification to the client, rather than its sound, is the most important feature for creating a therapeutic effect. For this reason, observation of the muscular and servo characteristics of the modification, as produced by the child, is at least as important as the sound of the modification. If the blends in pullouts are accompanied by obvious tension (indicated by a slight jaw snap or jerk or perhaps even eye movement), the child is probably not draining as much tension as possible out of the production. He should therefore be encouraged to repeat the production—or, even better, to try to drain out more tension on the next one. In speech modification, movement is the enemy of tension. A slightly exaggerated mouth movement may help the child to make the pullout more satisfying.

Slow Bounces

Dr. Dean Williams was an advocate of the use of slow bounces as a stuttering modification and pseudo-stuttering technique (Williams, 2003). Many children who stutter benefit from them; others do not. It does not hurt to experiment and see if the child you are working with is one of those who can achieve a greater feeling of control by using slow bounces. Like other techniques, slow bounces must be taught and practiced thoroughly in low-pressure situations in the clinic before being used in real-life situations. If the child starts using them to avoid stuttering, they will probably not "work," and he will be reluctant to consider doing them any more. If the bounces are not produced softly or easily or slowly enough, they may actually trigger real stutters. Therefore, some desensitization practice is a good idea before they are tried. This is only logical, because slow bounces are not just modification techniques but pseudo-stutters as well.

Even if they do not benefit the child in real-life situations, slow bounces are good tools for increasing awareness of tension on the one hand and smooth and easy mouth movement on the other. They can be useful in helping the child to slow down repetitions that are extremely rapid. They can also be used to transform the use of the schwa vowel in

repetitions to a more appropriate form for the stuttered word ("thuh—thuh—tha—thanks").

Teaching Slow Bounces

Slow bounces are actually repetitions of initial sound stretches. As such, they must be initiated very slowly and gently. If voiced, they should incorporate a gentle onset as well as continuous voicing, as much as possible.

On the word "baby," a slow bounce would be represented "bbaybbaybbayby" rather than "bbay bbay bbayby." The lack of pausing indicates that the voice is "on" continuously through the production. If a schwa vowel is allowed, it should be rapidly transformed to the proper vowel sound for the word, as in "bbuhbbaybbayby." Of course, for the /b/ sound, the clinician will model light lip contacts, gentle onset, and exaggerated but smooth and natural mouth opening in the transition to the vowel.

When slow bounces are used in pullouts, they can be used to relax tense prolongations, slow down rapid repetitions, or repair hard productions in cancellations (see the following subsection). They are highly confrontational and may be difficult for some children to use effectively.

It would be preferable to use the appropriate vowel sound, rather than the schwa vowel, as well. If the schwa vowel is used, part of the practice must include moving from the /uh/ sound to the proper vowel for the word; otherwise, the child may have difficulty doing this in real life. When slow bounces are used as pseudo-stutters, they are an extremely obvious form of advertising stuttering. Therefore, they should be taught in an open manner in the clinic, focusing on projecting the voice, maintaining strong eye contact, and using slightly exaggerated articulation. Watch carefully for evidence that the child is timing the bounces. This is often indicated by head bobbing. Such timing may mean that the child is planning, or waiting for, a totally fluent production after a given number of bounces is performed. If so, and if this fluent production does not happen, he may begin to feel that bounces are not working. Again, slow bounces are intended to increase confrontation of stuttering, provide stronger feedback of speech gestures, and (in some cases) serve as a pullout technique. If they are used to avoid stuttering or used as a timing gimmick, they are being misused.

Cancellations or Repairs

Hard-easy contrast drills and pullout practice are essential preparation for cancellations or repairs. They are often easier than pullouts for children to perform in real speaking situations, so they may actually be the first stuttering modification activity that is transferred.

Like the pullout, cancellations are usually easier to teach when fake stuttering is used in the clinic. But also like the pullout, it is essential that real cancellations be performed many times in the clinic before the child is asked or expected to do them in real life. As we will soon see, time pressure is a key issue associated with performing cancellations.

A *cancellation* requires the speaker to stop completely after a stuttered word, or after a phrase on which the first word was stuttered, identify the sound that was stuttered, evaluate the source or characteristics of the stuttering, plan a way to perform the sound in an easier (though not necessarily fluent or even more fluent) way, and then actually repeat the word using the planned modification. This may sound impossible at first, but because each person's stuttering tends to be the same on given sounds, just identifying the sound will soon enable the child to go through the remaining steps quite rapidly before doing the repair.

One reason why it is so important to begin teaching cancellations on fake stutters is that many (and perhaps most) children have difficulty at first identifying stuttering moments to cancel. It is also easier to reinforce the concept of completing the stuttered word before attempting to cancel the stutter.

Why Are Cancellations So Important?

The tension, forcing, and pushing involved in many stuttering events tends to be positively reinforced when these strategies result in getting through the stuttering moment and progressing to subsequent sounds or words. Because of the momentary release of tension that can result, it is commonly the case that a rush of fluent syllables or words (or even whole phrases) will result from these strategies. When this is repeated several thousand times each day, the stuttering (which is actually a behavior that constitutes a response to an internal event of disruption) is deeply reinforced. If the child simply stops in the middle of the stuttered word or phrase, the behavior will not be penalized and the repair,

which must involve the entire utterance (including the fluency reward), will not be complete. For example, on the word "thanks," a cancellation that stops after "thu-thu-thu" may not allow the child to cancel the jaw tension that is present on the subsequent /a/ sound. Additionally, if the stuttered utterance is not completed before stopping, avoidance may be reinforced.

Triads

Triads are excellent ways of teaching and practicing the discipline of cancellations in the clinic. Although they can—and should—be performed in ways that are best for the individual child, a good basic concept would consist of the following steps (see Figure 10.1).

1st production—hard attack, "push" through word (use pullout if stuttering is induced)

2nd production—easier attack, deliberate movement, slow rate, proprioceptive monitoring

3rd production—normal fluency, with very low tension, normal volume (if stuttering occurs, counsel that this is not a problem or have child repeat all steps)

Figure 10.1 Triads

The first (hard) production can be used to induce real stuttering in the clinic if such induction has previously been difficult. Care should be taken to ensure that the child is desensitized enough to open stuttering so that the experience will not be negative. If real stuttering does occur and tends to be perseverative, incorporating a pullout as a part of this production may be advisable.

The second production should be very deliberate, with a purposeful prolongation on the first sound and throughout the word. The child should be encouraged to *feel* his speech, using points from the teaching of normal speech discussed earlier. Exaggerated articulation is beneficial as well.

If the child has practiced sufficient voluntary and deliberate modifications during the second production, the last relaxed, normal production should be relatively fluent. Ask him how it feels. If he relates that there was a "flip" of fear or apprehension just before, that should be seen and discussed as something positive: he felt that he was going to stutter, but did not.

Proprioceptive and Tactile Monitoring

The preceding techniques all involve increased proprioceptive monitoring to a certain degree. Pullout and cancellation practice help the child become increasingly aware of the feel of moving slowly and easily through stuttering events. Putting together increasingly complex or lengthy proprioceptively and tactilely monitored utterances is an important subsequent step. At first, the clinician may target carrier phrases in simple games or activities that help the child be successful. As continued progress is made, increasingly complex games and activities should be used.

The older child may benefit considerably from the use of a delayed auditory feedback (DAF) device. This should be used deliberately with the objective of increasing the child's ability to feel the movements and aerodynamic characteristics of his speech, not just as a way of inducing greater fluency. Reading should be done using three- or four-word utterances in a very slow, very deliberate, fluid manner, focusing on smooth transitions between sounds (*co-articulation*). DAF can be used while reading or when speaking in conversation. Remember though, that the child will hear others' voices delayed during conversation, and this may require him to turn the device down or off when others are speaking.

CHAPTER 11: *Transfer and Maintenance*

Although transfer and maintenance are often discussed together (as they are in this chapter), they remain quite separate issues that require different approaches for facilitation.

Transfer refers to the generalization of modified communication styles and speech techniques from within the clinic to settings and situations outside the clinic. Transfer activities occur as an integral part of the therapy process, under the guidance of the clinician. This process lays the foundation for subsequent long-term maintenance of modified communication behaviors. The difficulty of transfer activities is usually hierarchically structured to build the child's confidence in his ability to employ techniques across various settings, while benefiting from the clinician's leadership and support.

In contrast, *maintenance* refers to the continued development of communication competence after direct therapy has been largely concluded. Before the maintenance phase begins, the child has experienced success in transferring techniques across settings and has gradually learned to become his own therapist. For maintenance to succeed, transfer must have become a natural part of the child's experience.

Intensive stuttering therapy programs, which usually last several weeks, require a somewhat different view of transfer and maintenance. Because they are generally not long enough to complete the transfer process during the program, transfer is partially amalgamated into the maintenance phase. Also, if the intensive program is a long distance from the child's natural environment, transfer of techniques to home and school will not even begin until after the program itself concludes. Therefore, the child may assume greater responsibility for transferring and maintaining changes in new settings. The likelihood that a child will be able to accomplish this level of self-therapy should be a factor in the decision as to which type of therapy to pursue. Fortunately, intensive therapy programs increasingly incorporate a long-term transfer and maintenance component to assist in the transition between environments. For example, the maintenance program of weekly visits described by Boberg (1981) is based on a long-term therapy program. The degree to which an intensive program is able to provide specific information regarding transfer and maintenance can assist the clinician in determining if an intensive program would benefit a particular child.

Transfer during Therapy

Although transfer of new speech behaviors to the child's speaking environment is important, it is not necessary to begin this process immediately in therapy, before new techniques have been properly learned. Parents often expect homework after only one or two sessions. To satisfy this desire, the clinician may assign some stuttering identification tasks instead. Indeed, homework assignments should reflect as closely as possible the clinical activities taking place at that point in the therapy process.

Early in therapy, transfer should aim to introduce an attitude of inquiry and curiosity about stuttering into the child's environment. Initially, inadequate desensitization may prevent significant inquiry from being conducted, for the willingness to confront stuttering is often a gradual process. Although full acceptance of stuttering may never be achieved for some children and adults, it is enough to initiate and encourage this process throughout therapy.

The transfer process is sequential and hierarchical, but also iterative, as it builds momentum during the treatment phases of identification, desensitization, modification, and stabilization. Because the process is iterative, it is sometimes tempting to begin activities that appear to offer high payoff too early. However, a lot of frustration for clinicians, parents and children can be alleviated if the sequential nature of the transfer process is respected and emphasized. A child who is unable to talk about his stuttering with anyone at school is very unlikely to perform stuttering modification activities there. It would be pointless to expect this child to carry out modification transfer assignments in school in the absence of a support structure, even if that performance would facilitate desensitization. However, the clinician can usually identify an environment or situation in which the child is comfortable discussing stuttering (e.g., talking with a special friend). Such an activity would provide a more appropriate starting point for the process of transfer. Specific transfer activities for each stage are described in more detail in the handouts located in the Appendix. General strategies are provided in the following sections.

In addition to the conscious transfer of behaviors, we have also observed a great deal of automatic transfer during the treatment process. This is particularly the case with very young, preschool children. This relatively automatic transfer appears to follow from the child's observation of clinician modeling and practice with easier and less effortful speech in the clinic. It may, in fact, be a part of the increased fluency associated with the recovery process or an unconscious application of strategies that seem to be advantageous.

Transfer of Identification

Efforts to make stuttering a subject of inquiry and investigation can dramatically change the child's attitudes toward his dysfluency. Investigating when and how stuttering occurs can be a first step in this process and provide information that the clinician can use in designing a transfer program and selecting specific activities for the child. Examples of specific outside activities include making lists of stuttered or fluent sounds, writing about situations when stuttering was severe or when speech was easy and fluent, and identifying people or communication situations associated with less or more fluent speech.

A possible clinical or parental concern during this transfer phase is that by consciously associating specific sounds, situations, and listeners with fluent or nonfluent speech, the child is being taught habits that may become ingrained and therefore more difficult to change. For example, if he identifies /f/ as being a particularly difficult sound, the clinician or parent might worry that a specific anxiety of or expectation about the sound is being be created. In short, some parents may fear any process that draws attention to the child's stuttering.

In fact, consciously identifying stuttering behaviors and environmental factors begins an important aspect of the behavioral change involved in the transfer of stuttering therapy: changing stuttering from something that is hidden, unconscious, and automatic to something that is examined and modified in a conscious and deliberate way. This transformation is an essential aspect of any therapeutic or change process, and it can actually undermine or mitigate the development of habitual fears of sounds, situations, and

communication partners. This change in perspective is actually the foundation for the transfer process, not its nemesis.

Transfer of Desensitization

Although the identification of stuttering behaviors is desensitizing to some degree, it does not directly confront those aspects of stuttering to which children are most sensitive: the reactions, comments, and judgments (real or imagined) of listeners. Of course, the clinic is the best place to begin desensitization procedures, but testing and reducing the child's worries and fears by speaking with people outside the clinic should begin as soon as possible. For example, the child could talk with his family and friends about stuttering. This could be accomplished by having him complete a questionnaire about his stuttering, and then comparing his responses to those of several listeners. Example questions are:

- What do you think causes stuttering?
- Have you ever stuttered or had a difficult time with your speech?
- Are you nervous about giving talks to groups?
- How do you feel when talking to a person who stutters?
- Do you think it's OK to say a word that a stutterer is stuck on?

There are many more that could be asked, of course, but the best questions are those that help to expose differences or inconsistencies in the child's knowledge of how people respond to or think about stuttering. Usually his perceptions about stuttering are more severe than those expressed by listeners. The point is not to have a debate, but to raise awareness of how he perceives communication.

Role of Peer and Support Groups during Therapy

Feelings of isolation and inferiority to others are often products of the child's sensitivity to stuttering. Therefore, encouraging children to participate in some kind of support group, or offering outside activities with other children who stutter, is a valuable transfer strategy. The clinician can create such a group using other children who stutter from the private practice or school caseload.

To decrease the chance that the children will feel that participation in the group shows that they are abnormal or not as good as other children, the concept of a team can be used. Peer group activities can include games, outings, and even drills of speech techniques. All of these activities are beneficial by decreasing the sense of isolation and difference that a child who stutters may be experiencing. The idea that the child is part of a "speech team" may make being part of a support group more acceptable to some children. There are many teams in sports, politics, business, and in the school.

Transfer of Modification

Generally, transfer of actual speech modification techniques (e.g., prolongations, easy onsets) is how most people define *transfer*. Without adequate attention to identification and desensitization, however, it is unlikely that meaningful generalization of modification skills will ever be adequately achieved. To ensure that the treatment process is one in which the child experiences success, it is important to develop a hierarchy of speech situations in which to use modifications. It is also important to document those situations in which the child is actually making or using modifications.

When failure is experienced (as it will be at some point for every child), this can be viewed as an opportunity for learning, through enhanced identification and desensitization. For example, if the child tries a cancellation or repair while giving an oral report in school (a difficult situation that would normally be high on a hierarchy list) and experiences an unexpected loss of control, this can be discussed in the clinic. Questions such as "What happened?," "How did it feel?," "What speech movements or secondary movements did you make?" can enhance the identification of stuttering behavior in that situation.

Creating a Stuttering Hierarchy

Ask the child to mark a piece of paper (or page in a notebook) with "easy" at the top and "hard" at the bottom. Ask him, "Do you notice that speaking can be easier sometimes, depending on where you are and who you're speaking to?"

This will often result in an interested response if it has been a concern to him. Then ask, "When is it the easiest to speak?" or alternatively, "Who is the easiest person to speak with?" Once the easiest speaking situations have been identified, discuss and have the child identify and write down the hardest ones. Then fill in the list with additional situations that he encounters. Besides providing the outline for a transfer plan, this exercise is extremely valuable for the child's understanding of the situational nature of stuttering. It also gives the clinician an important (and appropriate) window into the child's experience and communication challenges.

Selection of the appropriate speech styles to use in modification transfer should be dictated by the child's abilities, sensitivities, and needs. It is critical to select activities that will result in success of some type. For some children, this may mean that fluency-enhancing speech behaviors are all that can be transferred at first, and perhaps for a long time. It is important to realize that, from the point of view of most children, fluency-enhancing speech behaviors are virtually a sort of pseudo-stuttering. It is probably best to start with easy stretches and/or slow bounces, inserted in speech in a manner that will not be highly noticeable for listeners or highly confrontational for the child. For some children, this is all that is required to motivate them to begin transferring more and more behaviors. Others, no matter how hard we try or how much we encourage and lower the bar, will find it impossible to perform transfer activities with any consistency. Most children's transfer abilities will fall somewhere between these two extremes.

Transfer of Stabilization

This phase of transfer provides the rationale for decreasing frequency of therapy near the end of treatment. When intervals between therapy sessions are increased, the child is encouraged to take greater responsibility for maintaining his increased fluency and determining what he needs to do when dysfluencies arise. The common experience of fluency stability is that the roller coaster of fluent and dysfluent speech that occurred before treatment is replaced by a much less radical variation. In fact, this variation can often take the form of just having a bad day every once in a while. The child's response to a bad day can make all the difference in stabilizing fluency. This requires counseling and the teaching of self-diagnostic and self-help skills, often called "learning to be one's own therapist."

Counseling for Stabilization Transfer

If the preceding transfer stages have been properly conducted, stabilization will primarily involve instilling the prospective, executive skills of "remembering to remember." That is, the child will know what to do to get back on track when he has a difficult day or experience, but he may not always remember that he knows. Counseling for this can take advantage of transfer failures to help the child learn how to create solutions to difficulties—to problem-solve—when he is on his own. As therapy nears an end, the clinician may want to use occasional discussion points, such as "What would you do if . . ."

- You are having a bad day and you have a presentation coming up?

- You stuttered on your name when asked to introduce yourself?

- You start noticing that you are beginning to anticipate words or sounds on which you might stutter?

- You have a really important date coming up and the person does not know that you stutter?

- You did really well while performing in a play, but somehow cannot feel that that's an important accomplishment?

By providing the child with the opportunities to think about these challenges, the clinician can help ensure that the child has the problem-solving ability that the stabilization period requires.

Activities for Each Stage of Transfer

The following subsections review some activities for each of the stages of transfer: identification, desensitization, modification, and stabilization.

Identification

Identification is the stage or process during which the child's fluent and dysfluent speech, and the associated compensation and escape behaviors are explored outside the clinic. Here are some identification activities:

- Draw a speech person with speech helpers labeled

- Play reporter, writing down "speech news" consisting of people the child spoke with and what happened

- Watch news and sports casters and note how they open their mouths, how much they look at the camera, and so on.

- List other people's speech problems

- List hard sounds or words

- List easy words

- Tape-record speech samples

Desensitization

Desensitization transfer is important to the process of reducing the stuttering child's speech anxieties and negative emotional states that are associated with stuttering. Here are some desensitization activities:

- Talk to a relative about stuttering

- Talk to a friend about stuttering

- Talk with a teacher about stuttering

- Hang a poster of famous people who stutter in your bedroom

- "Adopt" a famous person who stutters and learn as much as you can about him or her

- Write a letter to the person about stuttering. If the person is alive, send the letter to him or her

- Make a class presentation about your famous person

Modification

Modification transfer involves the shaping and change of the child's abnormal behaviors and speech gestures in response to the fear or perception of disrupted fluency. The following are some modification transfer activities:

- Play board or card games while using fluency-enhancing techniques

- Develop a situation hierarchy to guide the progression of transfer activities

- Beginning with the least difficult situations, deliberately use fluency-enhancing, stuttering modification, and pseudo-stuttering speech styles in as many real-life situations as possible

Stabilization

Stabilization transfer is a continuing activity involving the consolidation of the new behaviors the stuttering child has learned to respond to the threat or occurrence of stuttering. The following are some stabilization activities:

- Use fluency-enhancing techniques as a habitual technique when playing games

- Use "chunking and stretching" speech or very slow, deliberate proprioceptive speech when reading in class or in public

- Insert voluntary stuttering or modified stuttering behaviors into everyday speech

- Continue open advertising of stuttering by discussing it with family and friends, even if the stuttering has been substantially eliminated

- Participate in stuttering support group activities

Maintenance after Therapy

When we speak of maintenance with regard to stuttering therapy, we refer to the maintenance of behavioral change, not just the maintenance of fluency. Even for the child who has graduated from therapy, fluency may vary from day to day, and even from situation to situation within parts of the day. The behavioral change that we hope will be maintained for graduated children first involves attitudes and beliefs regarding occasional dysfluencies. A complex of attitudes and beliefs that reflect the child's confidence in his ability to manage speech communications indicate that behavioral changes are being maintained.

It is important, then, to think of maintenance as embodying a range of possibilities with regard to fluency, not just "fluent speech" as is sometimes said. It is true that many children will essentially recover naturally fluent speech during therapy and will be able to maintain this fluency throughout life. It would be a mistake, though, to suppose that this will be true of even the majority of children who are seen for therapy after the age of four or five.

Role of Support Groups after Therapy

Support groups may be formal, such as the National Stuttering Association, Friends, or an Internet discussion group; or they may be informal or ad hoc, such as groups organized by a therapist, by a school, or by a group of adolescents or parents. All

such groups have the potential to offer real benefit to children and teens in maintaining the behavioral changes begun in stuttering therapy. In fact, involvement in such groups is itself a behavioral change for most people who stutter, and thus can provide its own benefits by being a model for increased involvement in other group activities and clubs.

Ongoing Maintenance Activities

Because maintenance is, by our definition, something that happens after regular therapy, the activities suggested here are more general in nature than others in this book. These activities are things that the child and adolescent can do to manage fluency on his own. Of course, with younger children, parents and teachers can support these activities. If the child received therapy in private practice outside the school (something that is more and more common in many areas), the school SLP can be a resource, as long as consultation with the private clinician is obtained. Parents should also be encouraged to consider the private SLP as a continuing resource for maintenance as well as for the resumption of therapy, should maintenance problems occur for any reason.

Measuring Maintenance

Child follow-up reflects a "going the extra mile" attitude that children and parents may appreciate. It can also provide the clinician with feedback on therapy that can help her improve services. Handout G: Follow-Up and Fluency Maintenance: Parent/Child Perceptions is provided in the Appendix to assist in collecting data useful in evaluating maintenance after therapy.

Practice Activities

If the child has been scrupulous in practicing fluency and change behaviors during therapy, more opportunities for success can be expected after treatment as well. In fact, almost any activity in which the child engages can be considered an opportunity for practice and success. Most people who have experienced the type of therapy recommended in this book report continuing improvements in the ease and effectiveness of their speech communication for many years after the end of formal therapy. The key is to focus on communication as the goal and the measure of success, rather than the absence of dysfluencies.

Among other things, *cluttering* has been simply defined as "disorganized speech." However, the presence of cluttering behaviors may be difficult to identify, because they can take many forms and frequently coexist with other speech-language disorders (Weiss, 1964). As a result, most definitions emphasize the coexistence of language and learning problems with cluttering, and the clinician will often find that the person whose speech dysfluency is diagnosed as cluttering has a history of academic problems, a diagnosis of attention deficit/hyperactivity disorder (ADHD) or another attention disorder, and a family background that features similar difficulties. Indeed, cluttering is sometimes defined as the speech that is characteristic of many people with such challenges (Myers & St. Louis, 1992).

However, not all people with learning disorders clutter. Thus, a definition such as the one provided by St. Louis, which stresses the importance of speech rate articulation and fluency problems, is useful:

Cluttering is a syndrome characterized by a speech delivery rate that is either abnormally fast, irregular, or both. In cluttered speech, the person's speech is affected by one or more of the following: 1) failure to maintain normally expected sound, syllable, phrase and pausing patterns; 2) evidence of great-than-expected levels of disfluency, the majority of which are unlike those typical of people who stutter (St. Louis, 2002).

Because of the strong organic and probably hereditary basis of cluttering (Kidd, 1984), it is clinically useful to attempt to meet with all members of the child's immediate family during the diagnosis phase. The speech environment of, and speech demands on, the clutterer are also important. If other family members use rapid speech rate or poor pragmatics (lack of turn-taking, failure to stay on topic, etc.), this may aggravate the clutterer's difficulties, deprive him of constructive communication models, and indicate that transfer will benefit from speech outside the family. In some cases, the clinician may find it necessary to provide counseling for the family, aimed at more effective communication.

Differential Diagnosis: Identifying and Quantifying Cluttering Behavior

A diagnosis of cluttering may be difficult to make at the first evaluation session. If the clinician suspects that cluttering may be involved, it is best to reserve judgment until the child has been seen for speech therapy several times over a period of days or even weeks.

There are perhaps as many manifestations of cluttering behavior as there are of stuttering. The severity of cluttering may be more difficult to determine, however, because there are no well-defined cluttering behaviors (except for rapid speaking rate) that can be quantified (Daly & Burnett, 1996; Georgieva, 1996). In subsequent therapy, one of the clinician's challenges will be to help the child identify the behaviors that serve as markers for the presence of the individual's cluttering. These markers can become as therapy tools and cues that, when learned by the child, indicate when behavior changes should be made.

Clinical experience indicates that the various manifestations of cluttering behavior fall into two broad categories. One category is cluttering that relates primarily to motor speech. This is evidenced primarily by articulatory difficulties—in particular *overarticulation*, which refers to "articulating over" syllables rather than exaggerating articulatory movements. A person who is overarticulating the word "business" may say "bihness" instead, omitting the /z/. The other category is more language-related, involving disruptions in speech due to problems with expressive language generation and word finding. Finally, there are cases of cluttering in which it is difficult to tell which element (speech or language) is the locus of the behavior. Figure 12.1 lists the characteristics of cluttering.

One of the more severe manifestations of cluttering is a behavior that appears to resemble an auditory (Wernicke's-type) aphasia, with speech that is rapid, unrhythmical, incoherent, filled with inappropriate sounds, and relatively empty or devoid of meaning. A primary difference from the idealistic, fluent aphasias is the presence of articulatory lapses, including underarticulation (in which syllables are left out, as in "booful" for "beautiful") and stuttering-like

Figure 12.1 Characteristics of Cluttering

- Rapid rate
- Overarticulation
- Inappropriate word segmentation
- Excessively dysrhythmical or monotone speech
- Excessively garbled or ungrammatical syntax
- Insertion of a very high number of inappropriate words or sounds

repetitions or prolongations that seem to be caused by the rapidity of speech, as if the person's speech mechanism appears disrupted, jammed, or broken, or (in the case of prolongations) is waiting for the person's brain to catch up.

At the other extreme, cluttering behavior may be barely noticeable, involving little more than slightly rapid speech rate, lack of rhythm or inflection, insertion of many interlocutions, or stuttering-like repetitions caused or aggravated by word-finding problems or difficulties with expressive grammar or language generation.

In between the extremes is a wide array of behaviors that characterize most clutterers. These can include combinations of rapid rate, overarticulation, inappropriate word segmentation, speech that is excessively unrhythmical or monotone, excessively garbled or ungrammatical syntax, insertion of a very high number of inappropriate words or sounds ("like," "uh," "and," etc.), and speech-motor breakdowns that can look virtually identical to stuttering, including whole and part-word repetitions, prolongations, and even blocking behavior. A curious behavior that we have noticed in several children is the insertion of inappropriate midword pauses or breaks, associated with breathing that looks disordered.

Stuttering can co-occur with cluttering, but it is important to make a distinction for individual children so that appropriate therapy techniques can be used. Slower rate and increased attention to modifying speech are usually effective in beginning to resolve the speech-motor breakdowns that characterize cluttering. (Indeed, such improvements may be an important diagnostic marker.) However, trying to correct speech or focusing on avoiding speech-motor breakdowns will usually not eliminate stuttering. Indeed, these activities may actually increase the severity of stuttering.

Other Co-Occurring Conditions

In addition to stuttering, cluttering often co-occurs with several other conditions, including ADHD and learning disabilities (LDs). Indeed, it may be possible to say that cluttering, because it is a symptom of another disorder, *always* has a co-occurring diagnosis. When diagnosing cluttering, it is important to consider such conditions, but because stuttering can also coexist with them, the differential diagnosis of cluttering would not be definitive.

Therapy Strategies for Cluttering

Structure and a methodical approach are important for cluttering therapy. However, for those clutterers who have attention problems, variety and frequent changes between structured activities are also encouraged.

Diagnosis will often extend well into the therapy period. Indeed, diagnosis may virtually never end in some cases, because of the impenetrability and changeability of some cluttering behaviors. One of the clues that cluttering, rather than stuttering, is the child's primary challenge is that the child rapidly learns and successfully begins using the "easy speech" techniques taught early in the treatment regimen. For stuttering children, such speech modifications are often intimidating, and their use too early in the therapy process can sometimes precipitate stuttering blocks. For many children who clutter, initial speech sounds are not the issue. Their "stuttering" may be precipitated by a very rapid speech rate or lack of attention to the content or objective of their utterances (such as beginning a sentence about a character before realizing that he does not know the character's name). For a cluttering child, slow-rate speech techniques and stretches on initial sounds may promote immediate relief from dysfluencies.

Because cluttering and stuttering may co-occur, it is vital to use fluency-enhancing speech behaviors whenever modification or drill activities are undertaken. This is particularly important because cluttering therapy, to be effective, requires the child to increase his awareness of speech behaviors. If the child has a predisposition to stutter, cluttering therapy that does not incorporate fluency-enhancing behaviors may result in an increase of stuttering.

The primary strategies for cluttering therapy are those that provide scaffolding for increasing the order and organization of speech. These include activities to slow the speech rate, increase the rhythm and stress of speech gestures, and increase the variety of speech loudness or pitch. The clinician should provide constant modeling and feedback that supports these changes.

Increased Awareness and Kinesthetic Monitoring

It is usually very difficult for people who clutter to realize or to become aware when their speech is becoming unintelligible. It is not difficult to understand why this would be so: speech becomes automatic and it is not usual for speakers to consciously monitor their speech. At the same time, speakers naturally have an interest in being intelligible or understandable. If people who clutter could improve their intelligibility simply by trying harder, they would probably do so. Auditory feedback, which is the primary monitoring system used by most speakers, is highly automatic and does not provide clutterers with cues about the specific types of breakdowns that they are having.

Clinical experience has shown that an increase in kinesthetic monitoring and a focus on the *feeling* of speech movements is a useful way of increasing awareness of speaking rate and rhythm. This may be supplemented with videotapes showing the positive effect of speech changes provided by such monitoring and demonstrating that novel and possibly exaggerated speech movements do not look strange. Of course, the clinician needs to "put all of these movements into her own mouth" to provide the child with a strong model of target behavior.

Delayed Auditory Feedback in Cluttering Therapy

Early in therapy, the clinician should obtain samples of the child's oral reading and expressive speech while he is using a delayed auditory feedback (DAF) device. Although a few cluttering children may not benefit from the use of such devices, most—particularly those who stutter as well—will find that DAF supports behavior modifications such as slow rate, pause insertion, and increased kinesthetic monitoring. Although it is not known with certainty why people who stutter feel less vulnerable to stuttering, and are usually more fluent when speaking with DAF, the important effect for

cluttering is the slowed speaking rate and the increased phonatory freedom that results. This can give the clutterer a chance to experience a different speaking rate in an automatic way, rather than having to slow down deliberately. The slower rate allows the speaker to monitor speech movements and to experiment with changing them to increase articulatory accuracy and completeness of articulatory gestures, including more deliberate beginnings and endings of words and co-articulatory movements that are slower and easier for listeners to understand.

Some children who clutter may have particular difficulties with sound and syllable awareness. Language may then become a stream of sounds that do not resolve into discrete words and phrases. DAF reading can help such children by reinforcing the sound and feeling of how individual sounds (*phonemes*) are combined to form a syllable and how syllables are combined to form a word. It is quite difficult to deliberately slow down speech movements if one does not understand the concept of syllables. For example, "un-der-stood" is much easier in both concept and performance than "uunnnddeerrssttooodd," particularly when it is desirable to speak in a more rhythmic manner. Some children simply do not know how to split words up into constituent syllables. Specific activities for DAF practice in the clinical setting are provided in Goal 16 (Part 2) of this book.

Emotional Factors in Cluttering

Many people who clutter have difficulty monitoring and becoming aware of their speech behavior, but that does not mean that they are insensitive to or unaware of the effects of their speech on other people and the listener penalties that can result from breaking the rules of speech communication. These rules include conventions of speech such as insertion of pauses, use of changes in rhythm and stress to emphasize meaning, and—most important for the clutterer—rate of speech. Because many clutterers have attention problems, they may also have difficulty with pragmatics as well. This includes communication behaviors such as turn-taking and staying on topic that require a relatively high level of attention and patience.

An example of how emotional factors may complicate cluttering and make it more severe is provided by the case of

Alan, a 10-year-old boy. Alan was an extremely bright child in many respects, but his speech was characterized by inappropriate word and phrase breaks (and deletions) that made him moderately to severely unintelligible at times. He was fascinated by the minute details of trading-card games and wanted to discuss them with children who were not as familiar with the cards as he was. Alan tended to use discussions of the cards as a way of communicating with his peers, whether or not they wanted to discuss them at that moment (an example of a pragmatic problem). When Alan attempted to discuss the cards, his listeners often had difficulty understanding what he was saying, because of his rapid rate and the inappropriate word and phrase breaks ("I'm afraid you . . . on't have the ....ay to und...and what I'm saying."). After a while, they would lose interest and begin to act bored or walk away (listener penalty). Alan's strategy for dealing with this was to try to provide more information by talking faster, which just made the situation worse. To help Alan begin to modify his behavior, the clinician encouraged him to talk about his feelings in the clinic. He revealed that he felt abandoned and hurt when people walked away from him and that this made him feel angry toward some people. Alan's feelings about listener penalties had never been acknowledged before by anyone outside his family. A problem-solving approach was then used to help him identify different strategies he could use to keep the attention of his friends. These strategies were consistent with the clinical behavior modification goals, such as inserting pauses or stretches to help him talk more slowly. They also included communication therapy (e.g., inserting pauses and using slower speaking rate while asking questions of his listeners) and discussions and role-playing associated with pragmatics, such as turn-taking, topic maintenance, interviewing or asking questions to stimulate discussion, and the like.

Adolescents and teens may also have emotional reactions to listener response and reaction. Indeed, though older children may have better communication skills to express these emotions, their feelings may be buried under many layers of discounting and even denial that such feelings are important. These feelings may then be expressed as hostility toward work colleagues, teachers, and family members. Should it become apparent that emotions are preventing or interfering with speech behavior modification, a referral to a psycholo-

gist or a certified counselor specializing in personal development may be beneficial.

Cluttering-Specific Therapy Goals and Activities

Specific goals and activities for cluttering treatment are designed to implement a general strategy of deliberate, step-by-step behavior modification, while employing fluency-enhancing speech techniques. A list of suggested therapy goals for cluttering is provided in Figure 12.2, with detailed activities provided in Goal 16 of Part II.

Figure 12.2 Cluttering Intervention

- Slowing rate
- Increasing the use of rhythm, pitch changes, and pauses to reinforce meaning
- Identifying marker behaviors that indicate the presence of disorganized speech
- Word finding and vocabulary enrichment
- Increasing awareness of structure and form in language
- Increase proprioceptive awareness of speech using delayed auditory feedback

It is important to change activities frequently in this type of therapy, because even activities that children with attention disorders enjoy can become boring and unstimulating for them. However, it is also important to provide focus. Therefore, several activities may be selected that work on a limited number of targets in several ways. For example, a session focusing on pauses could start with a simple card game, during which pauses are inserted in carrier phrases. A series of different, increasingly complex activities may be selected, culminating in a monologue or conversation in which pauses are deliberately inserted. Tangible rewards for each pause can be very effective for children under 10 or 12 years of age.

All DAF activities should also be conducted in an identical way without use of the device before the end of a treatment session. This will demonstrate to the child that he is capable of making modifications on his own, and will provide experience in what the modification feels like in a real speaking situation.

Strategies for Transfer of Cluttering Modification Behaviors

Most clutterers will have just as many problems as stutterers do in transferring their new speech behaviors from the clinic to real communication situations. However, the reasons may be somewhat different. Whereas stutterers may be reluctant to try new behaviors because they may stutter or sound different from others, clutterers may have difficulty perceiving when to employ the new behaviors. They simply may not have sufficient awareness of when their speech is breaking down or becoming difficult to understand.

One possibility for helping clutterers become more aware of when their speech is breaking down is to identify key marker behaviors of which the clutterer can be made aware. For example, if the person habitually breaks words or phrases in inappropriate places, working on developing an awareness of when such breaks are occurring may provide the child with a cue to employ a modification technique, such as inserting pauses or stretches to slow the speech rate. Jerky breathing or perhaps a sound made when gulping air might be such a marker for some children. Making the clutterer more aware of his behavior may seem to be the opposite of the desensitization that occurs in stuttering therapy. However, stutterers, though possibly more aware that they are having difficulty, may be just as unconscious of specific behaviors and of the frequency of their dysfluencies. Of course, care must also be taken to avoid aggravating any stuttering that may be present while awareness is being increased.

It is often easier for children to make behavior changes when they are actively doing something, rather than simply trying not to do something. For example, it may be much more difficult for children to "just slow down" than it is for them to add pauses or word-initial or word-final stretches that tend to slow their overall speech rate.

Clinical Outcomes and the Course of Cluttering Therapy

As in other types of speech therapy, it is sometimes the case that children or parents terminate cluttering therapy sooner than the clinician would recommend. Sometimes termination may be forced by the cessation of insurance benefits or other circumstances.

Even more than stuttering, the efficacy of cluttering therapy may be measurable more by indirect means (such as child satisfaction and evidence of reduced handicap) than by a quantitative reduction in specific cluttering behaviors. However, one clear and objective indication of change may be provided by the child's ability or increased ability to identify marker behaviors that signal speech breakdowns.

The experience of those who provide cluttering therapy is that the disorder can be very persistent and difficult to eradicate. Though many children may become proficient at cluttering modification techniques in the clinic, it is common for them to have difficulty attaining sufficient increased awareness of speech breakdowns to improve their communication during demanding situations. For clutterers (unlike stutterers), these situations may not include high-stress situations, but rather may include everyday communication situations in which they feel comfortable and at ease, and are therefore not prompted to monitor their speech as closely.

Stuttering therapy can take time, so anything the clinician can do to encourage children, parents, and teachers to allow time for therapy to work will facilitate its effectiveness. We have found that providing examples of stuttering recovery experiences, and even relating our own experiences at times, can help allay fears and reduce impatience. We can also connect parents new to therapy with other parents who have gone through the therapy process with their children. However, people often want to know for certain what "happens" when children who stutter "recover" or "get better." Though we cannot know this specifically for any particular child, we do have more than 100 years of clinical experience as a profession to draw on to provide helpful and reassuring information. And though we do not know specifically what happens inside children who stutter when they start speaking more fluently, there are some helpful hypotheses and an increasing array of hard experimental evidence that can help explain the process of recovery.

One of the best aids to helping children and parents understand the therapy process is a consistent story or "road map" that can be referred to when triumphs happen and when difficulties are encountered. Just as stuttering has a varied developmental course, the road to greater fluency varies for different people. Still, there are a number of similarities in these experiences from which we can learn.

Difficulties of Explaining Stuttering Persistence and Recovery

At one point or another, most older children and parents of those children will ask the clinician for an explanation of how therapy works to resolve stuttering or why, when other children have made rapid progress and moved out of therapy, their child is continuing in a longer therapy regimen. A perceived lack of sufficient progress in therapy can lead to impatience and a tendency to blame the child for not "using his techniques" properly or trying hard enough. Occasionally, lack of progress can be attributed to lack of motivation or traced to a concurrent attention problem (such as ADD or ADHD), but often people just expect too much of therapy too soon. In addition, some cases of stuttering are simply more severe and more impenetrable than others. Although

the neurological factors underlying some of these differences are not yet known with certainty, we will discuss some possibilities that should be considered.

Many models or explanations of stuttering used by clinicians are not sufficiently developed to provide logical explanations of the recovery process. For example, we know that there are clear neurological differences in the way the brains of people who stutter work during speech. However, telling people that stuttering is caused by a neurological deficit or "flaw" does not provide a useful explanation of the demonstrated benefit of fluency-shaping or other speech modification activities. The problem is compounded by the notion that stuttering is genetic in origin. How, some parents or children may wonder, could talking in a different way for a few months result in a repair of genetically determined neurological functions? And how, in a preschool child, could praising and rewarding fluent speech result in the complete cessation of stuttering in many cases? If fluent speech is a skill like hitting a baseball, why does intentionally pretending to stutter (missing the ball on purpose) facilitate fluency? The answer is that it isn't like that for children who stutter.

The explanations that are the most difficult to square with the recovery process are those theorizing that a so-called hard-wired—inborn or congenital—structural or organic problem in the brain is solely responsible for stuttering. Such explanations, while providing people with a convenient impersonal scapegoat for a child's dysfluencies, can also be impediments to persistence or progress in therapy. For example, parents who hear that their child's brain may be different from a fluent person's may conclude that there is no point in seeking therapy, or, when the child encounters difficulties (as they usually do), may not wish to keep investing in a cause that looks hopeless to them. Also, totally organic (or inborn) explanations do not provide a convincing explanation for the roles of fear, attitude, and other emotional factors in stuttering persistence and recovery, or of the importance of addressing these in therapy and in the home.

Another common explanation for how recovery happens involves the theory that stuttering is caused primarily by an imbalance in brain chemicals called *neurotransmitters*, such as dopamine. In this case, the explanation would be that, for stuttering recovery to occur, the chemical imbalance has to be addressed, perhaps with medications. However, this does not explain why people who take medications for stuttering usually achieve only modest improvements in fluency, or even *reduced* fluency (Maguire, 2003). Nor does it explain why thousands of children who stutter have recovered just as much, or even more, fluency without taking any medications at all (Conture, 2001).

In contrast, there are explanations of stuttering recovery that rely on so-called psychological or cognitive factors. In these explanations, stuttering occurs because of the secondary benefits to the child, a problem with assertiveness, a tendency to hold back, or some other reason that is largely unrelated to speech. The problem here is that persistent stuttering may be attributed to the person not wanting to be fluent. Just as explanations that attribute stuttering solely to neurological factors explain everything in terms of physical characteristics, psychological explanations of stuttering recovery make little or no room for neurological characteristics or classical conditioning that may underlie behavior and that may require speech modifications to begin to resolve. Parents may be told that if the child could simply learn to let go, he would be able to regain his fluency. Faced with demands he feels he cannot possibly satisfy, the stuttering child may become embittered and simply give up.

Perhaps the most common, but most difficult to explain, of the theories of stuttering recovery are those that view stuttering therapy as an education process. These are most often marked by the notion that stuttering recovery involves "relearning how to speak." As many people who stutter can speak fluently when they are alone, and would not really be allocating new neurological resources to speech, it is difficult to see how such relearning could take place.

A Useful Model for Explaining the Recovery Process

Behavioral researchers are increasingly finding that human behavior is too complex to explain by focusing on only one aspect or factor. When we say that a disorder is neurological in nature, that does not mean that it is totally caused by a genetic factor or even (in the case of injuries) totally by a physical trauma. The child's neurology is also strongly influenced by his environment, his own behavior, and his internal response to his behavior and the environment. All aspects of the human organism and the behaviors that express humanity are interrelated. Disordered behavior itself can cause neurological changes that may become permanent over time. Conversely, modifications in behavior can actually change some neurological characteristics. That is what we believe happens as a result of stuttering therapy.

Our model of stuttering is derived from clinical experience, our observations of stuttering behavior and the process of recovery from stuttering, and our interpretation of the findings of recent research in the areas of this disorder, speech science, and experimental psychology. It is useful in explaining the major features of the therapy and recovery processes, including the development of seemingly spontaneous temporary fluency in some children, the persistence of chronic stuttering in others, characteristic responses to the various types of therapy, its situational nature, the tendency to relapse, and the tendency of stuttering responses and reactivity to persist, even in many people who have regained virtual fluency and are in recovery from the disorder.

This relatively new way of looking at stuttering assumes that it does not primarily involve a neurological flaw or a disease process, but is a specific manifestation of normal and universal human processes of reactivity and self-protection. Further, it assumes that the observed physical characteristics are the result of that process of reactivity and self-protection, and are not in themselves the cause of stuttering, except as they may serve to support or create conditioned cues that trigger stuttering events. These physical characteristics may include the changes in brain activity and structural differences that are being discovered by brain scan research. In our view, these physical markers may be largely the result of changes in function and behavior associated with continued stuttering. This is indicated by experimental findings showing that the brain function of people who stutter can be changed by traditional stuttering therapy (De Nil, Kroll, Kapur, & Houle, 2000).

An Explanation of Stuttering

Our model of stuttering views the core phenomenon of stuttering as a self-inflicted disruption, inhibition, or disabling of language and speech-motor functions and awareness. This inhibition is implimented unconsciously or automatically for the purpose of preventing speech in the presence of speech-related threat situations. Very quickly after it begins in early childhood, this disabling or inhibitory reaction can be triggered by speech-related gestures that have been classically or operantly conditioned (closely associated with tension or with unpleasant difficulties or breakdowns in speech that are threatening to the child's sense of self control and well-being). Over time, the resultant behavior changes have a profound effect on the neurological circuits involved in speech communications.

The observed primary stuttering behaviors (prolongations, repetitions, and blocks) may result directly from the disruption of neurological processes required to generate fluent speech. Secondary behaviors of stuttering (at first, tension, forcing, and avoidance; later, fear and anxiety) may be viewed as responses or reactions to the presence of the disruption or attempts to communicate in spite of it. The onset of the phenomenon can be sudden, but its permanence is reinforced over time through the continued processes of fear and threat conditioning. Table 13.1 crudely illustrates how speech behaviors and environmental stimuli can become associated with feelings and reactions through the conditioning process. The child's reactions and compensations in the continued presence of the phenomenon can eventually result in long-lasting functional and structural changes in the neurological makeup of his speech system. The permanence of these changes is not known; however, research indicates that longer times before intervention are associated with a higher likelihood of the development of chronic stuttering (Yairi, et al., 1996). It is also known (as mentioned earlier) that stuttering therapy can result in sufficient reversals in neurological function to allow the recovery of fluent speech communication (De Nil, et al., 2000; Boberg et al, 1983). Theories that explain the extinguishment of conditioned reactions (LeDoux, 2001) indicate that this process occurs through inhibition of the conditioned responses by increased

TABLE 13.1 Conditioning Process in the Development of Stuttering Blocks

Activity	Child's Response External	Internal	Listener Response	Conditioned Behaviors
Small speech error	May not notice	Covert repair	May not notice	None
Second speech error	Notices problem	Covert repair attempt fails	May not notice	Awareness of problem
Third speech error	Concern; confusion	Covert repair attempt fails	Notices concern	Concern; confusion; attention from listener
Fourth speech error	Concern; increased speech tension; awareness of hesitation	Covert repair attempt results in hesitation	Notices concern and tension	Concern; speech tension; attention from listener
Fifth speech error (prolongation)	Frustration at speech block; attempt to push through hesitation	Speech disruption	Expresses concern or looks worried	Concern; tension; feeling of blockage; listener worry seen as anger or criticism
Sixth speech error (stuttering block)	All of the foregoing, plus fear of loss of control; spasms, tremor	Inhibition of speech	All of the above, plus may look away or express fear	Concern, tension, listener displeasure or penalty, frustration, fear, feeling of loss of control, spasms, and tremor

inhibitory activity in other areas of the brain. This may be supported for stuttering therapy by studies that reveal higher brain activity in formerly hypoactive areas for at least a year after the completion of successful stuttering therapy (De Nil, et al., 2000).

It is important to note that this model has little in common with popular theories that stuttering is caused solely by a panic reaction, by common flight-or-fight responses, or by assertive–aggressive conflicts. Such theories require that stutterers have a common psychological profile that is significantly different from fluent speakers (something not yet demonstrated by research). They do not explain stuttering that occurs in the absence (or fluency that occurs in the presence) of such reactions, responses, and conflicts—something commonly observed in people who stutter. It is consistent with an inhibition or freeze response, which helps explain the lack of high arousal (fear or panic) in most people who are stuttering (Alm, 2004).

Explaining Stuttering Development

The resulting model of development has several stages. It begins with the original dysfluencies that result from successful or attempted covert repairs of developmental phonological or motor-speech errors (which may be outgrown) and early experiences of control loss during speaking events; progresses to the experience of traumatic speech events by the person who stutters; and moves to consolidation of conditioning in the teenage years and adulthood.

Any theory of stuttering must explain why behavior that could be interpreted as severe or advanced occurs shortly after onset; why some children naturally recover fluency in spite of these severe symptoms; and why some children respond to therapy in a more positive way while others exposed to the same techniques do not. Individual differences and responses to conditioning may help explain these features.

An interesting anecdotal speculation that may show how individual differences affect stuttering is made by Guitar (1997) in his assessment and treatment of the stuttering of two young boys, "Adam" and "Bob." Because of its relevance to the present model, the passage is extensively quoted here:

> *Kagan and colleagues . . . hypothesize that some children are born with a greater reactivity to uncomfortable and unfamiliar experiences. Such children respond to threatening stimuli with heightened activation of the limbic system—a part of the brain that mediates emotions and behavior. This heightened activation causes many responses throughout the body, including increases in muscle tension, particularly in the larynx. Gray (1987) provided a neuroanatomical basis for Kagan's theoretical perspective by suggesting that limbic circuits may respond to fear and frustration with muscular contractions that produce tense and silent immobility ("freezing"), an innate response in most species that can be easily classically conditioned. Moreover, innate flight/avoidance responses may be elicited under threatening conditions and may alternate rapidly with "freezing" responses.*

Guitar sees the primary or "core" stuttering response in some people who stutter to be a freeze or flight-avoidance response, and this is in general agreement with our fear conditioning model:

> *It may not be too great a leap of imagination to reconceptualize the essential elements of chronic stuttering—core, escape, and avoidance behaviors—as manifestations of these three responses to fear and frustration: freezing, flight, and avoidance (Guitar, 1997, p. 282).*

It is important to emphasize that caregivers should not be told that one temperamental trait or characteristic of this type (i.e., inhibitive personality) is proposed as a cause of stuttering. Nor should it be said that all children with any one type of temperament are predisposed to stutter. Given the wide range of personalities and character traits associated with people who stutter, it is more likely that there are a number of very specific neurological characteristics involved and that the effect of these characteristics may overlap, as well as interacting with the person's environment, to predispose him to stuttering.

Explaining How Therapy Works

This model helps us explain the efficacy and inconsistency of the large variety of therapeutic approaches for treating stuttering, including the recent encouraging successes with early intervention and treatment of very young children (2½ to 3 years) using contingent rewards for fluent speech. It also indicates that many modern treatment approaches, (though successful in improving fluency,) may not succeed in quite the manner claimed by their purveyors.

For example, fluency shaping, voice-shaping treatment approaches, or so-called speech reeducation approaches are claimed to work simply by replacing a dysfluent speaking behavior with a new or "relearned" speaking behavior devoid of the "bad habits" that supposedly characterize stuttering. The mechanism for such relearning has never been explained. Our model theorizes that these methods are most likely extinguishing classical and operant conditioning by (1) eliminating internal and auditory cues of incipient stuttering; (2) eliminating conditioned tension that may trigger a disruption of speech-motor and language coordination; and (3) demonstrating fluency and lack of fear due to the effect of fluency-enhancing behaviors, thereby stimulating cortical areas capable of inhibiting conditioned reactivity. The latter effect can be accomplished by having the child repetitively produce gentle onsets, fluent stretches, or speech characterized by continuous voicing, or by using the highly exaggerated and heavily self-monitored speech gestures that Charles Van Riper called for (Van Riper, 1973). Behavior modification draws on the brain's memory resources, which seem to replace heavily conditioned stuttering trigger behaviors (involving tension, restricted movement, and clonic and tonic tremors) with movements that were formerly associated with fluent speech.

Our use of an integrated approach of fluency shaping and stuttering modification is inspired, in part, by the clinical observation that many stutterers do not succeed at mere fluency shaping, at least in terms of achieving the degree of control that these programs require for success. Such failures may be attributed to lack of motivation or lack of readiness to change on the part of the child. Although these judgments may indeed be correct in many cases, it is highly possible—based on this model—that there are also many children who

have extremely strong conditioning and reactions to their dysfluencies that are simply more difficult to extinguish. In children who had severe experiences of trauma during stuttering episodes, whose stuttering was not treated (or was not treated until later in childhood or in adulthood), or who lack the ability to focus on fluency targets and ignore habitual subcortical fear reactions, several months, or even years of fluency shaping (or, for that matter, stuttering modification) may simply not be sufficient to fully extinguish the reactions associated with stuttering. This is made more difficult by the fact that only one or two failures of the fluency-shaping techniques to produce the expected fluency may be sufficient to undo the entire fluency program.

Likewise, cognitive therapy or psychological approaches are often said to work by correcting false thoughts or negative thinking about one's ability to speak openly in public, or by showing the child that stuttering is caused by attempts to control speech, which interfere with the normal, automatic nature of fluent speech. That dynamic is similar to the child's attempts to control core dysfluencies in the earlier phases of this model. A common feature of cognitive approaches is the notion that conscious control of speech is the problem and that the child simply needs to let go and speak in a more automatic manner. However, in the context of the present model, such directions do not account for strong reactions, and failure to include emotion and conditioning is often a limitation of cognitive approaches. In fact, one of the pitfalls for stutterers undergoing therapy is so-called spontaneous fluency, during which the child is able to produce fluent speech due to temporary relaxation of the stuttering reactions. Without access to behaviors used to induce operant fluency (which typically include slow rate, conscious monitoring of proprioception and tactile feedback, and continuous voicing), the child may be vulnerable to relapse when conditioning is re-stimulated. In fact, a sober appraisal will show that all cognitive therapy approaches invariably induce operant fluency in the clinic and in a group situation, and then attempt to generalize it to various other situations, either during therapy sessions or by the child in life. If the operant fluency merely involves a distraction of some kind, it will not work for long, even for those with moderate reactivity.

The more successful cognitive therapists (as well as stuttering therapists who use cognitive counseling techniques) encourage children to use their operant fluency in a number of situations, varying from easy to difficult, practicing positive replacement thoughts and self-images. This is really a behavioral extinction technique in which speech drill and articulation practice occurs and is probably a key (but unrecognized) component if the therapy is successful. In our experience, pure cognitive therapy, even if it includes coincidental speech drill, is rarely successful in permanently increasing the fluency of severe reactive stutterers.

Stuttering modification therapy—developed by Charles Van Riper and refined by many other clinicians over the past five decades—is a direct application of operant fluency or modified speech to extinguish conditioned learning (Van Riper, 1973). The course of this therapy, encompassing the behavioral steps of identification, desensitization, modification, and stabilization, is specifically targeted at a model of stuttering similar to that proposed here, if lacking the anatomical details. Because it provides the person who stutters with specific techniques for modifying dysfluencies, stuttering modification may be the therapy of choice for severe cases in which cortical inhibitory control is not able to extinguish the stuttering reaction. In fact, there is clear clinical evidence that most successful fluency-shaping therapy actually involves a form of stuttering modification. One of the more popular recent books on stuttering describes the difficulty of using slow speech and fluency-shaping targets in public (Tunbridge, 1994). The author is only one of many who points out the necessity of the stutterer desensitizing himself to using modified speech, which is basically the same process used in stuttering modification therapy.

This model, therefore, indicates that a combination of fluency-shaping and stuttering modification therapy should be used to treat most moderate to severe stuttering behavior, except for very young children in whom the reactive subcortical response is not overly conditioned; these children often respond well to nonoperant or indirect treatment approaches. This treatment advice (if not yet this particular theory supporting it) is the emerging consensus among legitimate practitioners of stuttering therapy.

Testing the Model

This model was developed to help explain observations of, and experience with, the success and limitations of therapy techniques described in this book, and was configured to explain widely observed clinical results. Because the model is descriptive in nature, it is not necessary for it to be validated before one can confidently use the techniques we teach. The techniques are effective and have been developed and refined over the last 80 years by a variety of clinicians. However, other existing conventional explanations of stuttering do not sufficiently explain how and why the integrated approach to stuttering therapy is effective. On the one hand, they do not explain how stutterers can recover their fluency if stuttering is caused by an inborn structural or functional neurological flaw. On the other hand, they do not explain why—if stuttering is a psychological or mental disorder—relapse is so common, even in people who have largely recovered their fluency, or why the tendency to stutter can be persistent in such people, even as they conduct their lives as essentially fluent speakers. We hope this model will help to begin the process of explaining these factors and contribute to making therapy more effective for all people who stutter.

PART II

A NOTE TO THE CLINICIAN

As stated in Chapter 1, we often use the word "child" in a generic sense, realizing that many of the activities described in this and other sections are applicable to both young children and older adolescents. Other times, depending on the chosen goal and the activity described therein, our usage of the word "child" more specifically pertains to, for example, preschool-age children, older school age, and so on. Ultimately, it is up to the discretion of the clinician to tailor each activity to the interests and cognitive functioning of the children and adolescents with whom she works and to determine if a particular activity is well suited for each client.

We also want to alert the clinician to the fact that there are many activities listed in each category that may also be appropriate to implement when working on another goal described in this book but are not specifically restated elsewhere. Again, it is up to the professional to identify the appropriate goals for her clients and then choose the individual activities that best support these goals. Ultimately, there are an infinite number and variation of activity possibilities for each goal beyond those listed. The activities provided in this resource manual represent only a sampling of what is possible. The clinician is encouraged to rely on her experience and creativity to expand what we have offered here.

GOAL 1:

Parent and Caregiver Involvement

Rationale

As the child is in therapy only two to three times weekly, it is important for the parents to participate in the treatment process to assure maximum progress. Parental communicative style and communicative feelings of guilt, fear, and anger must be dealt with through the intervention process. Most experts on stuttering do not believe that primary caregivers cause stuttering. However, as Shapiro (1999) cautions,

> It is important for them to understand the factors that facilitate and those that inhibit a child's communication, specifically speech fluency. Therefore, during the assessment session, we discuss, demonstrate, and then direct parents in how to reduce the counterproductive communicative demands placed on the child while enhancing the facilitators of fluency, and address the feelings and attitudes of all people involved (p. 263).

As indicated by Shapiro, and supported by our experience, the environment created by the caregiver can affect the child's fluency in either a productive or a counterproductive way. For this reason, helping parents understand more about the dynamics of fluency and stuttering, and environmental factors conducive to both, may be as important as working directly with the child. In addition to Shapiro (1999), other professionals also promote caregiver involvement (Conture, 1997; Gregory, 1989; Guitar, 1998; Meyers & Woodford, 1992; Ramig, 1993; Starkweather, Gottwald, & Halfond, 1990; Zebrowski & Cilek, 1997).

Activities and Suggestions

Refer to Figure G-1.1, which outlines the information and activities presented in this section.

Information for Parents

1. Schedule regular parent-clinician conferences or maintain consistent communication with parents. During these

Support

The following citations provide support in the literature for our inclusion of this goal and the suggested activities addressing parent and caregiver involvement in the treatment process.

Botterill, Kelmaii, & Rustin (1991) ► Stuttering arises out of a complex interplay between the child's environment and the skills and abilities the child brings to this environment. Intervention programs should incorporate a dimension of environmental change that will facilitate fluency development.

Conture (1990) ► "All the good that is done in therapy can be offset, in a relatively short time, by parents who cannot, or will not, understand their role in their child's speech development" (pp. 87–88).

Conture (1997) ► The parents' role in therapy is critical, for they are often a child's most important listeners and conversational partners.

Gregory (1991) ► Parents need to understand the stuttering problem, its variability, factors associated with this variability, and how the child responds to fluency disruptions.

Gregory & Gregory (1999) ► When providing information to parents, include frequent pauses so that parents may interject questions or feelings. Also try to relate additional information to comments or concerns expressed earlier by a parent. Caution parents against using labels for their children, such as "shy" or "aggressive." Such labels may unwittingly reinforce these behaviors. In fact, both shy and aggressive children may be reacting to their dysfluencies when they exhibit inhibitory or aggressive behaviors.

Gregory & Hill (1993) ► Success of therapy depends to a great extent on the commitment of the parents.

Guitar (1976) ► Although parents should be supportive of the child during therapy, they should not function as clinicians.

continues

Support *continued*

Kelly (1995)
The speech of parents is usually more linguistically complex, more fluent, and faster than that of their children. Kelly reports that fathers, speaking either to children who do or to those who do not stutter, "produced nearly double the number of words, syllables, and morphemes than mothers" (p. 96). Fathers also exhibited shorter response time latencies, regardless of a child's fluency level. Such behavior may contribute to perceived time pressure by the child, especially by those who stutter.

Kelly & Conture (1991)
Stuttering results from complex interactions between constitutional and environmental factors. Intervention with children who stutter should include attention to these factors. Therefore, establishment of parent-child fluency groups may provide an opportunity for clinicians to assist parents to better understand the disorder and ways they can help their child.

Lincoln & Onslow (1997)
Tracked speech fluency of 43 children between the ages of 2 and 5 years who had received therapy. Therapy consisted of a parent-administered operant program. Follow-up showed that *all* children had maintained near-zero levels of dysfluency 1 to 7 years later.

Logan & Caruso (1997)
Noted that although some parents may realize that their child is struggling with dysfluencies, they are reluctant to enroll their child in speech intervention. Presumably they fear that bringing the unusual speech pattern to their child's attention will somehow make it worse.

Manning (1996)
Instead of bombarding parents with information about stuttering, clinicians should attempt to listen to parents and follow their lead by addressing concerns and providing information to specific questions. Once the parents become more informed, they will be more likely to provide insights and suggestions.

Perkins (1992)
Because parents are a major part of the environment that influences the child's speech, their direct involvement in working with the child is critical to effective treatment.

Ramig (1993)
Describes the three roles of parents during the treatment process as: (1) subjects of educational counseling, (2) facilitators of communicative interaction with the child, and (3) observers and participants in the treatment process. "Involving parents in the intervention process is an important step toward facilitating the changes for improvement in the young child who stutters" (p. 226).

Ramig & Bennett (1995)
"[T]he child experiencing the daily negative impact of stuttering can be helped to cope more effectively if the parents have a better understanding of the problems adversely affecting the child and family" (p. 139).

Shapiro (1999)
One part of the family cannot be understood in isolation from the whole family (which may include the extended family, such as grandparents, aunts and uncles, etc.). Parts of a family are interrelated such that change in one part affects change in other parts of the system. An attitude of sharing both burdens and successes is reflected in well-balanced families. The characteristics of the family therefore form an integral part of intervention.

Starkweather (1987)
Introduced the Demands and Capacities model, which asserts that impaired fluency represents an incongruity between the child's current abilities and environmental demands. For instance, some children may experience wider discrepancies between their own speech and that of their parents.

Van Riper (1973)
"Parents feel a profound sense of guilt" (p. 418).

Wall & Myers (1995)
The clinician should assure parents they did not cause their child's stuttering. There are many things they can do to enhance their child's fluency.

Zebrowski & Schum (1993)
Discuss the counseling aspects involved when working with children who stutter and their families. Acknowledging the attitudes, beliefs, and feelings of the family unit is an important component of the intervention process.

Information for Parents
1. Schedule regular conferences or communications
2. Explain the importance of parental involvement
3. Discuss normal dysfluency versus stuttering
4. Suggest or supply helpful books and videotapes

Activities for Parents
1. Modeling appropriate speech
2. Assessing caregiver's attitudes
3. Scheduling talking time
4. Participating in parent support group
5. Using restimulation techniques
6. Documenting changes in a diary
7. Quizzing the parents
8. Confronting voluntary stuttering

Figure G-1.1 Outline of Parent and Caregiver Involvement Information and Activities

meetings, parental fears and feelings (e.g., guilt and anger) should be assessed and managed appropriately. Parents must be given the opportunity to express their feelings.

2. Explain the importance of parental involvement. Be sure to provide illustrative examples of how parents can effectively contribute to the therapeutic process. In addition, Logan and Caruso (1997) stress that it is important for the clinician to reach some agreement with the parents about:
   a. How effective certain types of intervention may be (direct, indirect, or a combination)
   b. What side effects, if any, these interventions may have
   c. What the consequences of inaction may be (Ramig et al., 1988)

3. Discuss normal dysfluency and normal language development, focusing on the following developmental areas necessary for success in speech therapy:
   a. Motor coordination and timing
   b. Linguistic and cognitive development
   c. Emotional understanding or maturity (Ramig et al., 1988)

4. Provide the parents with information they can take home. Booklets, pamphlets, and videotapes are invaluable sources of information (see Handout I: Available Resources in the Appendix). Assess the parents' acceptance of their child, and the environment they provide for him, in a nonthreatening way. Suggest to the parents ways in which they can help change the environment to

help their child, such as by reducing conversation rate, reducing time pressure, modeling turn-taking, talking openly about stuttering (Starkweather, 1997), and "[r]educ[ing] the pace of activities and tension of everyday life" (Shapiro, 1999). Although parents should encourage the child to participate in activities in which he is likely to succeed, to increase self-esteem, it is important not to overschedule the child.
   a. If the child is preschool-age, *Stuttering and the Preschool Child: Help for Families* (Stuttering Foundation, 2001) is recommended. This video helps families understand stuttering and demonstrates how they can help their child. In addition, clips of professionals working with preschool children are highlighted.
   b. If the child is a teen, he and his parents should view and discuss the video *Stuttering: Straight Talk for Teens* (Stuttering Foundation, 2003). This film provides information, demonstrates treatment, and encourages teens to help themselves make changes.
   c. Provide the parents with the book *If Your Child Stutters: A Guide for Parents* (2003) and the video *Stuttering and Your Child: A Videotape for Parents* (2001). These sources will help answer many of the parents' questions. They can also be given to teachers along with the brochure, *The Child Who Stutters at School: Notes to the Teacher* (2003) (all from the Stuttering Foundation).
   d. Further information is available at the Stuttering Homepage, at www.stutteringhomepage.com; the Stuttering Foundation Web site, www.stutteringhelp. org; the National Stuttering Association Web site, www.westutter.org; and at the Web site of Friends: An Association of Young People Who Stutter, www.friendswhostutter.org)

Activities for Parents

1. Early in the intervention process, the parents should become familiar with the preferred speech model to be used with their child. Often the clinician will instruct the parents to slow their speaking rate and increase pause time. Parents need to practice these changes with the clinician to ensure consistency across environments. Such feedback, even if brief or periodic, assists in increasing parents' understanding of the difficulty in changing speech patterns. The parents are encouraged to observe and then participate in activities so they can carry out similar activities at home.

2. Ask parents to assess how they are responding to their child's dysfluencies by completing either the "Parent Attitudes Toward Stuttering Checklist" (in Crowe & Cooper, 1977) or the "Child Management

Questionnaires and Checklist" (in Zwitman, 1978). These checklists are helpful in facilitating parental awareness and change.

3. The clinician should encourage the parents to schedule "talking time" (Botterill, Kelman, & Rustin, 1991) during which the parents commit to spending three to five minutes, four to six times per week, communicating with their child. This should be carried out in a quiet room to avoid interruptions. During talking time, parents do not make demands or comments on the child's speech. Conversely, in their article, Rustin & Cook (1995) also recommend having the parents set aside time for their child when they can enjoy each other's company with *no* emphasis placed on the child's talking. The child should know that it is acceptable if he does not want to talk during this time. For very young children whose body tension increases rapidly with excitement, the clinician can encourage the parents to initiate quiet-time activities that involve storytelling in the arms of the parent, to encourage rest and listening skills.

4. Evening parent support group meetings present an opportunity for involvement for those who cannot attend in-school therapy sessions. Bennett (1990) discusses how a specific school district organized such meetings, complete with babysitters and translators, to discuss pertinent issues about stuttering, environmental factors that influence speech, and treatment considerations. This allows parents to share their feelings and attitudes with other parents in an accepting, warm environment. Parents should feel welcome to express their feelings about the treatment process.

5. When a child stutters more severely, the parents or teacher can use a restimulation method. That is, the adult restates what the child has said so he can hear it stated fluently (Dell, 2000).

6. Dell (2000) encourages parents to keep a diary of their child's stuttering to document cycles and changes in fluency. By keeping a diary, parents will feel an increased sense of participation by providing information on possible environmental influences that may be beneficial in therapy.

7. Under the guidance of the therapist, the child reads an article about stuttering and develops a list of questions and answers. Later, the child reads the article to his parents and gives them a quiz. The parents' answers provide a way of discussing aspects of stuttering and treatment and can be discussed further with the therapist.

8. To illustrate the fears and embarrassment associated with stuttering, invite the parents to voluntarily stutter, using the same strategies expected of their child. Encourage parents to experiment with stuttering during a support group meeting or even in public settings (e.g., ordering food in a restaurant).

Teacher and Peer Education

Rationale

The teacher often plays an important and influential role in the life of the child who stutters. Her understanding and support of the child and the upheaval stuttering can create in the school environment is most important to the child's social and emotional health. In contrast, a teacher's lack of understanding of how to most positively react to the child and his stuttering can become a memorable nightmare in the child's school and life experience. As a result, one of the major responsibilities of the clinician is to help educate teachers and other school personnel on how best to interact with and facilitate the child's classroom and overall school experience (e.g., Conture, 2001; Manning, 1996; Ramig & Bennett, 1995; Shapiro, 1999; *Stuttering: straight talk for teachers* video (Stuttering Foundation video no. 2002).

Helping children respond in a constructive manner to teasing and other forms of harassment and intimidation from others is an important responsibility held by the speech-language clinician (Manning, 2001; Ramig & Bennett, 1995; Shapiro, 1999). Not only can teasing cause life-long problems for those harassed, but caregivers and their legal representatives have made a significant mark in the pocketbooks of some school systems where evidence revealed that teachers, principals, and other staff did not do enough to remedy the problem once it was brought to their attention.

Activities and Techniques

Refer to Figure G-2.1 for a topic outline of the information and activities presented in this section.

General Guidelines

1. A clinician should collaborate and consult with the child's teacher as much as possible. Some basic guidelines are:
   a. Educate the teacher by providing information about stuttering, such as handouts, brochures, books, and videotapes. These materials can help her to "see through the eyes of the child who stutters" (Shapiro, 1999, p. 353). Many suitable brochures, books and

---

Support

The following citations provide support in the literature for our inclusion of this goal and the suggested activities addressing teacher and peer education.

Chmela & Reardon (2001) → Educating others about stuttering involves meetings or classroom presentations about stuttering to increase the child's ownership of the problem and develop self-advocacy skills (p. 126).

Chmela & Reardon (2001) → Create flowcharts to illustrate a teasing incident and generate positive reactions.

Dell (2000) → Provide teachers with information about stuttering, answer their questions, and reach a consensus regarding how to deal with stuttering in the classroom.

Langevin, Bortnick, Hammer, & Wiebe (1998) → For children who stutter, the incidence of teasing and bullying is higher: 81 percent of the children who stutter reported that they were bullied at school at some time, as compared with 49 percent to 58 percent of non-stuttering children. Fifty-six percent of children who stutter were teased or bullied about their stuttering once a week or more often, as opposed to 32 percent of nonstuttering children. Unfortunately, parents are not always aware of the harassment experienced by the child. Reportedly, imitation of stuttering and name calling were the most frequently reported types of harassment.

Lass, Ruscello, & Schmidt (1992) → Teachers' perceptions of stutterers included many negative personality stereotypes, indicating that their perceptions of stutterers were similar to those of other groups, including speech-language pathologists.

Lees (1999) → Teachers can change their interaction styles in several ways, including slowing their rate of speech, calling on the child early to speak, avoiding exclusion of the child from classroom activities, and building up the child's confidence.

continues

Support *continued*

Lass, Ruscello, & Pann-backer (1994) School administrators' responses to a questionnaire describing persons who stutter reported overall negative personality traits (e.g., shy, nervous, quiet). These results were similar to previous results from teachers, special educators, and speech-language pathologists.

videotapes are available from the Stuttering Foundation (see Handout I: Available Resources in the Appendix). A highly recommended video is *Stuttering: Straight Talk for Teachers* (Stuttering Foundation, 2002). For an additional explanation of education and stuttering, see Marty Jezer's account of his school days in *Stuttering: A Life Bound Up in Words* (Small Pond Press, 1998).

b. Explain possible causes and situations that exacerbate or reduce stuttering.

c. Discuss the treatment process and the teacher's role in it.

d. Ask the teacher to talk privately with the child about his dysfluency problem and let him know that she

---

General Guidelines
1. Classroom information for the teacher
2. How to interact with and react to a student who stutters
3. Class presentation on stuttering
4. Having the teacher attend therapy
5. Maintaining contact with teachers
6. Using information about stuttering in the classroom
7. Clinician in the classroom

Teasing and Bullying
1. Child's comfort in the classroom
2. Zero tolerance for teasing and bullying
3. Responding to teasing and bullying
4. Famous stutterers
5. Practicing responses
6. Role-playing
7. Talking with parents
8. Reenacting and discussing alternative behaviors
9. Drawing a picture

Figure G-2.1 Outline of Teacher and Peer Education Activities

---

accepts his stuttering and supports his efforts in therapy. This is also a good opportunity for the teacher to get feedback about how the child wants the teacher to deal with his stuttering in and out of the classroom.

e. The teacher should not, unless requested by the child, be instructed to interrupt the student's speech or tell him to use therapy techniques during class. For additional communication strategies, see the handouts for teachers in the Appendix (Handout I).

f. Talk about the teacher's role in facilitating fluency and how her observations of the child in class may assist (e.g., What is the child's communication style? Is silence common, or does the child initiate speech easily and frequently? What about turn-taking behaviors? Is topic maintenance a problem? Is the child using fluency-enhancing techniques?):
  (1) Provide the child with more opportunities to speak on more fluent days.
  (2) Expect the child to participate in regular class assignments and projects, but allow flexibility and anticipate adjustments.
  (3) Provide support and praise for each small success.
  (4) Prevent singling out a child who stutters.

g. Provide a brochure that gives guidelines to the teacher who is having difficulty with knowing what to do about a child who stutters in the classroom. A good one is "The Child Who Stutters at School: Notes to the Teacher," by the Stuttering Foundation (2003).

h. Prepare a joint presentation to share information with classmates, which may be prerecorded on videotape. Utilize Bill Cosby's book, *The Meanest Thing to Say* (Cartwheel Books, 1997), which addresses teasing. Guide small-group discussions about various situations for children with special needs. The National Stuttering Association publishes a helpful guide to delivering classroom presentations about stuttering (NSA, 2000).

i. Meet with the classroom teacher (and with the child when appropriate) to discuss his stuttering in the classroom. The clinician's objective is to learn about the teacher's beliefs about stuttering and the child's stuttering in class, specifically. This is a good time to discuss stuttering with the teacher and explain what the child is working on in therapy. Discuss classroom collaboration at this time and what the teacher can do to help.
Further details on collaborating with teachers may be found in Shapiro (1999), Zebrowski and Cilek (1997), or Ramig and Bennett (1995).

2. Teachers can provide information about how the child speaks and behaves in class. When the child stutters during class, the teacher should react calmly, patiently, and objectively, which will show the other students that stuttering is not something to deride. The teacher should let the child finish what he is trying to say and put a stop to any teasing or bullying in the classroom (Dell, 2000). During the transfer process, the teacher may wish to discreetly reward the child's efforts to use fluency and stuttering modification techniques in the classroom.

3. The clinician can be a guest speaker in the child's class and discuss what stuttering is, why it happens, and how to interact with someone who stutters. The classmates can be given tips on listening, such as not telling the child who stutters to "slow down," not speaking at a slower rate so as to imitate stuttering, and not interrupting or finishing what the child is saying. Often, informing the audience will educate them and direct their interest to helping, rather than hurting, their fellow classmate. Additionally, to better understand stuttering, the clinician can bring devices, such as a delayed auditory feedback machine, into the classroom for other classmates to use. Instead of teasing the child, they will better understand the nature of stuttering and become interested in how he speaks. In demonstrating how stuttering occurs, the clinician may bring professionally produced videos of other children in therapy into the child's classroom to illustrate what he does in therapy to help his stuttering. Videotaped endoscopies (Ramig & Smith, 1999) comparing a normal speaker with a stutterer can illustrate the differences between the two, if appropriate.

4. To better involve the teacher in the child's intervention, ask her to attend a therapy session to observe what the child is doing. If the child is resistant to talking in class, the teacher will be able to see and hear him talk in therapy. Also, inviting the teacher to a therapy session will allow the child to discuss his wants and needs regarding treatment with her. If the teacher is willing to be involved, techniques that are already successful in the child's therapy will be recommended, such as slowing down his rate, using easy onsets, and so on. Before the child agrees to involve his teacher, he will need to understand what it may be like to work with her—similar to working with her as another clinician. The teacher and child can role-play together in the therapy room to demonstrate for the child how this will work in the classroom.

5. The clinician should be in contact with the teacher on a regular, weekly basis to discuss the child's progress.

6. The teacher can encourage the child to write reports about famous people who stutter. Reports, bibliographies, or stories about stuttering can also be included in the teacher's curriculum. Many are listed at www.mnsu.edu;

www.stutteringhomepage.com. Look for "Famous Pws" link. To teach the students how speech is produced and performed, the teacher can discuss the speech process and the speech system and what can happen when interferences are caused by tension, blocking, and the like.

7. Teachers are encouraged to use the speech-language pathologist in the classroom during activities in which cooperative teaching is appropriate.

Teasing and Bullying

1. The clinician is responsible for making the therapy room a comfortable place for the child to discuss his feelings. The child should feel that the therapy room is a safe place to talk about stuttering and that no one will humiliate him for reporting episodes of teasing and bullying. When the clinician inserts voluntary stuttering in her own speech, she should assure the child that she does so to help him better understand his stuttering so that she can help him change it—*not* to mock him. Van Riper (1973) referred to this as having the clinician put the child's stuttering into her own mouth. Shield's "An Interview with Caroline: You Can Do Something about Teasing!" is a helpful resource available at www.mnsu.edu; www.stutteringhomepage.com. Look for it in the ISAD 2002 conference papers.

2. The clinician should involve the parents and teachers in curbing any harassment the child may encounter at school as a result of stuttering. The teacher should reassure the child that he can come to her for help when he is harassed. Telling a teacher, as well as his parents, can often eliminate teasing and bullying in the classroom. If teasing or bullying occurs between classmates and the student who stutters, the clinician should task the teacher to confront the perpetrators and address the issue.

   The classmates doing the teasing or bullying need to realize that this problem is no worse than other problems that many students confront, such as reading, writing and arithmetic struggles. The child's classmates and peers must be made to understand that such teasing is unacceptable and will not be tolerated. Teachers can use this opportunity to reinforce the idea that teasing of any kind is unwelcome behavior. Some students who stutter prefer to speak to their classmates directly, and the clinician can be of assistance in such a presentation.

3. Roth and Beal (1999) suggest that in response to teasing and bullying, the child can avoid, ignore, inform, confront, or use wit. Avoiding may not be the best strategy, because he may have to make sacrifices to avoid being teased. Instead of trying to resolve the problem, he can involve an adult in terminating the harassment. The child can confront the bully by

casually confirming that he stutters. The victim of teasing can use wit, by saying something like, "Oh, do you stutter, too?" or "You don't stutter the same way I do. Try it like this . . . . "

Whatever the strategy that the clinician and child decide to use, they can role-play situations in the therapy room where they take turns teasing each other and responding. Teach the child why others tease, why children react to stuttering, and how to stop reacting. As an activity in therapy, brainstorm and write down all the ways one can react to teasing.

Other possible responses to teasing or bullying can include the following:

a. "Yes, I stutter, and I am working on getting my speech better."

b. "When kids make fun of me, I just ignore them and walk away."

c. "You know who Bo Jackson [or other famous person who stutters] is? One of the greatest football/baseball players in history. He stuttered too!"

d. "That's just one of the differences between you and me." (This may get the person doing the harassing to wonder what the other differences are, and if they are good or bad differences.)

e. "When I'm teased, I say 'I can't help it,' and then I ignore them. I just forget about it."

f. Just one thing to remember—if somebody makes fun of you for stuttering then their problem is much worse than yours.

g. "Yes, I do stutter, and that makes me unique" or "If you don't like the way I talk, don't listen to me."

h. "When I get teased about stuttering, I just say, one of the ways I dealt with teasing is that I did a report about stuttering and presented it to my class in fourth grade. I'm glad I don't have to hide anything anymore."

i. "Just because I stutter does not mean I'm not smart. If you stuttered and I didn't, how would you feel if I made fun of you?"

The preceding excerpts are adapted from the "Just for Kids" Web site at www.mnsu.edu.

4. Share with the child information about famous and successful people who have stuttered or do stutter. In addition to gaining the insight that many persons who stutter are famous and well respected, the information

can provide the material for teasing comebacks ("Yeah, I stutter, but Samuel L. Jackson did, too, and look at him! He's a Jedi!").

5. After providing the child with examples of teasing responses, let him practice a few favorites for use in the future. It may be helpful to have younger children practice their responses using puppets. Additionally, if not already expressed to the clinician, the child may convey through the puppet his feelings about teasing during the role-play.

6. Lew (2001) suggests using role-playing with a child for situations in which he is often teased or bullied. For example, if a child gets teased frequently on the playground, particular strategies to counteract the teasing or bullying should be rehearsed. When a child is harassed about his stuttering, he could say, "Sometimes I just get stuck on my words" or "I bet I can stutter better than you just did" (Lew, 2000).

7. Ask parents to sit down with their children and discuss the many reasons why classmates tease and how they were teased when they were young. It is important to acknowledge and validate the child's feelings and hurt about the teasing or bullying, but also to help the child keep it in perspective, realizing that the person doing the teasing or bullying often has problems that he may be avoiding or trying to solve by hurting others (Lew, 2000).

8. When a young child experiences teasing or bullying, videotape him reenacting what occurred (with the clinician or a group member as the teaser) and how he reacted. Have the child watch the tape and discuss the alternative ways he could have reacted. After he chooses what he thinks is the best alternative, videotape him again reacting in this new way (Murphy, as cited in Guitar, 1998).

9. To work through the child's fear of teasing, have him illustrate on paper how he felt at the moment of teasing. Talking through the drawing with the child can help him express his feelings and can be helpful in letting go of hurtful remarks.

10. An excellent, detailed guide that provides information for parents, teachers, speech-language pathologists, school administrations and children is *Bullying and Teasing: Helping Children Who Stutter*, available from the National Stuttering Association (2004).

GOAL 3:

Success in Working with Younger Children

Rationale

Working with young children who stutter is highly recommended by the vast majority of speech-language clinicians specializing in fluency disorders. The first several pages of activities pertain to working with children individually. The next several activities offer suggestions for working with children in a group environment (e.g., Bloom & Cooperman, 1999; Conture, 1990; Ramig, 1993; Rentschler, 2001; Starkweather & Givens-Ackerman, 1997).

Group intervention environment can be very beneficial for children who have already worked individually with a supportive clinician and have learned basic coping strategies they can then practice with other children who stutter. This intervention setting should involve no more than three other children who are also working on their stuttering strategies, in an environment that approximates more closely their everyday speaking interactions. Benefits include helping the child feel less alone in dealing with stuttering; it can also reduce cost if parents are paying for treatment (Ramig & Bennett, 1997b).

Activities and Techniques

Refer to Figure G-3.1 for an outline of the information and activities presented in this section.

General Guidelines

1. In working with children, it is imperative to make the environment enjoyable, one where they feel supported and wanted. Van Riper (1973) suggests an activity that plays into helping the younger, more reticent child speak in a comfortable environment. In this activity, the clinician and child each has a box of toys. While each participant plays with his or her toys, the clinician slowly changes from playing alone to more cohesive play. While playing, the clinician does not expect the child to speak; this usually happens naturally as the clinician begins to vocalize her play with car or animal noises. The clinician uses "self-talk" strategies as they play together and this, it is hoped, will give the child leeway in verbal play. As the activity progresses, the clinician begins to draw the child out by asking

Support

The following citations provide support in the literature for our inclusion of this goal and the suggested activities for success when working with younger children.

Barbara, Goldart, & Oram (1961)
→ Within a controlled environment that permits the examination of stuttering, group therapy facilitates a sense of belonging, an atmosphere of unity, feelings of respect for others, and a spirit of acceptance and support.

Fawcus (1970)
→ Adult groups contain from 8 to 12 members, but smaller groups organized by age are recommended for children. Group therapy is considered to provide interpersonal relationships, realistic stress, and the opportunity for positive reinforcement. Results of the programs are considered promising.

Gottwald & Starkweather (1995)
→ Early intervention for stuttering has been proven to have dramatic and lasting results in remediation of the disorder. Part of therapy should focus on reducing the child's environmental demands through education, affective support, and behavior change facilitation.

Leahy (1994)
→ Speech-language pathologists who were involved in group therapy experiences considered people who stutter in a more positive light than those who rendered only individual treatment.

Leahy & Collins (1991)
→ Feedback provided by persons who stutter suggests that group therapy had a positive effect on personal behavior and facilitated transfer and maintenance of speech fluency.

Onslow, Packman, & Harrison (2003)
→ In the Lidcombe Programme, the parent gives verbal contingencies during conversational exchanges with the child. The SLP ensures that these parental verbal contingencies are neither constant, intensive, nor invasive, and that parents instead provide positive support for the child who stutters. This approach is individualized for each family and, as with any treatment for a childhood speech or language disorder, it is essential that the child enjoy the treatment and find it to be a positive experience.

General Guidelines
1. Warming up to therapy
2. Modeling of normal disfluencies
3. Appropriate language models
4. Desensitization and children
5. Confrontation: When fluency shaping fails
6. Contrasting smooth and bumpy speech
7. Analogies
8. Individualizing treatment
9. Quiet time
10. Setting talking-time rules
11. Token reinforcement
12. Linguistic hierarchy

Reinforcing This Component
1. Puppets and dolls
2. Wordless picture books
3. Support of new interests
4. Tag game
5. Imitation
6. Fluency-initiating gestures

7. Involving others
8. "Show and Tell"
9. Collaborating with the teacher
10. DAF and continuous phonation
11. Fluency-enhancing conditions
12. Picture cards
13. Flashlight game
14. Carrier phrases in gaming
15. Barrier games
16. Musical chairs

Working with Children in Group Intervention
1. Team practice
2. Timelines
3. Talk show
4. Imaginative dialogues
5. Mock interviews
6. If I had a million dollars . . .
7. Phone calls
8. What price fluency?
9. Writing a storybook

Figure G-3.1 Outline of Activities for Working with Very Young Children

questions requiring one-word responses. As the child begins to interact more, the clinician asks more questions and makes more statements.

Van Riper (1973) suggests another game to encourage talking and fluency by challenging the child to "Say the Magic Word." The clinician is always encouraged to offer opportunities for the child to express himself, whether it be fluently or stuttering. A major goal of these activities is to encourage the reticent child to talk and feel comfortable with the clinician.

2. The clinician should model easy, normal disfluencies as well as occasional stuttering dysfluencies. According to Peters and Guitar (1991), these models should have the following qualities:

   a. Only one or two repetitions of a word or syllable are used (like-like this, rather than like-like-like-like this).

   b. Between repeated words or syllables, airflow and voicing should be continuous, loose, and easy—not broken, tight, or tense.

   c. When the clinician models short prolongations, her voice should be very relaxed, and she should make smooth transitions from the first sound into the rest of the word (luh-luh-like this, without tightening any part of the speech mechanism).

   d. Voluntary dysfluencies produced by the clinician should be slow (most of all, the modeled speech with the child should be slow). The clinician

should be careful not to overdo modeling of the child's stuttering.

   e. Listen to how frequently the child stutters and model at about the same frequency or less.

   f. Speaking slower is a common characteristic of fluency-shaping methods. When producing these sounds, the clinician helps the child use speech that incorporates an exaggerated slow pattern. Slowed speech should focus on prolonging and stretching the sounds of words while maintaining normal stress, intonation, and juncture.

3. Van Riper (1973) argued that it is very important for the child's acquisition of normal fluency to be filled with unhurried, simple speech and language patterns. Incorporating rhythm and timing techniques into games will help the child practice these patterns in a relaxed environment. Begin with single words, then phrases, and then short sentences, depending on the age of the child.

4. Desensitize the child to fluency disrupters. For example, if the child's fluency breaks down when he is interrupted, gradually begin to interrupt him until just before he begins to stutter. (The signs will depend on the child: some may become less spontaneous and free-flowing and may sound somewhat halting or jerky; others may speak more rapidly or begin to "push" their articulators or have more abrupt onsets of phonation). Once this point is reached, let the child return to a

fluent state for a few minutes and begin to interrupt again until right before the child is going to stutter. Continue this pattern, gradually increasing the number of interruptions as the child becomes more tolerant of interruption (i.e., it takes longer to bring the child to the point of almost stuttering). Continue to desensitize the child to the major fluency disrupters that have been identified by the parents and the clinician. These disrupters can be introduced in a positive way, such as playing a game where the clinician and child take turns trying to make each other stutter (e.g., making funny faces, pounding on the table) when the other is speaking. By using stresses and pressures more and more like those in the child's environment, and pressing the child to greater and greater resistance, the clinician makes therapy a confidence-boosting experience and helps pave the way for long-term fluency.

5. When fluency-shaping strategies are not working well, some children require direct work on dealing with the stuttering moment. Specific to these cases, and once rapport and a positive comfort level have been established, direct confrontation can begin. This confrontation should be gradual but direct (Dell, 2000). The clinician can model pseudo-stuttering in her own speech and discuss nonchalantly how and why specific pseudo-stutters are used. In a relaxed manner, the clinician can then invite the child to implement pseudo-stuttering and begin working with him to identify and modify the difficulties in his speech.

6. The clinician can teach the child to substitute normal nonfluencies for stuttered speech. First, the child is taught to differentiate "easy" or "smooth" nonfluencies from "bumpy" or "hard" stuttering. Once differentiation is accomplished, have him practice making the stuttered speech easy by substituting less tense, more normal disfluency. The clinician provides modeling for the child if needed (Gottwald & Starkweather, 1995).

The child needs to be involved in activities to contrast between smooth and easy speech. He can pick various items out of a box as he names them with slow and easy speech. The clinician can first demonstrate this activity and then gradually include the child.

7. Guitar (1998) suggests using analogies illustrating strategies to overcome fears. For example, ask the child to think about a person who may be afraid of bugs, the dark, or some other fairly common thing. Discuss how people can overcome their fear and what rewards they get for accomplishment. Examples as simple as being afraid of an animal act as a "pep talk" for the child and can help him reduce his fear of stuttering.

Gregory and Hill (1980) recommend comparing easy, smooth speech with visual cues children can more easily identify with, such as rolling a ball or car across the table without any intervening obstacles.

8. Any activities used should correspond to the individual child's interests and skills. Children enjoy activities ranging from finger-painting to playing with puzzles or building blocks to reading storybooks. Through experimentation and time, the clinician can make appropriate decisions as to what is most interesting for each individual child.

9. For very young children whose body tension increases rapidly with excitement, the clinician can encourage quiet-time activities, such as storytelling as they sit together in a comfortable chair or couch. This activity is one parents should be encouraged to do as well. It is important that the adult speech model reflect slower talking, pausing, and slightly exaggerated inflection.

10. The clinician may want to set up "talking-time rules" that will help control the time pressure demands that may develop in therapy (Kelly & Conture, 1991). It is important to establish clearly defined turn-taking rules under which only one person may talk at a time and each person is given a turn to talk. When the child is in a therapy session, he must be treated the same as he would be in his classroom. Interruptions and undesirable behavior should be minimized. Teaching the child to raise his hand, or say, "Excuse me," to indicate his desire to talk is appropriate and encouraged.

11. The more drill-like the therapy, the greater the need for token reinforcement to provide motivation. Conversely, the more game- or play-oriented the therapy, the less the need for token reinforcement (Guitar, 1998).

12. The following activities were suggested by Guitar (1998) as a way of working a child through a fluency hierarchy: Single-word-level slow speech → carrier phrase + word-level slow speech → sentence-level slow speech → sentence-level normal speech → two- to four-sentence-level normal speech → conversation-level normal speech.

Reinforcing This Component

1. Another game can be played that shows the difference between smooth, easy speech, and bumpy, hard speech. After the child learns the difference between the two, he is asked to identify each when the clinician tests his knowledge. Activities with puppets mimicking the two styles of speech may create a more enjoyable experience for the younger child. To illustrate the differences between hard and smooth (or soft) speech, the child can work with smooth and bumpy surfaces or objects. The clinician may also set up an activity in which hard or soft toys provide cues for the type of speech the child will use. The smooth and hard items are hidden behind a partition; the child

chooses an item and speaks with the type of speech the item represents, and the clinician guesses the method he is using. Reversing the roles is important to provide the child with experience in feeling and observing the differences between the two types of speech.

Gentle onset, slowed speech rate, and smooth, continuous transitions from one sound and word to the next, and more appropriate turn-taking between speakers and listeners, are all concepts that can be incorporated into a game through the use of puppets or dolls to help generate conversation and enjoyment for the child (Gottwald & Starkweather, 1995). For example, puppet names can be stretched out and the puppets required to talk to each other using slow speech. When playing games, slow speech words (e.g., "Now it is my turn.") are used in transition, helping the child practice his easy, reduced speaking rate. When confronting the child's stuttering, Dell (2000) suggests having him identify what he does when he stutters, thus pointing out the ways he can make changes. It is helpful for the child to find a median between the tension he creates and the tension that is appropriate when grasping onto a word he is struggling with. Illustrating with dolls or puppets lets the child point out the tensions in the puppet's "stutter." By manipulating the puppet's tongue getting stuck in a word, the child can come to understand how he might be jamming this articulator during a stuttering moment. The clinician and child can each have their own puppet, and time can be taken to use the puppets for expressing the struggles in "getting stuck."

2. Wordless picture books, such as those by Mercer Mayer, for example, can be used with preschool and non–reading-age children. The books tell a story with no words involved, which encourages the child to create stories of his own and, by doing so, facilitates verbal exchange between the clinician and child. When using wordless picture books, the clinician is allowed to be creative as well by making up her own story, while adding theatrical expressions that will, it is hoped, contribute to a more fun and relaxed learning environment. When the child sees that there is no teasing or correcting, he usually cooperates and tells his own story to the therapist. These books can also be used for practicing easy onsets, light articulatory contacts, and other techniques.

3. Facilitate the child's sense of personal worth by helping him develop new interests and abilities to enhance his image with friends and classmates. Provide positive reinforcement throughout the treatment sessions. Use puppets to role-play situations and activities he can engage in with his peers.

4. A tag game is helpful for the child to listen and identify stuttering qualities. He "tags" the clinician after hearing

her stutter. This game gives the child a playful, supportive, and positive outlook in seeing that stuttering can be confronted and that learning can be fun.

5. Young children are prone to imitate adults and sometimes even enjoy making a game out of imitation. Starting with single words and gradually moving up to more complex linguistic levels, the child can practice the learning of slower speech through imitation. He can mimic the clinician in activities that encourage relaxation and smooth movements of the speech mechanism. The clinician might model loose contacts and produce difficult words that the child will need to work through by using therapy techniques. A young child may be prone to refuse activities such as imitation in easy stuttering or dysfluencies. If so, the clinician can illustrate a story that involves characters with names such as "Mickey" and another named "Mmmmmmickey." This game can help the child more comfortably practice using easy repetitions or prolongations.

6. Cooper and Cooper (1985) use pictures of cartoon characters to teach children fluency-initiating gestures. Fluency-initiating gestures were developed to teach children a slower rate of speech, easy voice onset, and smooth transitions between sounds and words. These authors recommended that children learn to keep phonation continuous while making light articulatory contacts.

7. Parents, siblings, teachers, and friends can join the child in one or more therapy sessions to create a realistic setting he can practice in. Involving other people in the therapy room should be in the appropriate context and time.

8. Situations such as "Show and Tell" can be role-played in intervention so that the clinician can encourage the child to use fluency strategies to perform successfully in a previously demanding speaking situation (Gottwald & Starkweather, 1995).

9. The clinician is encouraged to collaborate with the classroom teacher and help the teacher use a fluency-enhancing speaking and interacting style, as well as to assist the teacher in developing curriculum methods that support fluency.

10. Shames and Florance (1980) use delayed auditory feedback (DAF) to help the child learn two important skills: control of rate and continuous phonation. They begin with DAF set at its maximum delay and instruct the child how to use rate control and continuous phonation to produce slow, prolonged, stutter-free speech. Gradually, they increase the child's speaking rate by systematically reducing the DAF delay times.

11. When working with younger children, it is helpful to incorporate the following to facilitate fluency: choral speaking, singing, recitation of nursery rhymes, and rhythmic speaking.

12. Working with picture cards that enable the child and clinician to create stories can reinforce smooth, easy speech. Picture cards that facilitate fluency can be made or bought commercially. The pictures should involve objects that can be named with single words and should include all word-initial phonemes in the language. When practicing slow speech, conversation can be initiated by the clinician using sequence cards that create a story the child needs to "solve" by placing the cards in order.

13. In practicing easy prolongations, Guitar (1998) prefers a game called "Flashlight," which is intended to advance one's level of difficulty by having the child say a word for a longer period of time. He finds that using a carrier phrase plus a word is helpful in making the activity more complex. For example, "I see the _____," or "I think he is a _____." The game begins with introducing the child to different picture cards, placing the cards around the therapy room, turning the lights off, and working together to identify the objects. Once the child identifies an object with the flashlight, say the phrase together using slow, relaxed speech. To avoid having the child associate objects with specific carrier phrases, vary them, and later advance the level of efficiency for a challenge.

14. Use carrier phrases when playing games such as "Memory" or "Concentration" to help encourage the use of slow speech rates. The child, clinician, or parent is required to say a carrier phrase plus a word before turning over the chosen card. Useful games such as "Go Fish" and "Old Maid" require players to use a carrier phrase when taking their turns. Another activity is for the clinician and child to make an art project together, focusing on slow and easy speech methods to request materials and discuss the projects they are making. A game of "Go Fish" can be played in which each player fishes for magnetic cards with pictures on each. For each card the player catches, he names it using both hard and easy speech. The player with the most fish wins.

15. An activity Guitar (1998) suggests for taking slow speech to the sentence level is called the "Barrier Game." During the game, a barrier separates the clinician and child so the two cannot see each other's sheet of paper on the table. The clinician asks the child to draw an object on his paper while the clinician draws the same object, and vice versa, for a few turns. Through this activity, the child indirectly hears the slow speech being used and mimics the same speed and manner of speech.

Working with Children and Adolescents in Group Intervention

1. With group intervention, musical chairs can be played with the intention of using easy bounces or stretches in every round. Each chair in the circle has a different card with a word written on it. Each time the music stops, the child reads his word with target speech strategies.

2. Divide the group into teams of two for speech practice (described in Fraser, 2002). Each team will role-play, one person acting as the client and the other as the clinician. In this activity, the child is able to apply what he learned from his clinician in individual therapy to a more advanced speaking environment.

3. Group members can get to know each other better by sharing their individual life stories while practicing their speech techniques (Rentschler, 2001). Each child receives a large piece of paper, a pencil, an easel, and tape. The child is asked to draw a line horizontally across the paper to represent a timeline. A line drawn off of the main line is meant to represent an event that occurred in this particular person's life. Additional lines represent events such as a major world event that took place just before the child's birth, something that happened in elementary school, an event that occurred in high school speech class, first job interview, "who you are now," and "where you want to be in five years." Each member of the group is given time to tell his life story using specified speech strategies.

4. As a group, all members can take part in a "Talk Show" (Rentschler, 2001) and practice using extemporaneous speaking. One child is selected as the host; the others are the participants and audience. The host is given a card on which is written a premise that the child will discuss. The host introduces one of the guests and interviews him for five minutes, and then moves to the next.

5. Within the group, the members can tell a story with the goal of engaging all the children in imaginative dialogue (Rentschler, 2001). One member starts a story, on any topic; as the story travels around the circle, each member adds new information with the reminder to retell the first half of the story.

6. Mock interviews can assist in practicing strategies and techniques within a group. Taking turns, each member is directed to the front of the room while the other members interview him and ask questions pertaining to his life story. The member in front answers questions while keeping his focus on correcting his speech as needed.

7. In a group discussion, give the group a scenario such as, "If I had a million dollars, I would . . . ." Have each child write down a response and then share each other's thoughts and ideas.

8. With the group broken up into two small teams, one practices making phone calls while the other team members watch and observe. As the phone calls are made, the other team members can comment on the strategies used, and what they liked about the use of techniques. Then have the callers share their feelings with the group.

9. Rentschler recommends emphasis on the value of fluency when in a discussion group. An indirect question could be, "What price is a child willing to pay to be fluent?" Once the child has determined a price, ask him to decide what price might be too high to pay for such a skill. Engaging in this particular activity stimulates thoughts and feelings related to stuttering and gives children a chance to openly discuss any ideas.

10. The group members can interact as they write a storybook for children concerning the positive aspects of being a stutterer and how stuttering affects their lives everyday. The story could include pictures to accompany the narrative. As children contribute their own ideas to the story, they share their concerns and feelings about stuttering, as well as confronting it with peers who stutter.

Determining What Is Interfering with Normal Speech Production

Rationale

From the beginning of treatment, it is important for the clinician to empathize with the child and determine his motivations and feelings regarding therapy. As the clinician gains a better understanding of the child's specific needs, she can begin to clarify his specific strengths and challenges. This process continues throughout many sessions, and never truly ceases.

In addition, the clinician may share specific information with the child to increase his level of understanding about stuttering. For example, we have found it very useful to explain how stuttering and its concomitant behaviors prevent air from moving effortlessly through the vocal mechanism during speech. This goal is largely achieved through an appropriately detailed lesson on the anatomy and physiology of normal speech production. The negative feelings that often accompany stuttering can be acknowledged here for the first time—though certainly not the last—as tension and stress usually aggravate stuttering, making fluent speech difficult if not impossible. However, before strategies to manage physiological tension and emotional stress can be successfully learned, the child needs a clear understanding of the adverse effects of stuttering on speech production.

Activities and Techniques

Refer to Figure G-4.1 for an outline of the information and activities presented in this section.

Teaching Normal Speech Production

1. To illustrate the respiratory, laryngeal, and articulatory subsystems of speech, use a large, poster-board representation of a person that includes attachable manipulatives of the diaphragm, lungs, vocal folds, tongue, lips, and teeth. These pieces should have Velcro backing that allows the child to place them in their proper locations. Facial characteristics should match the gender of the child.

Support

The following citations provide support in the literature for our inclusion of this goal and the suggested activities for determining what is interfering with normal speech.

Conture (1990) → It is important for the child to understand how respiration, phonation, and articulation work together to produce speech. Analogies are useful when working with school-age children.

Dell (1993) → Emphasize fluency. In reality, a child may only stutter on 2 to 10 percent of words. He may not even realize how much of the time words are fluently spoken.

Healey (2004) → Discuss the differences between normal fluency, normal nonfluencies, and stuttering. Use voluntary stuttering to produce imitations of the child's stuttering pattern. Focus on physical sensations and emotional feelings.

Manning (1996) → "An understanding of the anatomy and physiology, as well as the acoustics, of the speech production system will enable the clinician to apply her knowledge in the assessment of what the stuttering speaker is doing to make the process of sequencing from one speech segment to another so difficult. As the treatment progresses, it will become important for the client as well to take this perspective about his speech production system" (p. 91).

Nelson (1998) → "First, study how fluent talking is done. Don't just enjoy fluency when it occurs. Learn from it. What does fluent talking sound like, look like, physically feel like in your body? What does it emotionally feel like in your mind?" (p. 26).

Ramig (1998) → "Paying attention to how we physically use our tongue, lips and voice box as we produce sounds can help us understand how we often create more stuttering" (46).

continues

Support *continued*

Van Riper (1973)

→ "Whatever the stutterer is doing that is inappropriate to the normal production of the sound, syllable, word, or utterance should become a vivid error signal so that it can be altered in the direction of the normal production" (p. 312).

Zebrowski & Kelly (2002)

→ Use pictures, diagrams, and models to augment a basic description of the parts of the speech mechanism, including lungs, larynx, and speech articulators. "In showing and discussing the speech mechanism with our clients, we are helping them to begin to objectify speech" (p. 127).

Explain how airflow is manipulated by the various parts to produce speech and how the child can exercise control over these by himself. Later, he can use this teaching aid to explain the process to his parents or others. To enhance interest in the topic, this representation may

Teaching Normal Speech Production
1. Make a poster-board representation of the subsystems of speech
2. Adapt terminology to the child's level of understanding
3. Watch a videotape that describes the speech production mechanism

Comparing Fluent and Dysfluent Speech
1. Compare the differences between muscle tension during normal and dysfluent speech using progressive relaxation
2. Demonstrate the basic mechanics of appropriate airflow by blowing bubbles through a bubble wand
3. Contrast fluency and stuttering using analogies

Reinforcing This Component
1. Play a "Catch the Stuttering" game
2. Create original artwork or literature that explains these processes
3. Publish a document on normal speech production and stuttering
4. Work with the classroom teacher to co-teach anatomy and physiology of speech

Figure G-4.1 Outline for Activities to Determine What Is Interfering with Normal Speech Production

resemble a cartoon, story, or action figure that the child admires or even the child himself (see Figure G-4.2).

2. Realistic models and pictures from textbooks or from the Internet may help mature children understand more precisely how the various subsystems of speech look and interact. To this end, plastic medical models of the larynx and articulators serve as excellent teaching aids. As with younger clients, explain normal speech operation in clear, concise language. Depending on the child's curiosity, it may be appropriate to provide greater detail and more professional terminology. The child should learn the material well enough to explain the process to another person using the provided material.

3. View a videotape that describes the speech production mechanism, emphasizing the structures underlying respiration, phonation, and articulation. For example, *Therapy in Action: The School-Age Child Who Stutters* (Stuttering Foundation videotape No. 79) addresses this topic. Afterward, discuss how disruptions in these areas may interfere with or cause a breakdown in communication.

Comparing Fluent and Dysfluent Speech

1. To illustrate differences in muscle tension during normal and dysfluent speech, teach the child to progressively tense and then relax different muscle groups. Ask the child to describe the differences between feeling tense and feeling relaxed. Progressive relaxation is initially more easily learned using larger muscle groups, like arms and legs, before targeting smaller laryngeal muscles, for example. In addition to facilitating awareness and recognition of tension in different areas, this exercise can demonstrate to the child that he possesses the ability to modify his motor behaviors.

2. Demonstrate the basic mechanics of appropriate airflow by blowing bubbles through a bubble wand. Point out that when the child relaxes and blows air through the wand at an easy pace, pretty bubbles are produced. In contrast, too much tension and blowing hard will cause the liquid soap to spray messily and prevent the smooth flow of bubbles. Likewise, too much air pressure when speaking will tense the vocal mechanism, producing deteriorated physiological conditions for fluent speech.

3. The differences between fluent and dysfluent speech can be compared using various analogies that help the child describe these feelings. For example, Conture's (1990) water-hose analogy compares areas where the water and air are turned off and what happens as a result. Just as a pinched hose will not permit the smooth flow of water, a closed larynx will prevent fluent speech. Also, when speech is fluent, with a constant airflow, it is like swooshing a basketball into a basket. If the basketball rim were made smaller, which is analogous to an increase in ten-

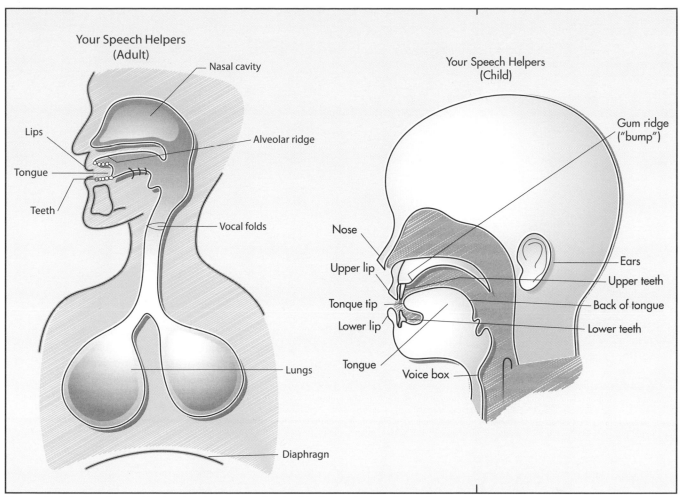

Figure G-4.2 Sample graphic showing the structures involved in the production of speech.

sion, the ball would no longer fit through. Finally, ask the child to generate and share his own analogies that contrast the two sensations.

Reinforcing this Component

1. Play a game in which each player catches the other player during a stuttering moment. The players should explain how normal speech fluency was interrupted and be able to reproduce the identified behaviors. Whether the stuttering is genuine or feigned is unimportant, for matter-of-fact pseudo-stuttering by the clinician can simultaneously target desensitization in the child. Picture cards that illustrate the location(s) of tension can be incorporated in the activity to facilitate learning.

2. For 10 minutes a session across several meetings, have the child work on a model, short story, poem, or painting that describes the way normal speech is disrupted during

fluency. For example, have the child look through magazines and cut out pictures of speech helpers (i.e., articulators) to make a collage. The child can explain the function of each helper as he pastes them onto a piece of construction paper. The finished product can be displayed in the therapy room or in the child's home as a meaningful reminder of what happens during stuttering.

3. In group therapy, children can collaborate to produce an informative publication that discusses the differences between normal speech and stuttering. If appropriate, the article can be published on a Web site or distributed at school to demonstrate to the child the importance of sharing such information with others.

4. Work with the classroom teacher to co-teach an anatomy and physiology lesson about the mechanisms involved in speech production. Refer to Chapter 5 "Working with Teachers," and the corresponding Goal 2, "Teacher and Peer Education," for additional collaborative exercises.

Establishing Fluency through Increasingly Longer and More Complex Stimuli

Rationale

For most children, fluency can be produced more easily when semantic and syntactic demands are lower (e.g., Conture, 2001; Gregory & Hill, 1999; Logan & Conture, 1997; Yaruss, 1999). For this reason, we have outlined numerous activities that can be implemented to first establish fluency at a simpler level before increasing linguistic demands and expecting higher levels of fluency. Usually, fluency is easier to accomplish when responding at the one-word level than when telling a story or asking questions. Logically then, structuring intervention that begins at the one-word level and then progresses to more complex levels is often helpful.

Activities and Techniques

Refer to Figure G-5.1 for an outline of the information and activities presented in this section. Although these activities are generally separated by linguistic complexity, many of the individual activities can easily be adapted to accommodate changes in complexity. In other words, a lower-level activity can be converted into a higher-level activity simply by incorporating a starter phrase. For example, a typical response elicited during a game of UNO (e.g., "Blue six") becomes "I have a blue six" during a later phase of therapy.

Word Level

1. *Memory games*, such as *Bingo* or *Concentration*, are useful in eliciting single-word responses. While using a stuttering modification or fluency-enhancing technique, the child names a picture after turning it over. The clinician models the same behavior during her turns.
2. Go Fish *and* Outburst *games*. These games use pictures or word cards to elicit single word responses that can be modeled and reinforced by the clinician. These games, like many listed in this section, also facilitate pragmatic skills such as turn-taking, and can be used in a group setting.

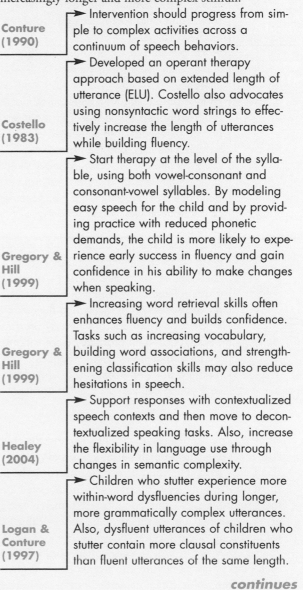

Support

The following citations provide support in the literature for our inclusion of this goal and the suggested activities for success in establishing fluency through increasingly longer and more complex stimuli.

Conture (1990) → Intervention should progress from simple to complex activities across a continuum of speech behaviors.

Costello (1983) → Developed an operant therapy approach based on extended length of utterance (ELU). Costello also advocates using nonsyntactic word strings to effectively increase the length of utterances while building fluency.

Gregory & Hill (1999) → Start therapy at the level of the syllable, using both vowel-consonant and consonant-vowel syllables. By modeling easy speech for the child and by providing practice with reduced phonetic demands, the child is more likely to experience early success in fluency and gain confidence in his ability to make changes when speaking.

Gregory & Hill (1999) → Increasing word retrieval skills often enhances fluency and builds confidence. Tasks such as increasing vocabulary, building word associations, and strengthening classification skills may also reduce hesitations in speech.

Healey (2004) → Support responses with contextualized speech contexts and then move to decontextualized speaking tasks. Also, increase the flexibility in language use through changes in semantic complexity.

Logan & Conture (1997) → Children who stutter experience more within-word dysfluencies during longer, more grammatically complex utterances. Also, dysfluent utterances of children who stutter contain more clausal constituents than fluent utterances of the same length.

continues

Support *continued*

Miles & Ratner (2001)
→ No statistically significant differences were found between two groups of parents (parents of a stuttering child and parents of a nonstuttering child) on any of the measures of language complexity, including syntactic complexity, lexical diversity and rarity, and conversational participation. When parental language scores were examined independently from child language scores, the "distance" between parental scores and child scores was equivalent in the two groups.

Perkins (1992)
→ People who stutter are more likely to be fluent when using short, simple utterances.

Peters (1991)
→ Incorporate linguistic hierarchies that progress from a single word, to a carrier phrase plus word, to a sentence, to two to four sentences, and then gradually progress into conversation. Manipulating clinician models, physical settings, and audience size are additional components of intervention with young school-age children.

Riley & Riley (1983)
→ Children stuttered more during longer or more complex sentences. Improving the child's sentence formulation skills through a gradual increase in length of utterance proved successful in facilitating fluency.

Ryan (1984)
→ Developed an operant therapy program (GILCU) based on gradually increasing the length and complexity of utterances. Ryan reported a 100 percent success rate for very young children using this approach.

Shine (1980)
→ Described stuttering as a discoordination between speech muscle and language encoding systems, in that muscle innervation may be too slow to keep up with the linguistic ideas the child wishes to express. Therapy should begin with simple responses and gradually move toward more complex utterances, to aid the child in organizing his motor-planning strategies.

Starkweather & Givens-Ackerman (1997)
→ Dysfluent children whose language development appears overstimulated can be helped by involving the parents in modifying their interactions with the child to include less talking and fewer direct, complex questions.

Stocker (1980)
→ Fluency in children deteriorates when increased communicative demand is placed upon the speaker. Stocker developed both a diagnostic and a therapeutic approach based on these findings.

Wall (1980)
→ Children who stutter tend to use the word "and" frequently but use other conjunctions and subordinate words less frequently. Some children may be at a lower level of syntactic development and consequently use "and" more frequently.

Yaruss (1999)
→ For some children who stutter, stuttered utterances are, on average, longer and more syntactically complex than fluent utterances.

---

3. *Animal Farm.* In this game, the clinician and the child take turns selecting animals out of a box and placing them on a farm. The child names the animals as he puts them on the farm. The child can also imitate each animal's sound (e.g., "Mmmmooo!" or "Nnnneigh") or give each animal a proper name (e.g., Elsie, Wilbur) using appropriate strategies.

4. *"Secret Grab Bag" games.* To elicit single-word responses, each player draws a picture card from a box and identifies its name, color, function, and so on. A motivating variation is to place a number of different objects in a box or bag and have each player reach in and feel an object in order to describe and identify it by touch. After the player states which object he is feeling, he pulls it out of the bag to confirm his guess.

5. *Word retrieval games,* of which there are several types, facilitate lexical access and organization by strengthening associations. The clinician should tailor the vocabulary to the development of the child.

   a. *Synonyms.* The child matches objects or picture cards that are similar (e.g., "large"/ "big" or "picture"/ "photo"). You can also group these items and ask the child to give two words to describe the groups (e.g., "lady"/ "woman").

   b. *Antonyms.* The child is presented with picture cards and responds by naming the opposite.

   c. *Serial cueing.* The clinician recites part of a sequence and allows the child to complete it (e.g., "Monday, Tuesday, _____," "one, two, three, _____,").

Word Level
1. Memory games (*Bingo* and *Concentration*)
2. *Go Fish* and *Outburst* games
3. *Animal Farm*
4. "Secret Grab Bag" games
5. Word retrieval: synonyms, antonyms, serial cueing, sentence completion
6. Classification games (categorization and association)
7. Rhyming games

Phrase Level
1. Word combinations
2. Carrier phrases
3. Memory games
4. Picture cards
5. "Tell Me What You Do with It"
6. "Simon Says"
7. Clinician-made board game

Sentence and Multisentence Levels
1. Verb cards
2. Jobs and occupations
3. Picture books
4. Sequence pictures
5. Reading activities

6. *Fokes Sentence Builder*
7. Guessing games
8. Question asking and answering
9. Conjunction review
10. Description activities

Story Level
1. Recounting of past events
2. Sequencing story cards
3. "What if?" questions
4. "Show and Tell"
5. Books with no words
6. Riddles and short poems
7. Felt-board stories
8. All About Me books
9. "Retell the Story"
10. Giving directions
11. Completing the story

Conversation Level
1. Role-playing
2. Problem solving
3. Opinions and refutations
4. Idioms, proverbs, and analogies
5. Joke telling
6. General conversation

Figure G-5.1 Outline of Activities for Establishing Fluency through Increasingly Longer and More Complex Linguistic Stimuli

d. *Sentence completion.* The clinician presents incomplete sentences or nursery rhymes that the child completes. Some examples are:
"The leaves fall from the _____."
"Turn the light _____."
"Please tie my _____."
"Open the _____."
"The time is 6 o'_____."
"Jack and Jill went up the _____."
Younger children may benefit from having several choices, such as: "We gave her a birthday _____" (choices: "carpet," "present," "toothbrush").

6. *Classification games.* Provide a more cognitively stimulating activity at the single-word level as the child classifies a number of different pictures or words. The clinician chooses a number of different categories, selected according to the child's age, and asks him to put each response item into the correct category.

a. *Categorization.* The child names five items in a certain class (e.g., animals, blue things, fruits, etc.) or lists ten items involved in certain activities (such as

what to take on a picnic, camping, etc). This can relate to classes of words (naming action words or things, proper names, etc).

b. *Association. Scattergories* (semantic) or *Boggle* (phonetic) are helpful games at the single word level. For more ideas, refer to Wiig and Semel (1980).

7. *Rhyming games.* The clinician says a word modeling easy speech and the child names a word that rhymes with it. A variation on this, which also builds phonological awareness, is to say a multisyllabic word and ask the child to omit the first or last syllable, just saying the remainder.

Phrase Level

1. *Word combinations.* Stringing words together in various ways is the beginning of phrasing activities. Word combinations, such as color + noun, adjective + noun, and number + noun, can be easily elicited through *UNO, Trouble, Bingo, Concentration,* matching, and sentence-building games.

2. *Carrier phrases* are easily elicited with games such as *Chutes and Ladders* and *Candy Land.* The child is instructed to respond at each turn with "I have a purple card", for example.

3. *Memory games.* Modify the child's response to include a carrier phrase, such as: "I have a _____.", "There is a _____.", or "This is a _____."

4. *Picture cards* can be used to elicit a wide variety of phrase-level responses. For example, the clinician may have the child use the cards in a drill activity to generate a phrase response describing the picture. The level of difficulty may be increased by having the clinician ask questions, such as "What is the boy doing?" or "Tell me what you do with it," to elicit a response.

5. *"Tell Me What You Do with It" games.* The clinician can have the child describe the use of a variety of objects, tools, or devices.

6. *"Simon Says."* Initially, this game can be modified by inserting a pause between "Simon says" and the command (e.g., "Touch your toes"). This modification reduces linguistic complexity and provides practice with pausing. Later, the game can be played normally to provide sentence-level practice.

7. *Board game.* The clinician can prepare numerous types of board games using poster board and construction paper. As an example, she can make a game board composed of different colored squares accompanied with a deck of corresponding colored cards that contain functional written phrases. Using dice or a spinner, each player travels around the board. After each turn, as the child lands on a color, he picks a matching card and reads the phrase written on the back of it.

Sentence and Multi-sentence Levels

1. *Verb cards.* Pictorial verb cards can be used in several ways; two examples are to have the child describe the action taking place in the picture or to have him form a complex sentence (or more) about two or more pictures placed side by side.

2. *Jobs and occupations.* Provide the child with pictures of individuals depicting different occupations and instruct him to explain what each person does.

3. *Picture books.* The child is requested to describe each picture with a sentence. Clinician modeling during this task may be necessary to obtain the desired response. This task may be introduced initially by having the child simply repeat back a sentence produced by the clinician.

4. *Sequence pictures.* The child is presented with sequence pictures and asked to arrange them in the proper order while providing a sentence for each picture.

5. *Reading activities.* While practicing easy speech on each word in the sentence, the child reads out of a textbook

from his classroom, or a favorite book or magazine from home or the library. Later in therapy, older clients can use fluency techniques on the first word of every sentence or insert pseudo-stuttering to practice pullouts when reading aloud. Using books from class can be a meaningful, functional practice of novel or difficult words in preparation for classroom discussion.

6. *Fokes Sentence Builder* (1976) is an older but excellent tool that can be utilized to gradually increase the length and complexity of the child's sentences while providing visual stimuli. This may also be used to elicit nonsyntactic word strings of increasing length.

7. *Guessing games.* With guessing games, one person provides clues describing a person, place, or thing. The other player attempts to guess the answer in the fewest number of clues. Similarly, a game of "20 Questions" limits the total number of clues before the players switch roles.

8. *Question asking and answering.* Activities that assist the child in maintaining fluency when asking or answering questions are pertinent to the school-age child who stutters. A fine commercial option is *Brain Quest* (University Games), a game for grades 1 to 6, which allows individual players to answer developmentally appropriate questions. Questions are divided into various categories, such as reading, math, vocabulary, social studies, science, and grab bag.

9. *Conjunction review.* Early in the intervention process, it may be beneficial to stretch connecting words, such as conjunctions, articles, and pronouns, instead of nouns and verbs. Children who stutter may be less likely to have difficulty with noncontent words. In fact, connecting words may be used appropriately as starter words to facilitate fluency. It is helpful to practice a wide variety of connecting words to avoid the overuse of "and" to connect series of phrases.

10. *Description activities.* Using picture cards, ask the child to describe a variety of attributes of a picture: "What does it look like?", "What is it for?", or "Where can it be found?" are questions that can elicit sentence-length responses. *Guess Who* (Milton Bradley) and *Mystery Garden* (Ravensburger) are excellent games for eliciting such descriptive sentences.

Story Level

1. *Recounting of past events.* It may be helpful in the beginning to ask questions that require sequencing and specific people or experiences to answer, such as:
   a. "What happened on your last birthday?"
   b. "What did you do in school today?"
   c. "What did you do over Christmas vacation?"

2. *Sequencing story cards or magazine covers.* Using "What's Missing?" or "What's Wrong with This Picture?" cards

or *Highlights for Children* magazine covers, ask the child to describe in two to three sentences what is missing in the picture or what is wrong with the pictures.

3. *"What if" questions.* require that the child propose answers to certain hypothetical situations requiring language reasoning skills (e.g., "What would you do if you saw smoke coming out of a building?").

4. *"Show and Tell."* A child may enjoy bringing objects or photos from home and describing them in therapy. The explanation can be structured like a classroom presentation so that the student can gain such experience in a comfortable environment.

5. *Books with no words.* Wordless books, like those by Mercer Mayer and others, are especially effective for a very young child or a dysfluent child who is exhibiting delays in reading development.

6. *Riddles and short poems.* In our experience, reading may facilitate fluency for some children who stutter. Reading materials that incorporate short, predictable rhyming patterns can assist in learning easy, yet deliberate phrasing while speaking.

7. *Felt-board stories.* Another creative activity is to provide the child with a felt board and felt cut-outs of different objects and people so that he can combine them to tell a story.

8. All About Me *books* and stories encourage the reader to relate to the ideas being portrayed while adding complexity to simple sentence structure.

9. *"Retell the Story."* Incorporating rebus stories, in which certain nouns and verbs are replaced with pictures, facilitates ease in language formulation, reading, and fluent speech production.

10. *Giving directions.* Obtain two identical sets of a variety of shapes or small objects. One set is for the child and the other for the clinician. Place a barrier between the clinician and the child. The clinician constructs a picture from a series of objects. Because the child cannot see the picture, he must ask questions about the objects (e.g., their shape, their position, etc.) to enable him to copy the picture accurately. Either a time limit or a certain number of questions should be used. Later, the clinician can make it more difficult for the child by shortening the time, decreasing the number of questions, or creating fluency disrupters that would help him practice using tools for modification. The child is expected to use his techniques throughout the game (e.g., stretching, easy onset of voicing, soft contacts).

11. *Complete the story.* Present the child with a starter sentence in a story and invite him to complete the story by generating a creative response. The clinician should individualize the story starter to the interests of each child. *Easy Does It—1* and *Easy Does It—2* provide good guidelines for addressing this component.

Conversation Level

1. *Role-playing* can be used in therapy to address numerous objectives, from desensitization to learning to handle teasing. It also can serve as a fun introduction to more advanced levels of linguistic complexity.

2. *Problem solving.* Present the child with various scenarios or problems and have him brainstorm and present possible solutions. Exercises of this type can help the child gain experience using strategies while thinking on his feet.

3. *Opinions and refutations.* Discussing topics that elicit strong opinions presents an additional challenge to the maintenance of treatment techniques.

4. *Idioms, proverbs, and analogies* offer brief, structured chances to practice that lack the pressure of joke punch lines.

5. *Telling jokes.* Maintaining therapeutic techniques when the joke teller himself laughs during the telling, as well as delivering an effective punch line, presents a rewarding challenge for many individuals who stutter.

6. *General conversation.* Discuss favorite activities, television shows, the family, what happened in school, and specific interests of the child.

Facilitating Adequate Breath Support

Rationale

Adequate breath support and respiratory management are important variables to be addressed with some children and adolescents who stutter. In response to their dysfluency, some children develop aberrant breathing patterns in an effort to control their stuttering. Behaviors such as talking with expiratory reserve air or during rapid inhalation are commonly observed in dysfluent children. For those children who exhibit difficulty initiating or maintaining airflow during speech production, direct techniques may be necessary to reduce respiratory and laryngeal tension. Although a few clinicians continue to advocate the curative effects of controlled airflow on stuttering, implementation of the following breath control strategies are invariably insufficient, by themselves, to effectively manage stuttering.

Activities and Techniques

Refer to Figure G-6.1 for an outline of the information and activities presented in this section.

Teaching Appropriate Respiration

1. Many children, especially young ones, do not require much respiratory work during therapy. However, some children may exhibit poor timing of the respiratory cycle that negatively affects their speaking pattern. For these children, increased awareness about breathing patterns may be required to facilitate change. One method for promoting change is to discriminate between diaphragmatic and clavicular breathing patterns:
   a. Have the child lie on the floor and place his hands below his sternum. He should feel his belly rise during inhalation and fall during exhalation.
   b. Have the child repeatedly inhale and exhale slowly and smoothly. Vary the rate and size of breaths, and describe the sensations between them. For example, slow, deep breaths feel relaxing, whereas quick, short breaths feel rushed.
   c. Help the child identify moments of quick, shallow breathing or examples of talking on exhausted breath (e.g., "Did you breathe deeply enough?" or "Are you talking with no air?").
2. For the child who forces words out using expiratory reserve volume, assist him in slowing down his rate of

Support

The following citations provide support in the literature for our inclusion of this goal and the suggested activities for success when facilitating adequate breath support.

Adams (1980) — Utilizing breath stream management within a hierarchy of linguistic complexity maximizes the child's chances of competently executing intricate laryngeal behaviors.

Bloodstein (1995) — "Antagonisms between abdominal and thoracic breathing, irregularities of consecutive respiratory cycles, prolonged expirations or inspirations, complete cessation of breathing, interruptions of expiration by inspiration, and attempts to speak on intake of air" often characterize stuttering patterns (p. 11).

Costello (1983) — Breath stream regulation may facilitate the reduction of hard contacts, glottal stops, and "bombastic" initiations of phonation that characterize the dysfluent speech of some children.

Denny & Smith (1997) — Respiratory control is "not dichotomous between voluntary and automatic, but forms a continuum" (p. 135).

Denny & Smith (2000) — In some stuttering speakers, atypical respiratory control occurs during the inspiratory phase, prior to sound production.

Dromey & Ramig (1998) — Sentences are spoken more quickly by stutterers at the lowest lung volumes than at normal conditions by normally fluent adults.

Fraser (2004) — "Although easy, quiet breathing is helpful in enabling the stutterer to speak more freely, it is not suggested that the stutterer try to consciously control the inhalation and exhalation of breath. Trying to consciously control breath can too often result in breathing abnormalities that include speaking at the end of a breath, gasping or hyperventilation with a resulting increase in tension" (p. 146).

continues

Support *continued*

Hoit, Solomon, & Hixon (1993)
➤ Voice onset times were longer at high lung volumes in five nonstuttering male adults. At high lung volumes, the diaphragm tends to flatten and pull the trachea and larynx back, exerting a force that may abduct the vocal folds.

Johnston, Watkin, & Macklem (1985)
➤ Stutterers may speak either at substantially higher or lower lung volumes than normal subjects, confining their speech to the inspiratory capacity or expiratory reserve volume.

Mallard, Hicks, & Riggs (1982)
➤ Although people who stutter may not regularly use easy onsets of phonation, they are equally capable of learning how to produce speech in this manner as people who do not stutter.

Mitchell, Hoit, & Watson (1996)
➤ Normal adult speakers tend to pause more and "waste" air during propositional speech, producing (1) fewer syllables per breath group (that is, more milliliters of air escaped per syllable), and (2) fewer syllables per second. However, the mechanical behavior of breathing was not affected by cognitive-linguistic load (between higher and less demanding speaking tasks).

Peters & Boves (1988)
➤ Examined the buildup of subglottal pressure prior to voice onset time and during phonation and articulation in adults who stutter. Deviant patterns of subglottal pressure occurred even in fluent speech of people who stutter as compared to nonstutterers.

Riley & Riley (1983)
➤ The reconstruction of the speech support process, including airflow management, is an elementary goal in any fluency shaping program.

Silverman (2004)
➤ Abnormalities observed in the breathing movements of persons who stutter during moments of stuttering usually are not present during silence. The same types of breathing abnormalities tend to occur during both moments of stuttering and expectancy of stuttering.

Wall & Myers (1995)
➤ With older children, breathing exercises should be used only if the clinician detects an aberrant pattern. For example, clavicular breathing creates tension in the upper chest and laryngeal areas, and can be replaced with a thoracic-abdominal pattern.

Wall, Starkweather, & Cairns (1981)
➤ Stuttering occurs with significantly greater frequency at clause onsets (i.e., boundaries) than at nonboundary positions of clauses. There was also an extremely high frequency of stuttering on the word "and."

Teaching Appropriate Respiration
1. Increasing awareness of respiration
2. Discouraging speech on expiratory reserve volume
3. Implementing relaxation exercises
4. Chunking of words into manageable phrases

Coordinating Respiration and Phonation
1. Teaching the concept of "easy voice"
2. Speaking after an /h/
3. Incorporating an "aaaahhh" or breathy "I" after an exhalation
4. Contrasting tense and easy voice onsets

Figure G-6.1 Outline of Activities for Facilitating Adequate Breath Support

speech to prevent a rush of words and in pausing to resist time pressure. A simple cue to the child to "pause for a second" may facilitate more appropriate breathing patterns. Runyan and Runyan (1999) suggest drawing a parabolic curve on a chalkboard or poster with a rising line for inhalation and a falling line for exhalation. Place an "X" on the line shortly after exhalation begins to show when speech should start. With practice, the child can eventually self-identify where on the curve he is beginning to speak. Healey and Scott (1995) recommend a simple line drawing of mountains or a playground slide to provide an easy way to help visualize the process of inhalation and exhalation (see Figure G-6.2).

3. At the beginning of therapy, lead the child in a brief stretching or yoga session to relax the body, focus the mind, and promote controlled breathing. This exercise can incorporate progressive relaxation to teach differentia-

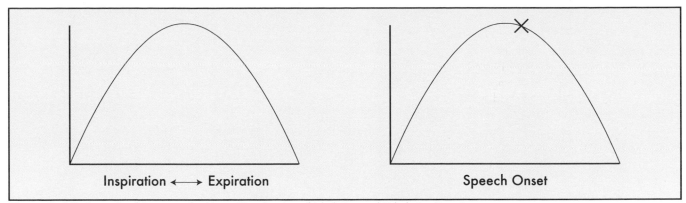

Figure G-6.2 Example of Diagrams for Use in Visualization of Inhalation and Exhalation Exercise.

tion between feelings of relaxation and tension (see Goal 4, "Determining What Is Interfering with Normal Speech Production"). These strategies can ultimately help the child reduce tension as he encounters it. The book *Instant Calm* by Paul Wilson (Plume, 1999) lists more than one hundred relaxation exercises.

4. Model appropriate "chunking" of sentences into short phrases to facilitate adequate respiration during speech. To indicate when to pause and inhale before continuing with speech, mark a series of phrases on a reading passage and have the child read it aloud. The marks will cue the child to pause and take a new breath before continuing. Inserting a pause between each phrase may help the child resist feelings of time pressure.

Coordinating Respiration and Phonation

1. Teach the child the concept of "easy voice." The clinician demonstrates a breathy initiation of phonation on a consonant-vowel (CV) combination. Instruct the child to feel how easy airflow lets his voice "turn on." The following hierarchy may be employed when teaching easy voice:
  a. Begin with passive breathing.
  b. Move to passive breathing with phonation. Have the child let out a small breath of air while beginning to move his articulators, and then begin phonation on this breath stream.
  c. Proceed to single-word production.
  d. Proceed to carrier phrase (e.g., "I see a _____.").
  e. Proceed to phrase and sentence levels (Ramig et al., 1988).

  Easy voluntary prolongations at the beginnings of phrases facilitate easy onset of voice, continuous voice

production, and reduced laryngeal tension by reducing subglottal air pressure prior to voice production.

2. If the child is having difficulty conceiving of regulation of breath stream, the concept of "speaking on an /h/" can also facilitate appropriate breathing. The child inserts a /h/ before vowel sounds and attends to the feelings of this "easy voice." Minimal pair contrasts, such as "hold/old" and "hat/at," further facilitate awareness of easy vocalization.

3. Wall and Myers (1995) provide a step-by-step method for incorporating longer phrases that begin with "a slow, easy sigh, something like a heavily aspirated 'ah.'" Incorporating an easy "aaaahhh" during exhalation relaxes the vocal folds and teaches the child to coordinate respiration and phonation. After practicing this a few times with the clinician's model, a breathy, voiced "ah" with an easy onset should result. Next, change the production into a breathy "I" and, while maintaining slightly loose airflow on the "I," elicit short phrases such as "IIIIII'm Jimmy." As shaping continues, the child learns to use the easy "I" at the onset of increasingly long phrases and sentences (appropriate to his linguistic ability). Later, as the clinician reduces the loose airflow of the modeled "I" to improve naturalness, the child usually follows suit.

4. Instruct the child to feel the clinician's larynx during the production of tense, hard voice onset and relaxed, gentle onset (vowels or CV combinations are appropriate). Then have him feel his own larynx during tense and relaxed productions. Alternatively, illustrate to the child the effect of incorrect airflow behavior by turning a radio on and off to emphasize the importance of correcting dysfunctional breathing patterns.

Controlling Speaking Rate

Rationale

Use of a slowed speaking rate is advocated by many authorities on stuttering (e.g., Bakker, 1997; Conture, 2001; Culatta & Rubin, 1973; Healey & Scott, 1995; Meyers & Woodford, 1992; Ramig & Bennett, 1997a; Wall & Myers, 1995). A reduced speaking rate helps enhance the spacing and timing of respiratory, phonatory, and articulatory movements necessary for the production of fluent speech. The ultimate goal of this activity is to enable the child to slow down his stuttering so that he can engage proprioceptive and tactile awareness to modify and move through the stuttering moment. A slightly slower overall speaking rate, which the child is able to modify when he needs to, will facilitate achievement of this goal.

Activities and Techniques

Refer to Figure G-7.1 for an outline of the information and activities presented in this section.

Teaching a Reduced Speaking Rate

1. Introduce the concept of a reduced, controlled speaking rate by assigning a meaningful name to it. Meyers and Woodford (1992) suggest naming the slow speech rate so the child will know when to utilize the activity. "Turtle Talk" and "Slow, Easy Speech" are popular names for children who stutter. "Slowed Rate," "Slowed Speech," and "Stretched Speech" are more appropriate for the older child.

2. Provide frequent models of reduced speaking rate. Emphasize smooth articulatory transitions, slightly prolonged consonants and vowels, and natural-sounding intonation and stress patterns. Conversely, let the child play "teacher" by catching the clinician when she talks too fast. After consistent modeling, reduce the frequency of modeling to assess the child's ability to self-monitor his own speaking rate (Ramig et al., 1988).

3. Starkweather and Givens-Ackerman (1997) advocate a three-stage method of teaching rate control (see Figure G-7.2). The first stage is learning to talk in "super slow motion." The second stage, rate control, involves gaining increased control by varying speech rate. In the third stage, cued rate control, the child learns to adapt his rate in response to moments of speech difficulty.

Support

The following citations provide support in the literature for our inclusion of this goal and the suggested activities for success when working to control speaking rate.

Bakker (1997) ➤ Technology may be applied to facilitate rate modifications using an auditory stimulus, such as a metronome. Computer software (e.g., *Dr. Fluency*, Sonido Inc.'s *Fluency Suite*, or Artefact's *DAF/FAF Assistant*) may also assist the child in modifying his speaking rate.

Conture (1990) ➤ Changes in speech production behaviors that are conducive to modifying the child's physical tension and rates of production should be incorporated into the treatment plans of children who stutter. These rate changes should be developmentally appropriate.

Gregory & Hill (1980) ➤ The combination of a slower rate with easy vocal onsets and smooth articulatory movements often facilitates fluency development.

Hall, Amir, & Yairi (1999) ➤ Among groups of (1) normally fluent children, (2) children who exhibited persistent stuttering, and (3) children who eventually recovered without intervention, no significant differences were found in articulation rate (as measured in syllables per second). Using a phones-per-second measure, however, revealed significant group differences between the control group and the recovered and persistent groups.

Healey & Scott (1995) ➤ A slower-than-normal conversational pace may have a physical and mental calming effect that is influenced by speech and nonspeech behaviors. Healey and Scott argue that it is essential for the clinician to control the pace of conversation during the treatment session.

Jones & Ryan (2001) ➤ Slower speaking rates of both the mother and child decreased the child's frequency of stuttering, which was not associated with reductions in either linguistic complexity or frequency of interruption.

continues

Support *continued*

Kloth, Janssen, & Kraaimaat (1995)	Pre-onset articulatory rate of high-risk children who developed into stutterers was significantly faster than that of high-risk children who did not demonstrate stuttering.
Max & Caruso (1998)	Increased fluency resulted from decreased speaking rate.
Meyers & Woodford (1992)	Contrast slow versus fast speaking rates during fluency therapy. Incorporate conceptually based therapy activities, during which children learn to experience "slow versus fast" through various motor, language, reading, and speech activities.
Perkins (1992)	A reduced rate of speaking facilitated the coordination of phonation with articulation while maintaining normal prosody. Use controlled prolongations to promote rate reduction.
Ramig (1984)	Some persons who stutter become more fluent, at least temporarily, when they reduce their speaking rate.
Shine (1980)	Reductions in speaking rate and vocal intensity may serve to modify physiologic and aerodynamic speaking variables that are compatible with fluency and incompatible with stuttering.
Wall & Myers (1995)	A slow-normal rate of speech may simplify motor timing which may reduce the number of repetitions and prolongations of sounds in the speech of young stutterers. Additionally, co-articulation may occur more easily when the speech rate is slowed.
Wall, Starkweather, & Cairns (1981)	Determined that sentence complexity did *not* influence rate of stuttering.

Teaching a Reduced Speaking Rate
1. Assign a meaningful name to the concept of a reduced, controlled speaking rate
2. Provide frequent models of reduced speaking rate
3. Teach the three stages of rate control
4. "Easy Relaxed Approach–Smooth Movement"
5. "Rainbow Speech" activity
6. Draw semantic maps to teach slow speaking rate

Contrasting Fast and Slow Speaking Rates
1. Contrast speech at a rapid rate and a slow rate
2. Provide useful analogies for fast versus slow speech:
   a. Contrast fast and slow vehicles
   b. Use speed bump analogy
   c. Compare fast and slow music to changes in speaking rate
   d. "Rabbit speech" and "turtle speech" analogy
   e. Additional analogies
   f. Stop-light analogy
   g. "Tigger" versus "Eeyore" speech

Reinforcing This Component
1. Play "Traffic Cop" by issuing people tickets for talking too fast.
2. Use old coffee can of yarn in reinforcement activity
3. Use tactile, verbal, and visible cues to improve rate monitoring
4. Use DAF to facilitate slow rate
5. Use a metronome to reinforce rate
6. Play "giving directions" game
7. Use a rubber band to stretch out speech
8. Assist in desensitization to time pressure

Figure G-7.1 Outline of Activities for Controlling Speaking Rate

Starkweather and Givens-Ackerman note, "With practice, children succeed at this activity and can slow down for a half-second to get through a particular sound at the beginning of the word and then be back to a normal speech rate before the word is finished. Listeners will hardly be aware that he is slowing" (p. 127). The authors suggest that the child verify this by interviewing several listeners (Ramig et al., 1988). He should not be expected to talk abnormally slowly indefinitely, but to implement a slowed, normal rate and to resist time pressure. This can be accomplished either by inserting pauses into his speech or by prolonging sounds in words. This technique should not be used as a means to avoid stuttering, however.

4. The "Easy Relaxed Approach–Smooth Movement" (Gregory, 1991) technique can be used for controlling speech rate in a school-age child. He begins by slowing his speech rate and reducing tension from the first sounds of a phrase and then the remainder of the phrase is produced at a normal rate.

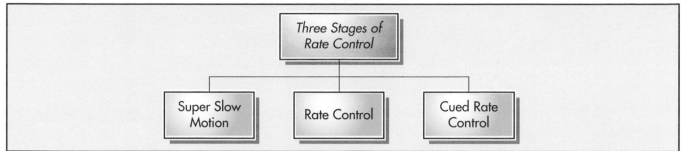

Figure **G-7.2** Three-stage Method of Teaching Rate Control (Starkweather and Givens-Ackerman, 1997)

5. Draw a picture of a rainbow and have the child prolong a word as he traces the shape with his finger until he gets to the end of the rainbow (see Figure G-7.3). This "Rainbow Speech" activity provides visual and tactile cues for the child to slow his speech rate. Its curved shape can also be used to illustrate breathing patterns or easy vocal onsets.

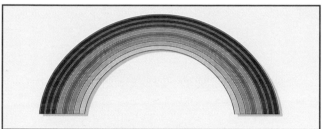

Figure **G-7.3** Rainbow Speech Activity

6. Draw semantic maps to teach the concept of slow speaking rate to older children. These maps show how slow rates are produced, how they change speech, and why they help to control stuttering. The child can draw his own semantic maps to individualize the learning (Healey, 2000). For example, in Figure G-7.4, the child is instructed to brainstorm specific benefits of using a slow rate and then use these to fill in the areas that radiate from the center of the map.

Contrasting Fast and Slow Speaking Rates

1. When appropriate, have the child contrast speech at a rapid rate and a slow rate. With a fast rate of speech, the child will underarticulate and chop up his words; in a slow rate of speech, he will overarticulate and smoothly pronounce words with ease. For more emphasis, he can watch himself in the mirror and see the difference. He can also close his eyes and feel the difference between the two rates. After some time, discuss his feelings about the exercise; ask if it was helpful in showing the differences.

2. A slow rate can be illustrated by giving the child analogies to adhere to which will be useful outside of therapy.

a. Vehicles can provide useful analogies for slow versus fast speech. Guitar's concept of slow "four wheel drive speech," rather than faster "two wheel drive speech," can be a helpful analogy for demonstrating how children may negotiate bumpy speech passages (1998, p. 13). Additionally, analogies between driving in a school zone as opposed to a highway or the obvious differences between a horse's canter and gallop clarify understanding of speaking rate. To further illustrate differences in speaking rate, watch scenes from a videotape or DVD in fast forward, normal play, and slow motion.

b. Illustrate the importance of slow speaking by describing a car slowing down in traffic. When a driver is operating a car at the speed limit on the highway and sees traffic or a bumpy section of road ahead, he is required to slow down. This helps the child understand that the speed of his speech may have to vary according to circumstances (Starkweather & Givens-Ackerman, 1997).

c. Slow and fast music can also be compared with differences in the child's rate of speaking. The child's awareness and control of speaking rate can be enhanced by focusing on a variety of music tempos as he concentrates on matching the beat he hears.

d. A turtle can be used to represent a slow talker, and a rabbit can represent a fast talker. In addition to using pictures, have him draw a turtle or a rabbit out of a bag and speak at the corresponding rate while identifying the item. Have the child hold a stuffed turtle when he hears slow music or a stuffed rabbit when he hears fast music. If the child uses "rabbit speech" at the wrong time, the clinician can model the more appropriate "turtle" speech (Roth & Worthington, 2000). Compile a photo album of fast and slow animals (e.g., cheetah, sloth) and describe or imitate their body movements. Be sure to use comparisons for slow-rate speech that the individual child finds to be positive, to help reinforce the behavior change.

e. Depending on the child's age, other items may be used to teach awareness of slow and fast speaking

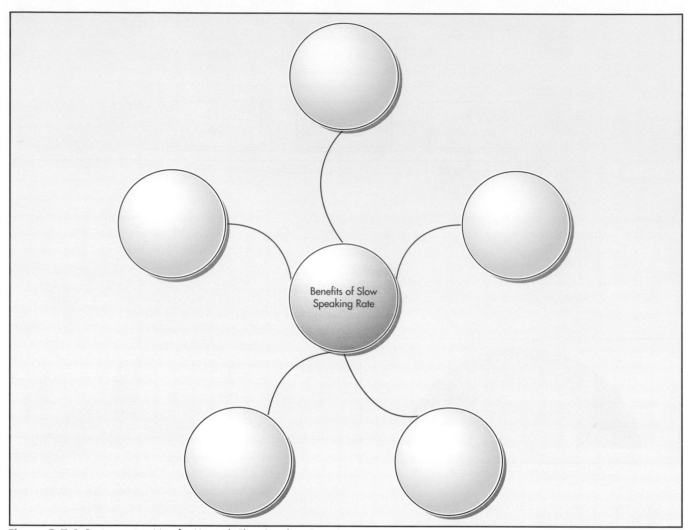

Figure G-7.4 Brainstorming Map for Use with Slow Speaking Rate Activities

rates (e.g., cars, balls, toy snails, etc.). With young school-age children, play a game using different hats to cue different rates of speech. The clinician initially selects a cowboy hat and models a slow speaking rate. The clinician then gives the child his own cowboy hat and they talk slowly together. Next, the clinician instructs the child to continue with his slow rate after she puts on a policeman's hat. They continue the conversation while she speaks at a faster rate and he continues to use "cowboy speech." Finally, a fireman's hat can represent the fastest rate, which will further challenge the child to resist the rate of others. The clinician can switch between the different hats (and rates) to either remind or challenge the child to maintain his own rate of speech.

f. It is helpful to reverse roles and have the child teach the clinician how to slow down stuttering. After the clinician says a word too quickly, he can demonstrate

how she could have said the word more slowly. It may be helpful to include a visual aid, such as a picture of a yellow traffic light, to indicate when the speaker needs to slow down. Either the clinician or child can point to the picture if the other's rate is too fast.

g. Read Winnie the Pooh stories or watch Winnie the Pooh videos. Imitate and contrast Eeyore's speech and Tigger's speech. By contrasting these two different speaking rates, the child may better comprehend the differences between fast and slow speaking rates.

Reinforcing This Component

1. Play "Traffic Cop" with young children to illustrate the consequences of going too fast when either driving or talking. In both school and home environments, deputize the child to issue tickets to others for talking too fast, or "speeding with their speech."

2. An old coffee can, yarn, and pictures can be used to teach a slower rate. The clinician draws a face on the can, punches 20 holes in the lid, ties knots on the ends of 20 pieces of yarn, puts the knotted sides in the bottom of the can, and leaves the unknotted ends slightly protruding through the holes. The child draws a picture and makes up a sentence about it, using a slow voice. While saying the sentence slowly, he pulls gently and slowly on one piece of yarn, until it reaches the knot. He continues until all the pieces of yarn are pulled out, so it looks like the coffee can has hair. The clinician can put a prize in the can and when the child finishes saying his 20 sentences using a slow rate, he can take off the lid and find it (Roth & Worthington, 2000).

3. While training the child to use a slower speech rate, provide tactile, verbal, or visual cues. Visual cues are helpful to remind the child to produce slow and fast speaking rates. The clinician can bring two fingers together when the child is producing a faster rate and spread them apart during slower speech. Other cues, such as touching the child's arm, holding up a start/stop sign, or ringing a bell, can likewise be used to cue the child. Consult with the child to determine which signals would be acceptable to use as slow-rate reminders. Low-visibility signals can also be employed by classroom teachers or caregivers to discreetly signal the child.

4. Utilize DAF to facilitate a slowed rate of speech. Begin at a very slow rate (about 250 ms) and gradually increase to a level reasonable for fluency (about 50 ms). DAF can be eliminated gradually from therapy as a slowed rate is consistently transferred to spontaneous speech.

5. To help keep a more steady rhythm in slow speech and to help the child experience the feeling of each syllable and its blending (co-articulation) into the next, use a metronome set at a low pace (two- to three-second intervals in between ticks is preferable). He can read a story at the set pace, making sure to stretch each sound into the next. One word should be said per tick; with time, the child will learn to hold onto his words and find a comfortable speed that is appropriate.

6. An activity called "giving directions" facilitates the practice of continuously speaking at a slower rate of speech. The clinician and child share a laminated street map of a preferred town, with clear landmarks such as parks, schools, buildings, and so on. The clinician will first model a slow rate of speech, giving the child directions to an unknown destination from a known starting point (e.g., "Go down Main Street two blocks, then turn right onto Canyon"). The clinician will speak slowly enough that the child can mark a path on the map with a dry-erase marker without asking her to repeat. When the clinician is finished, the child announces the destination where he has arrived, and can earn a prize for arriving at the right location. Later, he can take his turn giving directions to the clinician, focusing on keeping a slow, continuous, and deliberate rate of speech.

7. To emphasize slow movements, give the child a rubber band or a large stretchy ribbon used in physical therapy to stretch out slowly when speaking (Goven & Vette, 1966). Slow movement is important when learning the basics of articulating and maintaining a comfortable rate; thus, the clinician can use activities that involve slow movement, such as a card game that requires slow, thoughtful, and patient moves. The child will understand how important it is to take his time, as he may want to win the game, but only by using a controlled rate of speech.

8. The feeling of time pressure is the enemy of slower speech rates, particularly during stuttering moments. Whenever possible, identify activities that allow the child to feel and confront time pressure. Reinforce this by making sure that he understands time pressure as a feeling of impatience, which may include a fear that other people will criticize of us for being too slow. When playing a board game, count out moves on the board with a very slow rate, using continuous voicing. Ask the child to go slower and slower until he feels as much impatience as he can stand. Your acceptance and rewards may help desensitize him to time pressure in the clinic.

Establishing Light Articulatory Contacts and Movements

Rationale

Children, adolescents, and adults who stutter frequently produce hard articulatory contacts at the initial sound of words and within longer words (Conture, 2001; Dell, 2000; Gregory, 1991; Runyan & Runyan, 1999; Van Riper, 1973; Wall & Myers, 1995). Doing so often results in more severe and frequent stuttering due to tension in the muscles of articulation. Another result of this tension can be interference and impedance of airflow in the oral cavity. Thus, teaching the production of softer, loose articulatory contacts and movements can be helpful in reducing muscular tension and maintaining the normal flow of air and creation of voicing. Teaching lighter contacts can also aid the person who stutters in learning to reduce tension during the stuttering moment.

Activities and Techniques

Refer to Figure G-8.1 for an outline of the information and activities presented in this section.

Teaching Light Articulatory Contacts

1. Teach the child the concept of producing soft, loose sounds. Emphasize the feeling of loose articulatory movements and smooth, continuous airflow. How relaxed does the tongue feel? Does the jaw feel loose? Are the lips pursed or pulled back? "Soft sounds" can be taught at the phoneme level and incorporated into activities that follow a hierarchy of increased length and linguistic complexity, up through conversation. Squeezing or tapping the child's arm to show hard versus soft contacts as he speaks is helpful in teaching contrast between light and hard. Voluntary stretches, accomplished by lengthening or prolonging the first syllable of a word, involve soft, slow articulation of the consonant and prolonged phonation of the vowel. These stretches may be incorporated from the single-word level to conversational tasks.

2. Visuals are effective when demonstrating the differences between hard and light contacts. A plastic model of the speech mechanisms can be helpful in illustrating how to use the tongue and lips when speaking. For example, if the child is jamming his tongue to the alveolar ridge during the sound /t/, he may push his thumb hard against the model's alveolar ridge. He can then press his thumb

---

Support

The following citations provide support in the literature for our inclusion of this goal and the suggested activities for establishing light articulatory contacts and movements.

Conture (1990) ► Recommends making speech "visible" when learning easy onsets by using a volume unit meter to demonstrate how one can "make appropriate vocal initiations and transitions" (p. 196).

Gregory (1991) ► Advocates an easier initiation of speech with smooth movements from sound to sound.

Irwin (1980) ► Prolonging or "plasticizing" the first syllable of a dysfluent word may reduce the muscular tension in the speech organs.

Peters & Guitar (1991) ► Teach the fluency-enhancing behavior of "soft contacts" to some children. "By this, we mean that the movements of the articulators (tongue, lips, jaw) should be slow, prolonged, and relaxed. These articulatory movements should not be fast and tense" (p. 231).

Rustin, Cook, & Spense (1995) ► Children should "maintain the place and manner of normal articulation without slurring or omitting sounds." They should also produce all or some of the consonants within a word using lighter contacts between articulators, principally on plosive sounds (p. 64).

Silverman (2004) ► Stutterers may judge the severity of their stuttering in a particular situation as much (if not more) on how it feels as on how it sounds.

van Lieshout, Peters, Starkweather, & Hulstijn (1993) ► Persons who stutter demonstrated higher intensity and longer duration of muscle activity than nonstutterers in a simple lip-rounding gesture prior to initiation of a sentence.

Van Riper (1973) ► Light articulatory contacts reduce oral tension, especially within the context of the modification of stuttering behaviors.

continues

Support *continued*

Wall & Myers (1995) → Loose articulatory contacts are a useful technique in reducing muscle activity in the vocal tract, thereby permitting smoother movements while preventing the escalation of immobilizing tension.

Wood (1995) → During periods of stutterers' fluent speech, lingual palatal contacts of some phonemes consistently differed from those of nonstutterers. Stutterers produced greater articulatory variability; during successive repetitions, their articulatory patterns often became less similar to the target (or normal) configuration.

Zebrowski & Kelly (2002) → Illustrations, a mirror, a tongue depressor, and other such items may be used to facilitate understanding and production of light articulatory contacts.

Teaching Light Articulatory Contacts
1. Concept of soft, loose sounds
2. Visual presentation of speech mechanism
3. Labeling of light contacts
4. DAF
5. Differential contact

Comparing Hard and Soft Articulatory Contacts
1. Learning auditory discrimination
2. Labeling easy and hard stuttering
3. Demonstrating "hard" versus "bumpy" speech
4. Emphasizing kinesthetic awareness
5. Playing "smooth speech" versus "bumpy speech" game
6. Child versus clinician tests
7. Using manipulatives
8. Using analogies

Reinforcing This Concept
1. Cancellations
2. Varying or playing with speech
3. Triad drills
4. "Piano fingers"
5. Turning plosives into fricatives
6. Producing easy stuttering on cue
7. Negative practice drills
8. "Recipe Creations" activity
9. Adapting board games

Figure G-8.1 Outline of Activities for Establishing Light Articulator Contacts and Movements

---

softly against the ridge before practicing it with his own articulators.

3. As with slow rate, the concept of light articulatory contacts benefits from a name that is meaningful to the child. To explain the concept of light articulatory contacts, Healey and Scott (1995) suggest inviting the child to imagine things that touch lightly and softly, such as "leaves falling to the ground" or "a butterfly landing on a flower." Clapping the hands very lightly so that they just barely touch can be contrasted with a hard clapping motion and used as another example when teaching this concept.

4. A DAF device may be used with older children to facilitate light articulatory contacts through abnormally slowed rate. DAF provides an older child with the opportunity to practice easy onsets by slowing down the speaking rate (Bloodstein, 1995). The device can be used with a hierarchy from single words to reading and conversation levels.

5. The following excellent excerpt, from Dell, *Treating the School-Age Stutterer* (2000), describes a method of teaching light, loose articulatory contacts:

When you are stuttering hard on it, you will feel your tongue jammed up against the alveolar ridge. You will also feel air pressure building up behind your tongue. The air wants to escape but you are forcing it back with your tongue. Now gradually loosen the pressure on your tongue by reducing the force of the air pressure pushing up against it. Then gradually begin to relax the tension you have purposely placed on your tongue. When you remove some of this lingual pressure, you will probably hear a little burst of air escaping between the tongue and

the alveolar ridge. You then need to change these bursts into a small, steady stream of air. Once you have this steady stream of air, it is easy to add the voicing necessary and once again slide into the word but beware of prolonging the vowel. It should be "tttable" not "taaable."

Comparing Hard and Soft Articulatory Contacts

1. In an auditory discrimination exercise, have the child identify when the clinician is using hard or soft contacts. The child can also become the teacher, correcting hard onsets and modeling easy speech for the clinician (Ramig et al., 1988).

2. Dell (2000) provides three different phrases to help children discriminate between articulatory contacts: (1) the "regular fluent way," (2) the "easy stuttering way," and (3) the "hard stuttering way" (see Figure G-8.2). The clinician demonstrates one way of saying a word and asks the child to identify which way is being used. The child can

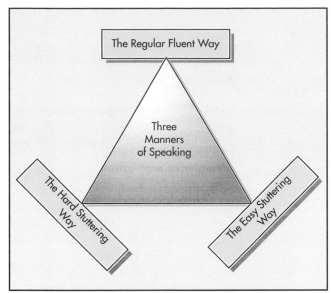

Figure G-8.2 Three Manners of Speaking to Help Children Discriminate between Articulatory Contacts (Dell, 2000)

take the clinician's place and practice using different ways to say one particular word. Place cards with the phrases in a hat; pull one card out and have him produce the style of speech that is chosen. One of three labels, for example, can be chosen to contrast easy and hard stuttering: "Easy and Hard Talking," "Easy and Hard Speech," or "Hard Stuttering Way" and "Easy Stuttering Way." Learning an easy phrase that child, clinician, teacher, parents, and friends can use consistently when in contact with the child encourages the learning procedure.

3. There are ways to use toys or demonstrations to help young children understand the differences between hard and easy speech movements. With the very young child, floppy rag dolls and puppets can be used to convey relaxation. Another involves the clinician assuming a relaxed, floppy posture while making movements to suggest muscle looseness.

4. Contrast drills are helpful activities to increase the child's kinesthetic awareness of hard versus soft articulatory contacts. Ask him to read aloud while alternating hard and soft productions of each word. Encourage the child to feel the difference by exploring the feelings associated with various speech movements and postures done in an "easy" way and in a "hard" way. Negative practice drills, in which he produces a very hard stutter and then reduces the tension first by 50 percent and then by another 50 percent, provide an excellent way to demonstrate this concept of hard versus soft speech production.

5. An effective method for distinguishing hard and light contacts is to work with a partner, while deliberately varying the forcefulness of articulatory contacts. One person speaks while the other identifies the hard and light

contacts in the speaker's speech. Having the child feel, hear, and see these differences helps kinesthetic awareness become more natural and automatic.

6. To explore the differences between smooth and bumpy speech, the child and clinician can take turns testing each other. Place two pieces of paper on the table with one labeled "smooth speech" and the other labeled "bumpy speech." The clinician says a word in one of the two ways and the child guesses which way it was said. If the child is correct, he gets to place a sticker on the appropriate paper. The clinician and child should also switch roles.

7. To understand the differences between hard and easy onsets, the child may benefit from working with hands-on materials that he can pull apart with ease. For example, two overhead transparencies, two magnets with different poles, two pieces of Velcro, or pull-apart toys with different degrees of looseness can be used to demonstrate and build understanding of the concept of light touches and easy onsets. The clinician can define the differences in loose and hard contacts and then give the child the opportunity to pick the material that best represents each type of contact.

8. There are many types of analogies the clinician can use to demonstrate easy speech to young children. Some examples include:

a. To demonstrate light versus hard contacts, one puppet with a large mouth (such as an alligator) can talk with light contacts and another puppet can talk with hard contacts. The child is asked to identify which type of contact each puppet is using.

b. For very young children, try dramatizing the effects of hard or tense speech on stuttering using a puppet or action figure of a dragon, which may be called the stuttering dragon. Demonstrate how the dragon gets stronger and starts flying around as long as the clinician is forcing her speech sounds and movements. Then show how the dragon becomes less active and goes to sleep when the clinician uses light articulatory contacts and loose sounds. The child and clinician can take turns being the dragon and the person who is speaking in different ways.

c. To practice easy speech, the child and clinician can play "I Spy" and take turns being "it. "When the clinician is "it," she says, "I spy something _____," and the child guesses what the clinician is describing; this continues until he can guess the correct object. Then the child can be "it" and describe an object to the clinician. Depending on the age of the child, use *Mad Libs*, where the clinician asks the child to supply a part of speech to fill in the missing spaces of a story without reading the story. When the story is complete, the child can read it using his easy speech strategies (Roth & Worthington, 2000).

d. The child and clinician can practice light contacts by playing a board game, such as *CandyLand, Chutes and Ladders, Junior Scrabble, Lotto, Junior Outburst,* or *Trouble.* To take his turn, the child has to say something using easy speech. This can also be done using games like *Jenga* or *Kerplunk.*

e. A young child can play with *Mr. Potato Head* and ask the clinician for each body part, using light contacts.

f. Ask the child to name all the items in a category (fruit, holidays, and cartoons) that he can recall, while using easy or hard speech.

g. The child and clinician can also play a number of games that involve requesting the identity or characteristics of certain items. *Memory, Go Fish, Guess Who,* and *Mystery Garden* all require one person to ask the other person if she has a certain card (or characteristic on a card), the child should do this using easy speech and light articulatory contacts.

h. When practicing initial-sound prolongations, have the clinician and child stretch Silly Putty as the child prolongs each sound. The child continues to stretch as long as he is pulling on the putty.

i. During a game of connect-the-dots, the child can follow the prenamed dots, identified by letters of the alphabet. As he moves from one dot to the next, he will slowly say "A—B—C . . ." and so on.

j. Westbrook (1994) describes "Jacob's Secret Speech Bracelet." In this activity, the child makes a bracelet, each bead of which represents a particular therapy strategy. The bracelet, worn all day, is a cue to transfer his strategies to other settings. Ramig and Bennett say that transfer also involves "the exchange of information regarding speech and stuttering; discussing and observing how television personalities speak; or rating others' speech on the components of rate, smoothness, volume, and pressure" (1997a, p. 307).

Reinforcing This Component

1. Cancellations may be employed to further facilitate awareness of light articulatory contacts. Immediately after the stuttering moment, the child should repeat the word with a light articulatory contact. "This technique allows the child to reattempt a word in which the articulatory gestures have not been smoothly produced" (Wall & Myers, 1995). Another version of this is to ask the child to rehearse or mime the word (without any sound) after catching a stuttering moment and then to say it smoothly (Ramig et al., 1988).

2. The clinician may demonstrate several types of stuttering behaviors and then demonstrate how she can manipulate or change them. The clinician may slow down a repetition, stretch out of a frozen articulatory posture or block, or do an easy repetition to ease out of a laryngeal block.

3. Triad drills are one way of facilitating comprehension of different ways of stuttering. Each point of a triangle represents certain ways of stuttering: hard bounce (HB), easy bounce (EB), and slide (S) and/or easy bounce, slide, and easy onset (EO). Starting with the first triad (HB, EB, S), the child learns how to change his stuttering patterns and gradually works toward the second type of triad (EB, S, EO). Multiple repetitions of triad drills will facilitate the development of monitoring and proprioception skills. For the younger child, Westbrook (1989) uses the analogy of energy to facilitate this concept. The child manipulates various levels of tension as a means of "conserving energy"; energy being on a continuum of 100 percent energy (hard speech) to 25 percent energy (easy speech).

4. Runyan and Runyan (1999) teach the child to keep the articulators moving by using "piano fingers." The child taps each finger on a tabletop as he says each syllable, helping him smoothly move from sound to sound.

5. When practicing loose articulatory movement with the /t/ sound, have the child begin instead with an /s/, using a light articulatory touch with the tongue to the alveolar ridge. Explore the subtle differences between the tongue postures used to create the /t/ (more pointed) and /s/ (flatter) while maintaining easy contacts.

6. Have the child produce easy stutters on cue. When the clinician provides a tactile cue, the child should insert an easy stutter. Once the child can do this, have him insert easy stutters during connected discourse without any cues. The clinician uses a counter to determine how many he inserted. The child can keep track of how many easy stutters he inserts during several sessions, with the goal of increasing the number (Dell, 2000). Another way is for both the clinician and the child to use counters to tally each other's easy stutters during a conversation.

7. Negative practice drills, in which the child produces a hard stutter and then slowly reduces the tension to produce an easy stutter, provide a way for the client to differentiate between hard and easy speech. Light articulatory contacts may also be applied with cancellations. When a child encounters a moment of stuttering, he is asked to repeat the word using a light articulatory contact. This will help him feel the difference between the contacts and movements in hard and easy stuttering.

8. An activity called "Recipe Creations" can be used to emphasize and practice behaviors such as reduced rate, easy onset, and light articulatory contacts. Following a written or picture recipe, the clinician and child discuss, plan, prepare, cook, and then eat what was made. While

reading and discussing the recipe, the child should be requested to focus on specific target behaviors. When eating what was created, both the clinician and child should use deliberately soft and easy biting, chewing, and swallowing movements. Recipes designed with children in mind include smoothies, ants on a log, rice cake faces, and so forth.

9. To demonstrate the differences between easy and hard speech, as well as how easier stuttering feels better than hard stuttering, play a board game with the child.

 a. The child and clinician navigate through the game using easy and hard speech depending on what is depicted on the game square. For instance, one section of the board might involve a rocky incline, which indicates that hard speech is needed to advance to the next square. Another part of the board could have a meandering stream to indicate that easy speech is needed. Throughout the game, the clinician can help the child determine the difference between hard and easy contacts and practice changing hard stuttering into easy stuttering.

 b. A game similar to *Sorry* can be used to work with smooth and bumpy speech patterns. Each player draws a word card. Under each word, there are instructions to read it with either bumpy or smooth speech.

 c. Any board game can be modified to focus on practicing hard and easy contacts by using one die and a spinner that has six different sections. The six divisions on the spinner could be *hard sticky, easy sticky, hard bouncing, easy bouncing, hard stretch*, and *easy stretch*. The die determines the roll of spaces on the board, while the spinner represents the kind of stutter to have. Each space has a specific word that is used for the hard or easy blocks, repetitions, or prolongations.

Facilitation of Oral Motor Planning and Movement

Rationale

Research supports targeting oral motor planning and coordination in stuttering therapy (Riley & Riley, 1986). Many people who stutter, both children and adults, often speak with reduced articulatory movement, reduced jaw opening, and increased velocity as movement occurs. Slowing the speaking rate while slightly increasing articulatory movement facilitates increased spacing and timing of articulatory movement, which can enhance fluency. Encourage and reinforce slight overarticulation during speaking activities once the child has established a reasonable level of fluency. If overarticulation is introduced too early, however, children may have difficulty focusing on both fluency techniques and the overarticulation. If the child exhibits severe groping and posturing behaviors, or other behaviors that may be signs of developmental dyspraxia, more direct dyspraxic treatment may be warranted.

Activities and Techniques

Refer to Figure G-9.1 for an outline of the information and activities presented in this section.

1. Kinesthetic feedback can be used to help the child feel the position and movement of his articulators. This kinesthetic awareness technique is commonly called *proprioception*, although that term more correctly refers primarily to awareness of the relative position of body parts. It may help the child to do this with closed eyes, to better utilize the sensory feedback and movement awareness to feel what his tongue, lips, jaw, and other articulators are doing when he makes various sounds.

2. Frick (1970) uses four techniques for motor planning: structuring, developing the child's awareness of a breakdown in planning, becoming aware of fluency, and improving motor planning ability (see Figure G-9.2).

   Analogies from sports and dance are used to visualize the structure and movements of fluent speech. The child signals the clinician when stuttered speech is anticipated and performs a self-appraisal of how this anticipation is cued: through anticipation of movement, auditory monitoring, or vision. The awareness of fluency is taught by exaggerating and feeling the movements of fluency and viewing them in a mirror. Finally, the child practices formulating a fluent utterance, signals the clinician when

Support

The following citations provide support in the literature for our inclusion of this goal and the suggested activities for facilitating oral motor planning and movement.

Ratner (1995) → Stuttering may coexist with other speech and language problems that involve difficulties with verb phrases; words starting with particular sounds; or complex, coordinated constructions acquired later in the developmental sequence. Ratner recommends strategies for dealing with these coexisting conditions.

Ingham (1984) → Cited Zimmerman's studies, which state that the articulator(s) of the stutterer have a much less synchronous relationship during fluent and dysfluent productions, compared with the articulators of nonstutterers.

Kelly, Smith, & Goffman (1995) → Utilized electromyographic (EMG) activity recorded from orofacial muscles during fluent and dysfluent speech. Some older children (who had stuttered for five years or more) appear to exhibit tremor-like oscillations similar to some adults who stutter. Tremor is "a general characteristic of motor disorders and indicates the operation of unstable systems" (p. 1032).

McClean & Runyan (2000) → Ratios of tongue speed to jaw speed were significantly greater in severe stutterers, compared with normally fluent speakers and less severe stutterers. In severe stutterers, these ratios were related to increases in lower lip and tongue speed and decreases in jaw speed.

Riley & Riley (1985) → Some children may not master the necessary motor aspects of speech in time for normal fluency to develop, thus requiring intervention. Oral motor coordination is characterized by three parameters: accuracy, smooth flow, and rate.

Riley & Riley (1986) → Incorporate an oral motor planning goal in therapy when indicated. An earlier study by Riley and Riley (1983) revealed that 87 percent of dysfluent children experience difficulty timing the laryngeal, articulatory, and respiratory events that support accurate syllable production.

continues

Support *continued*

Smith & Kleinow (2000)	➤ Suggest that the kinematic characteristics of stutterers' fluent speech generally overlaps that of normally fluent speakers; however, subtle differences in kinematic parameters reveal susceptibility to speech motor breakdown when performance demands increase.
Stark-weather & Givens-Ackerman (1997)	➤ For younger children, the coordination, speed, and speech control required to speak fluently are best practiced under those circumstances during which fluent speech is more likely to occur.
van Lieshout, Stark-weather, Hulstign, & Peters (1995)	➤ Longer words, words in longer sentences, words occurring early in a sentence, and words carrying a higher semantic load necessitated rate and timing adjustments in speech coordination.
Zimmer-man & Hanley (1983)	➤ Argued that inadequate central processing capacity is the "subsoil" of stuttering. As a result, stutterers may display limitations in their abilities to integrate motor speech output and its associated feedback.

ready, and carries out the fluent speech. To reinforce planning during continuous and spontaneous speech, Frick asks children to practice cancellations of entire phrases when motor planning breakdowns occurred (Wall & Myers, 1995).

3. Clusters of consonants are often challenging for young children who stutter. Syllable drills can provide massed practice to help master clusters. For example:

/strei/ → /stri/ → /strai/ →/strou/ →/stru/

Activities

1. Kinesthetic feedback and proprioception
2. Four techniques of motor planning
3. Teaching consonant clusters
4. Using DAF to teach proprioception
5. Deliberate variation of ingrained behaviors
6. Cueing for changes in pitch or volume
7. Keeping a journal of difficult sounds and words

Figure G-9.1 Outline of Activities for Facilitation of Oral Motor Planning and Movement Outline

Instruct the child to close his eyes in order to concentrate on the speech helpers and the movements occurring in his mouth. After practicing with syllable drills, pair them with words:

/strei/ → "straight"
/stri/ → "street"
/strai/ → "stripe"

After experiencing success, let the child choose combinations that he finds difficult (Ramig et al., 1988).

4. A delayed auditory feedback (DAF) device assists in slowing the rate of speaking and—apart from changes in speaking rate—has the effect of providing feelings of natural fluency in individuals who stutter. One way in which a DAF device may be used is to teach the child to follow the machine's delay, which reduces speaking rate. This effect can help children feel individual speech movements and raise awareness of the complexities of oral motor coordination and co-articulation. Highlighting how one sound blends into the next is particularly useful in heightening awareness of speech movements. After the child has mastered slow-rate speech using the device, he can attempt to "beat the delay" by talking at a more normal rate. In this instance, the speaker must ignore the delayed auditory feedback and concentrate on the kinesthetic movements of speech to avoid being "tripped up" or slowed down by the delay.

5. Deliberate variations, such as slowing down, easing out of, or changing the force and direction of speech movements can provide the child with a feeling of increased control over his speech. For example, if the child is exhibiting silent laryngeal blocks with complete cessation of airflow, suggest or demonstrate that he try to "bounce out of the hard speech" using deliberate jaw movements. Easily bow-bow-bouncing out of blocks helps the child mo-mo-move forward during moments of stuttering instead of succumbing to tense, silent blocks. If the child exhibits multiple part-word repetitions, slowing and stretching his words out may be particularly helpful in breaking the typical stuttering pattern.

Variation of ingrained stuttering behaviors is an essential prerequisite to successful modification and can be useful for oral-motor coordination. Activities such as singing, varying loudness, and changing pitch are additional ways to manipulate speech and understand their effect on oral motor movements.

6. Up and down arrows may be used to cue pitch or loudness changes during therapy activities. For young children, a toy car can also cue the child to increase volume as the child pushes the car up a hill.

7. Some children may enjoy keeping a journal of more difficult words or sound combinations. This also helps them

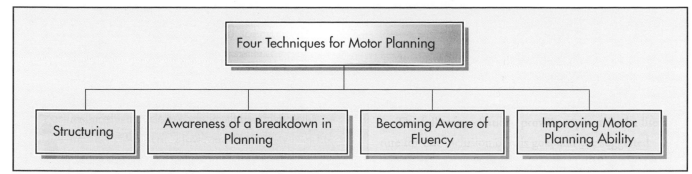

Figure G-9.2 Four Techniques for Motor Planning (Frick, 1970)

to self-identify what types of sounds are more challenging. By locating a pattern of dysfluencies, a child may feel more confident as he takes steps to better understand stuttering. Although he may identify cyclical variations in stuttering, he will also recognize an underlying consistency in his dysfluent speech.

Desensitization Intervention

Rationale

Incorporating desensitization is especially pertinent for children who are beginning to react negatively to their stuttering (as most will if the stuttering continues). Positive strategies to help desensitize children to the fear and expectancy of getting stuck are very important (e.g., Conture, 2001; Dell, 2000; Guitar, 1998; Ham, 1986; Manning, 2001; Ramig & Bennett, 1997a; Van Riper, 1973). In that regard, helping them become less sensitive to the stuttering moment can be highly beneficial to the significant reduction, and in some cases the elimination, of stuttering. The vast majority of authorities on stuttering realize that the child's inability "to say what he wants to say when he wants to say it" causes concern and eventually apprehension and fear of stuttering. If these feelings are ignored by the clinician, the child's stuttering can worsen as he attempts to avoid stuttering and the negative feelings associated with it.

Activities and Techniques

Refer to Figure G-10.1 for an outline of the information and activities presented in this section.

Learning to Accept Stuttering

During therapy activities, the clinician may model easy and open stuttering behaviors. Years of clinical experience indicate that open stuttering in a caring environment will help desensitize the child to stuttering. This approach will enable him to reduce his negative reactions to real stuttering moments, as well as assist him in changing stuttering moments. As the clinician stutters without struggle, tension, or negative emotions, the child learns a new way of reacting to his own dysfluent speech. As always, it is important to reduce or manage the tension one may produce when stuttering. Remind the child to relax and if necessary repeat a word on which he has stuttered in an easier manner. Emphasize that it is acceptable to stutter, but that it does feel better and we will be able to communicate more effectively if we stutter without as much struggle and tension and with fewer reactions.

Support

The following citations provide support in the literature for our inclusion of this goal and the suggested activities for desensitization intervention.

Gregory (2003) ➤ Hierarchies of stimulus conditions will gradually desensitize the client to sounds, words, and situations that were previously associated with stuttering.

Guitar (1997) ➤ Clinicians should teach children many ways to be open about stuttering, including humor, talking about stuttering with friends, and acknowledging stuttering in difficult speaking situations.

Ham (1986) ➤ Desensitization endeavors to change clients' reactions to normal nonfluencies, stuttering, people, situations, or specific words. Therapy should incorporate activities that reduce one's fears and anticipatory behaviors.

Healey (2004) ➤ Use voluntary stuttering to reduce anxiety, sensitivity, and fear of stuttering. Teach the child to stutter in different ways and play with stuttering.

Manning (1996) ➤ "As the client learns that it is indeed possible to stutter without losing complete control, he will begin to realize that he has some choices that were not apparent before. For example, he has the ability to alter selected features of his stuttering syndrome" (p. 157).

Peters (1991) ➤ Desensitization alters reactions to fluency-disrupting stimuli, such as interruptions, competition to speak, or excitement that may produce increased moments of stuttering. Reduction of negative feelings and attitudes and elimination of avoidance behaviors should be incorporated into the therapy plan of some children who stutter.

Ramig & Bennett (1997a) ➤ Desensitization is aided when the child can practice voluntary stuttering in a supportive, accepting, and caring environment.

continues

Support *continued*

Van Riper (1973) → Because the fears, avoidance and struggle associated with confirmed stuttering tend to grow stronger, no therapy can be successful unless it seeks directly to reduce these feelings. Additionally, it is essential to help the child to understand what he should do differently when he fears or experiences stuttering.

Silverman (2004) → Wolpe's reciprocal inhibition principle (1958) states that each time a person does not become highly anxious in the presence of a stimulus that ordinarily elicits a high level of anxiety, the link between that stimulus and the "old" response is weakened a little.

1. Knowing that others share difficulties with speaking may help a child to accept himself in spite of his present dysfluencies. Knowing that he is not alone in confronting stuttering reassures him that he can work to become a better speaker. Visit Web sites where the child can learn of many other children and adults who stutter, such as:

   a. The "Just for Kids" and "Just for Teens" Web sites maintained by the Department of Communication Disorders at the University of Minnesota: www.stutteringhomepage.com
   b. "Friends: An Association of Young People Who Stutter," www.friendswhostutter.org.
   c. National Stuttering Association: www.westutter.org

2. An excellent way to encourage the child to take responsibility for his therapy is to ask that he record his own speech, review it, and write down his feelings and responses. Keeping a regular journal, however, requires a level of maturity that some younger children may not exhibit.

3. Williams describes a technique in which the clinician explains the similarity between making simple mistakes in everyday situations and stuttering. Williams believes that by explaining stuttering as a simple mistake, the clinician teaches the child not to run away from his stuttering, but instead to confront it as he would any other behavior he wants to correct (in Guitar, 1998).

4. Videotaping the child using fluency-enhancing or stuttering modification techniques (including pseudo-stuttering) can help desensitize him to the use of such techniques outside the clinic. Audio and video tapes, used appropriately, can be excellent desensitization tools. A child may be surprised to realize that he does not stutter all the time. By listening to an audiotape of himself and counting fluent words, he will learn that the majority of them are said fluently, even when stuttering is severe. Listening to a tape also allows him to

Learning to Accept Stuttering
1. Visit stuttering Web sites
2. Keep a journal
3. Compare normal dysfluency and stuttering
4. Listen to self on audio or video tape
5. Self-rating by child
6. Encourage easy bouncing and stretching behaviors to vary stuttering
7. Use variations of real stuttering
8. Compete to exaggerate stuttering
9. Read or speak using easy pseudo-stuttering
10. Generate stories
11. Learn about famous people who stutter
12. Practice through gaming
13. Desensitize to stuttering in a variety of feared modes and situations
14. Practice eye contact
15. Use freezing
16. "Framing My Speech" activity
17. Build self-esteem

Disclosure
1. Write a letter about stuttering
2. Use art activities to promote disclosure
3. Match emotional faces
4. Engage in verbal disclosure

Reinforcing This Component
1. Teaching bounces with a bouncing ball
2. Teaching prolongations with a rolling ball
3. Animal talk
4. Counter-conditioning
5. Dealing with speech disruptors
6. Role-playing and speech disruptions
7. Scavenger hunt
8. Class presentations
9. Fluency disrupters
10. Addressing time pressure

Figure G-10.1 Outline of Activities for Desensitization Intervention

identify and study what he is doing when he produces sounds dysfluently. Encouragement and support by the clinician may also help promote acceptance of the fact that he does stutter, that it is all right to do so, and that he can bear it. The child's desensitization may be enhanced by watching other people stutter and identifying their stuttering behaviors and modification strategies. While identifying core and secondary behaviors, the child can learn to analyze moments of stuttering. The clinician can videotape herself pseudo-stuttering and have the child critique its realism.

5. Have the child rate his performance on an activity in therapy. As performance fluctuates, discuss with the child what is working and not working best for him. Let him know that his performance shows courage and that the clinician wants the best for him in therapy, school, work, and so on (see Stuttering Foundation video tape No. 89).

6. Have the child insert easy stuttering into his real speech, showing him that he has some control over his stuttering and a way to overcome his fears (Dell, 2000). To become familiar with the child's specific needs, it is essential to accompany him during situations where he pseudo-stutters when talking with strangers. After practicing, encourage the child to share his feelings about what occurred. When working with desensitization, the child needs to become familiar with his speech. Voluntary repetitions, also known as *slow bounces* (i.e., bay-bay-baseball), allow the child to focus on the feeling of the speech movements rather than how they sound. Voluntary prolongations also show the child that he can "play" with his stuttering.

7. After the child experiences success with easy stuttering, encourage him to use easy bouncing and stretching on real stuttering. By consciously manipulating some aspect of stuttering, variation facilitates feelings of increased control. For example, if the child is exhibiting silent laryngeal blocks with complete cessation of airflow, suggest (or model) that he try to "bounce out of the hard speech." If the child exhibits multiple part-word repetitions, slowing him down and stretching his words out may be particularly successful.

8. To confront the emotional component of stuttering, the child and clinician can exaggerate stuttering to become familiar with it. The clinician and child can even compete for who can stutter the hardest or for the longest amount of time.

9. The clinician instructs the child to read a passage using easy pseudo-stuttering on random words the clinician or child has marked. The clinician can suggest that the child practice this method at home when he reads his homework assignments. Later, to help normalize the child's feelings toward stuttering, the child and clinician

can reverse roles during practice of pseudo-stuttering. As the child, pretending to be the clinician, critiques the pseudo-stuttering of the real clinician, he can observe the forward flow of speech and hear how this sounds preferable to typical stuttering.

10. Encourage a child who has difficulty telling stories because of his stuttering to use his creativity by creating a spoken story, using flash cards as helpers. Offer cards with words or pictures; have him pick five cards and develop a story using the ideas on the cards. The child could also make his own cards with words or pictures of his choice. If he has difficulty at first, the clinician and child can take turns adding elements to the story using the cards as cues.

11. With the purpose of reassuring the child that his stuttering does not have to limit his options, the clinician can bring in pictures of famous people who stutter. Ask him if he recognizes any of them. If the child does not recognize some of them, the clinician should provide a brief explanation of who they are and why they are famous, emphasizing their contributions to humanity. If the child has not already guessed, inform him that these people all have stuttering in common. Some information about how stuttering did or did not affect their lives can also be provided. The child can make a collage to serve as a tangible reminder that stuttering need not limit his goals in life. The Stuttering Foundation and friends have posters of famous individuals who stutter available as well.

12. An alliteration game can provide an opportunity to practice stretches, pullouts, and voluntary stuttering. The game consists of the child and clinician taking turns rolling one die and picking a card from a pile of alphabet cards. The number rolled determines the numbers of words the player must say starting with the selected letter. This game can be targeted to any behavior; in this case, when saying the chosen word, he must voluntarily stutter and use a pullout to move through. If the player is able to successfully name a certain amount of words, he earns points equal to the number on the die. If the player cannot think of a word, the opponent has a chance to think of one instead. The player with the most points wins the alliteration game.

13. For an older child, Ham (1986) recommends two approaches to desensitization: (1) desensitization to stuttering by repeated exposure to stuttering in a variety of modes and situations, and (2) desensitization to fears by exposure to a hierarchy of situations, ranked for their anxiety-causing, stuttering potentials" (p. 134). This exposure to a "stuttering bath" may reduce spasm frequency, severity, and complexity while increasing tolerance and objectivity for some children.

14. Encouraging good eye contact can help reduce the feeling and appearance of uneasiness that can accompany stuttering. By focusing on something other than his speech, the child may find it easier to modify his words in a way that is natural and relaxed. At the same time, looking at his listener is a positive and outgoing activity that can change the way the child feels about himself when he is speaking. Furthermore, the clinician can model the difference between eye contact and aversion during stuttered speech. This may help the child see that listeners will view him as someone who is less anxious or afraid if he maintains eye contact. During conversation, test who can keep eye contact the longest when speaking. The clinician should take turns pseudo-stuttering with the child.

15. A method known as *freezing* helps the child stay focused on the feeling of tension when he begins to stutter and, subsequently, helps desensitize him to the time required to ease out of the tension and into an easy pullout. While looking into a mirror, the child freezes the position of his articulators whenever he stutters. The therapist may ask him to describe the feelings of tension. Also, the child can practice pulling out of moments of stuttering by relaxing the tense areas. Looking in a mirror helps to desensitize him to stuttering. Once the technique of freezing is learned, the clinician and child should cue each other to hold onto the tense freeze until signaled to release it.

16. When the child is willing to explore his feelings about his stuttering, try an activity called "Framing My Speech." Using a real, empty picture frame or one drawn on paper, ask the child to choose cutout, preprinted words that reflect how he feels and place them in his frame. For example, words that describe feelings, such as *sad, happy, mixed-up, tired, frustrated, surprised, bad, mad, upset, excited, proud, tense*, or *guilty* can be used when describing his speech.

17. Make a habit of encouraging the child to speak more freely and build his self-esteem and confidence during conversation by regularly initiating discussions in areas of interest to the child and listening intently, providing validating feedback. When he indicates he is finished, the clinician should offer praise of the positive aspects of his speech and communication. Validating the child's improvement communicates to him his success in therapy (Starkweather & Givens-Ackerman, 1997).

Disclosure

Acknowledging stuttering momentarily and matter-of-factly when the child is frustrated and embarrassed can help both the child and his listener feel more comfortable with the situation. Rehearsing or discussing ways this can be done can help the child be more spontaneous when appropriate situations for disclosure arise. As with other phases of therapy, disclosure often benefits from a graded, hierarchical approach. Many children, especially young ones, may display resistance to or a lack of interest in openly disclosing their stuttering to others. Initial, less direct activities can address important emotional issues and help convince the child of the importance of such exercises before more open forms of disclosure are introduced. Disclosure starts in the safety of the therapy room between the clinician and child by openly discussing stuttering and its emotional effects.

1. Ask the child to write a letter about his stuttering to a friend or family member. Whether the letter is actually delivered can remain up to the child, but the very act of writing to someone about a problem to which he is sensitive may open up lines of communication in the future. If the letter is delivered, the recipient should be encouraged to reply in a positive manner.

2. Encouraging the child to express his feelings about his speech using art can uncover both positive and negative emotions and help the child explore them. Through art, many express themselves in ways not explored before. A young child who is shy and having difficulty warming up to, or sharing feelings with, the clinician can be given an alternative to conversation. Paper, markers, and crayons can give him the opportunity to draw pictures about his feelings regarding stuttering. In a less confrontational setting , the clinician is able to talk with the child informally. Chmela and Reardon's *The School-Age Child Who Stutters: Working Effectively with Attitudes and Emotions* (2001) provides a well-planned strategy for using drawings and other creative activities to address these topics. Also, the Stuttering Homepage exhibits many samples of art by children who stutter (www.stutteringhomepage.com).

3. Healey offers activities for young children that involve the child in hands-on interaction while concentrating on his stuttering. The clinician gives the child several drawn faces expressing different emotions and asks him to match the picture to his emotions. Whichever the child chooses, he can express his feelings through drawing or clay figurines. Encourage him to select which face relates to his individual fear and permit him to scribble or stomp on the object chosen (see Stuttering Foundation video No. 89).

4. Although most listeners realize that the child stutters, very few directly address the issue because they do not want to embarrass him or appear insensitive. Additionally, the child himself usually goes to

behavioral extremes to avoid directly acknowledging stuttering. The child's own silence further confirms the listeners' decision to avoid the topic.

Verbal disclosure (i.e., stating openly that one is a stutterer) is a simple way of addressing the obvious: This person stutters. A brief disclosure indicates that stuttering itself is not taboo and helps place both the stutterer and listeners more at ease. Often, it serves as an opportunity to educate listeners about stuttering and how they can sensitively respond in its presence. Clinicians should be able to advocate and model self-disclosure for older children. Some children may want to inject humor into verbal disclosure, whereas others may not (Guitar, 1998).

5. Involving parents, siblings and teachers in the therapy process may help the child become more comfortable with his stuttering. Putting easy, voluntary stuttering in their speech when around the child will provide an environment in which stuttering is accepted. However, *restimulation* (i.e., deliberately modeling an easy form of stuttering after a hard block) should be avoided by family members if the child objects or if the clinician recommends against it.

Reinforcing This Component

1. When working with a young child who struggles with fluency, use a rhythmic method like bouncing a ball back and forth. The child can practice using easy bounces in his speech as he bounces the ball. The clinician can give the child words or phrases to say as he bounces the ball. A predetermined phrase, "bounce the ball," may be repetitively used in practicing easy repetitions in speech. As clinician and child create new words to say as the ball bounces between the two of them, take turns adding new information to create a story. Producing easy repetitions while bouncing the ball gives the child a cue to use bounces, as well as a sense of control over the stuttering. Desensitization to the stuttering will also be achieved through the intentional production of easy stuttering. In addition, by "stepping out" of the treatment room, this game will assist in the maintenance of new speaking skills. As with many other activities, a parent, sibling, or peer can be invited to join in on the learning experience for the stutterer.

2. Using the same rhythmic technique, the child and clinician sit on the floor a few feet apart from each other and roll a ball back and forth with an emphasis on voluntary prolongations or stretches. The child holds onto each initial sound prolongation as the ball is rolling and produces the word when the ball reaches the clinician. The activity targets not only modification of stuttering, but desensitization, transfer, and maintenance as well.

Another variation of this game involves practicing easy prolongations as the ball is rolled toward a target rather than a person. Involve a parent, sibling, or peer at home for personal communication.

3. Directed to young children, "Animal Talk" is a game focusing on desensitization while acting out the sounds of certain animals. Cards with animal pictures are used to indicate the animal to be acted out. Choosing a card, the player acts out the animal sounds with a stutter like the animal might possess. For example, if the player was acting like a mouse, he might talk and stutter in a high-pitched and quiet voice. In addition to targeting desensitization, this activity allows the child to practice varying and modifying his stuttering in a fashion that helps give him a feeling of control over how he stutters.

4. Use humor to confront stuttering in particular circumstances. Peters & Guitar (1991) suggest having a puppet show in which one of the characters goes into "wild gyrations of stuttering." A game known as "Catch Me If You Can" gives the child a chance to catch the clinician in a stuttering moment. When the child correctly catches his teacher, he earns a point; however, if he misses the stutter, the clinician earns the point. The player with the most points wins. Encourage the child to purposefully do things that show he is not uptight or frustrated when he stutters. In fact, give the example of Van Riper twiddling his thumbs when stuttering to show that he did not take stuttering too seriously. Brainstorm with the child to find a similar way to demonstrate that he is not ruled by his stuttering.

5. Van Riper often used counter-conditioning during games to help desensitize a child to stuttering. This technique involves interrupting the child during speech to teach him how to respond to interruptions and resist stuttering. To address loss of listener attention, the clinician can look away, stand up and get something, use a calculator, look at a magazine, open mail, or write notes while the child is talking. An example of a game he can play is "Can't Catch Me." The clinician can structure therapy activities that provide the child with opportunities to "catch" the clinician bouncing. The clinician reacts to being caught in a positive manner, which facilitates increased acceptance of the stuttering, as well as providing a model of easy stuttering. This activity may be expanded to include the clinician catching the child bouncing, the child imitating the clinician's bounce, or the child providing an easier way to say the dysfluent word. Refer to Figure G-10.2 for a sample dialogue of the child catching, correcting, and modeling an easier way of stuttering to the clinician. An activity wherein the child catches, corrects, and shows the clinician a more acceptable way of stuttering increases client learning and facilitates the reduction of anxiety so often

associated with stuttering. Further, as implied earlier, this exercise enables the child to positively react to his being caught by the clinician. By incorporating this activity with the previous one, the child positively reacts to being caught.

Child:	"I heard you bounce!"
Clinician:	"Good! What word did I bounce on?"
Child:	"Marshmallow."
Clinician:	"Good! Can you show me how it sounded?"
Child:	"Ma-ma-marshmallow."
Clinician:	"Good! Now show me an easy way to say that word."
Child:	"Mmmmmmaarshmallow" (the child produces the word with a stretch on the first sound and easily proceeds through the next sound).

Figure G-10.2 Example of Child Catching, Correcting, and Modeling an Easier Way of Stuttering

An updated version of this game starts with placing a jar of rubber balls (or pieces of a puzzle, stickers, etc.) in the middle of the table. The child is told he will be asked questions, but before he answers the question he must take a ball from the jar and bounce it five times. If the child does not, he will have to put all the balls he has earned back into the jar. The player to collect the most balls wins. The goal of the activity is to reduce anxiety by teaching the child to answer questions slowly and not to give in to time pressure (in Guitar, 1998).

6. Dell (2000) offers role-playing suggestions for disrupting speech while the child focuses his attention on using stuttering modification techniques. Activities include the clinician role-playing an impatient waiter or principal and the child pretending to give a report or talk onstage; also, therapy can go to the playground and individuals can shout to each other. The clinician tells the child that she is going to try to disrupt his speech, and that the child should try to maintain fluency during this time. The child earns points for reinforcing the maintenance of fluency. These activities should be done as a game or a challenge. If the child is failing more than being successful, he should be provided with another activity. Clinician and child together can identify words and environments that are particularly difficult for the child and work on the particular words in those specific environments, if possible.

7. Give the child a different speaking environment to work in by taking him on a scavenger hunt around the clinic. As he asks people for objects on the list, he will be encouraged to pseudo-stutter in a manner appropriate to his progress in therapy.

8. To help the child feel more comfortable working in his classroom setting, the clinician can work with the student to develop a classroom presentation about stuttering and why the child stutters. Topics can include the dynamics of stuttering, famous people who stutter(ed) (e.g., James Earl Jones, Charles Darwin, Winston Churchill, and Carly Simon), what it feels like to stutter, interesting facts (e.g., most stutterers can sing without stuttering), and how to listen and talk with a person who stutters. See Chapter 5 for additional suggestions.

9. It is important to address desensitization because there are many things outside the therapy room that will disrupt the child's speech and possibly his fluency. Exposure to these disrupters will make him aware of and help him become more familiar with his stuttering. Several fluency-disruption exercises can be employed, such as verbal or nonverbal interruptions, noise, fast speech rate, loss of listener attention, and time pressure. These disrupters should be used when the child is fluent and using speech modification techniques. For interruptions, the clinician can answer the telephone while the child is talking, have someone knock on the door and interrupt him, or put him in a group with someone who has poor turn-taking skills. For noise, the clinician can open the door, turn a radio on, or do therapy outside.

10. Desensitize the child to time pressure by:
   a. Hurrying him while he is picking out an activity
   b. Attempting to leave the therapy room while the child is talking
   c. Asking questions quickly
   d. Using an hourglass to limit the child's response time
   e. Having a group session where children race to come up with the correct answer

   After such activities, the child's reactions and feelings should be solicited and discussed.

Reduction of Avoidance Behaviors

Rationale

Avoidance behaviors must be eliminated because they facilitate progressive growth of the fear of stuttering.

Activities and Techniques

Refer to Figure G-11.1 for an outline of the information and activities presented in this section.

Identifying and Reducing Avoidance Behaviors and Related Fear

Note: Many of the activities described in Goal 12 can be modified for purpose of this section as well.

1. Younger children may not understand what the clinician means by *avoidance*, because it may be a strategy that just seems natural or logical to them. To begin a discussion of avoidance, try watching the end of a *Looney Tunes* cartoon together. When Porky Pig blurts out, "That's all, folks!" after a significant amount of stuttering, ask the child what Porky probably wanted to say. What if, instead of just wanting to say "bye-bye" or "goodbye," Porky was ordering "chocolate ice cream" and ended up ordering a flavor he didn't like?

2. The clinician and older child can discuss word, sound, and situation avoidances he uses, as well as why hc feels it is necessary to avoid. Discussing strategies to use in place of avoidance is important and should be practiced with the clinician demonstrating.

3. The older child can keep a log book of specific words and sounds he avoids and in what situations these avoidances occurred. This journal will help keep therapy time personally relevant and focused on those aspects he finds meaningful. Also, a hierarchy of feared words devised by the child can provide structure to the therapy plan.

4. After avoided situations are identified, Fawcus suggests ranking them hierarchically. "Although some clients may begin by confronting the least feared and avoided situation, other clients may choose to start much higher on their hierarchy list, particularly if the avoided situation is very meaningful." (1995, p. 82–83). Fawcus also suggests having the young client acquire a list of actual reactions to his stuttering by walking up to people and asking the time or directions.

5. After the child has identified specific avoidances he uses and how they may be affecting his speech, brainstorm

Support

The following citations provide support in the literature for our inclusion of this goal and the suggested activities for reduction of avoidance behaviors.

Bloodstein (1993) ► The client who thinks of himself as a "stutterer" expects to stutter. This anticipation to stutter is, at times, enough to produce stuttering. "Almost every stutterer has his or her own private list of difficult words" (p. 5).

Breitenfeldt & Lorenz (2000) ► "Getting the stutterer to give up avoidances is remarkably similar to getting the alcoholic to give up liquor or getting the drug addict to refrain from using narcotics. The similarity is this: Stuttering avoidances, narcotics and alcohol can be comforting on a short term basis. However, in the long run they not only hinder us in solving our problems, but actually make the problems more severe" (p. 43).

Fawcus (1995) ► In combating avoidance, it is important to help the client notice actual listener reactions so that he may more reliably predict how people will behave when he stutters.

Fawcus (1995) ► Avoidance behaviors insidiously maintain word and situation fear." Because the idea of eliminating avoidance can be threatening to the client, a clear rationale is needed to encourage adolescents to work on this aspect of stuttering.

Ginsberg (2000) ► Understand the complex interplay between behavioral, psychological, and demographic characteristics in individuals who stutter. Assessment of struggle, avoidance, and expectancy behaviors; exploration into shame and social anxiety; and information regarding affiliations with others who stutter provides an appropriate foundation on which to build individually tailored treatment programs.

continues

Support *continued*

Mahr & Torosian (1999)	Mahr and Torosian compared symptoms of anxiety between stutterers, social phobics, and nonpatient controls. Stutterers exhibited more social anxiety and avoidance than nonpatient controls. Also, there was no significant difference between the stuttering and social phobia groups on a measure of general anxiety. However, the majority of stutterers reported speech-related fear as their primary phobia. The authors suggest that stutterers in general do not suffer from social phobia, but that some stutterers may avoid social situations because of fear of stuttering.
Manning (1996)	"Decreased avoidance translates directly into decreased handicap" (p. 230).
Peters & Guitar (1991)	Emphasize the importance of reducing the child's negative feelings about his speech and of eliminating any avoidance behaviors.
Van Riper (1973)	Incorporate "easy stuttering" games into the therapy session to model an easier type of stuttering. Showing the child a different way of stuttering, without struggle and tension, helps reduce expectancy, negative emotionality, and struggle and tension behavior. Van Riper cautions, however, not to make the dysfluent child sound or word conscious, because each child demonstrates marked variation in the words and sounds he will have difficulty on at any given point in time.
Williams (1971)	Encourage the attitude that stuttering (i.e., getting stuck when speaking) is only a simple, harmless mistake, which is analogous to those made as part of everyday experiences.

Identifying Avoidance Behaviors
1. Discussing the characteristics of word and sound avoidance behaviors
2. Discussing avoidance
3. Keeping a log book of specific avoided words, sounds, and situations
4. Ranking avoidances
5. Discussing the consequences of using avoidance behaviors
6. Relating avoidances to past difficult experiences

Fears
1. Facing fears using puppets
2. Clinician insertion of pseudo-stuttering
3. Arachnophobia analogies and the like

Word and Situation Avoidances
1. Giving examples of avoidances via videotaped samples
2. Using flash cards
3. Counting interjections on an abacus
4. Playing "Catch the Interjections" game
5. Reading passages containing feared words
6. Identifying situation avoidances

Reinforcing This Component
1. Role-play feared word usage
2. Role-play feared situations
3. Engage in other activities to work on avoidance
4. Give a presentation using feared sounds and words
5. Wear anti-avoidance badges
6. Practice pseudo-stuttering
7. Become a "master of my stuttering"

Figure G-11.1 Outline of Activities for Reduction of Avoidance Behaviors

and discuss why they often work temporarily, but can exacerbate stuttering over time. Discussing the consequences of using avoidance behaviors can also help the child understand the importance of reducing or eliminating them. Through this exercise, the child should better understand how the long-term costs of avoidances outweigh the short-term benefits.

6. When encouraging a child to address his fears of stuttering, it is helpful to let him confront them by relating

them to past difficulties, such as getting back on a bicycle or horse after falling off. Emphasize that it is important to have a quick turnaround recovery so there is less time to dwell on the mistakes.

Fears

1. When a child fears certain sounds, words, or situations, using puppets can help him more comfortably express his feelings with less vulnerability. He may write a play incorporating his identified avoidances as part of the process of

helping him feel more comfortable with confronting his stuttering and reducing avoidances. Allowing him to read the play to the clinician can give the child yet another way to lessen avoidance and its associated negative feelings.

2. A first step in helping a child become more comfortable with his stuttering involves the clinician casually inserting easier forms of stuttering into her speech. Doing so helps the child come to understand that stuttering is not as bad as he thought. This also helps in creating an environment wherein the child feels the clinician enjoys hearing what he has to say, whether he stutters or not.

3. Comparing the child's fear of stuttering to other types of fears may help him realize that he needs to face stuttering to overcome it. The clinician can explain how children are often scared of monsters under the bed until the day they actually look and realize there are no monsters there. Explain to him that being afraid of words or situations is much the same. It is important to validate his fears, but it will be helpful to explain that people tend to be afraid of certain situations until they confront them and learn to cope with them. The clinician may demonstrate coping skills by providing activities to help the child overcome his fear of particular sounds and words. For example, if the child makes a telephone call in the clinician's presence and uses extensive word avoidances, they can discuss his phone call and work out different strategies for coping with his apprehension and fear the next time.

Guitar (1998) suggests using analogies in illustrating strategies to overcome fears. For example, ask the child to think about a person who may be afraid of bugs, the dark, or something similar. Discuss how people can overcome their fear and what rewards they get for accomplishment. Examples as simple as being afraid of an insect or animal can act as a pep talk for the child and can change his attitudes toward his fears of speaking and stuttering.

Word and Situation Avoidances

1. The clinician can show the child a video of another dysfluent person using word avoidances to demonstrate that listeners can often tell when this is happening. The child should be invited to comment on what he sees rather than having it pointed out by the clinician.

2. A major goal of therapy is to provide the child with positive experiences as he confronts avoidances. Flash cards with both familiar and some fearful words can be helpful as the child practices strategies to confront stuttering. As with most game-related activities described in this book, the child should enjoy the experience of playing the game.

3. To help eliminate "uh"s and "um"s used as avoidance behaviors, the clinician may use an abacus or counter to identify and count these behaviors. The clinician can work with the child to produce more fluent speech with fewer or no interjections, demonstrating that the child has the ability to say the feared words without the interjections. Catching an interjection and repeating the phrase without it can be helpful in reducing avoidance.

4. Playing games in which the child and clinician insert "uh" and "um" as often as possible while the other person "catches" them may assist him in identifying this avoidance behavior. Once he has identified this feature in his own speech, he can practice eliminating it. He must become comfortable and feel safe with his stuttering through the use of voluntary stuttering, triad drills, and easy bounces and slides. As he confronts the moment of stuttering openly and without fear, the use of this type of avoidance behavior diminishes.

5. If a child needs to be confronted with the words he fears (and the clinician is sure that the child can handle this), work with him to create a list of sounds and words he fears, and then write a story together that uses them as much as possible. If necessary, first begin by choral reading the story with the child, helping him move fluently through sounds and words with which he may otherwise struggle.

6. Along with facing one's fears, the child should be encouraged not to avoid a difficult situation by demonstrating how avoidance may make the situation worse. Use as an example of a car that is not starting on every single try. Without service, the car's condition may get worse—and if the car will not start in a difficult or dangerous situation, this may create a bigger problem. Even if the eventual outcome is unclear, it is better to fix problems now instead of when they get worse.

Reinforcing This Component

1. The use of a "Bath of Stuttering," a strategy created by Van Riper (1973), enables the child to achieve the milestone of confronting his stuttering moments and helps him move on to modification activities. Have him read a long passage aloud while combining real and voluntary stuttering on every word. Such constant stuttering can reduce anxiety and the tendency to exaggerate the power of stuttering.

2. Once the child has identified sounds and words he avoids, have him use these in a role-play situation. By becoming familiar with them, he will be better able to see that he can challenge his fear and, with time, see these sounds and words as manageable. Helping the child reduce his fear of situations can be reinforced by role-playing situations in the treatment room that induce fear for him. If the child is young enough, puppets can be used. The clinician and child can role-play the situation

as well, to practice what it might be like in real speaking situations. After a level of comfort has been reached, have the child face his fear, whether in the classroom or another public environment.

3. Consider the following list of activities related to reducing word avoidances:
   a. Talking to the child about avoidance behaviors and their effect on fluency.
   b. Discussing and helping the child identify the different avoidance behaviors he uses.
   c. Playing "catch me" games using various word avoidance behaviors.
   d. Watching videotapes with the child and asking him to point out avoidances.

4. A creative presentation can be used to address the child's fears of difficult sounds and words. The child gives a presentation on a topic relating to his fears and avoidance behaviors, making it personal and realistic, for himself alone. For example, the child may fear words with the sound /k/ or the word *coffee*, thus, the subject of the presentation may be coffee. After some practice, the child is encouraged to give the presentation to the clinician and then to a designated group. As he becomes comfortable with his speech corrections, he is better able to confront and start using his previously used avoidance sounds and words.

5. The child who wishes to do so can wear a name tag or badge stating the goal he wants to accomplish (e.g., "How's My Eye Contact?" or "Take Out the Garbage Speech". . . a picture of an eye or a garbage can makes the badge noticeable and humorous).

6. Encouraging the child to pseudo-stutter can help him become more comfortable with stuttering. Helpful activities include holding contests to see who can have the longest, hardest, shortest, loudest, or easiest stutter.

7. Dietrich (2001) details important steps in Goal #1 of her 10-goal intervention program called, "Tension Control Therapy." Goal #1 is called "To Become Master of My Stuttering" and is very helpful in guiding a child to slowly examine, confront, and change behaviors that may otherwise maintain or exacerbate stuttering. Many of the following steps also fit into other activity goals listed in Part II of this resource manual; however, many of the proclamations pertain specifically to ways to reduce

avoidances. Note that all statements begin with the words "I will" in order to reinforce the child's role in making changes:

To become master of my stuttering . . .

- I will explore and understand how I feel when my words get caught.

- I will explore and understand how my muscles feel when my words get caught.

- I will know my own style of stuttering better than anyone else who stutters.

- I will be able to imitate my own style of stuttering.

- I will become skilled with my muscles so I can "play" with the stuttering when it occurs—make it longer, make it shorter, and make it sound different.

- I will stop fearing stuttering and look at times of stuttering as chances to study the behavior.

- I will stutter openly and not try to pretend that I don't stutter.

- I will communicate with my listeners using good body language, especially when my words get caught.

- I will not avoid talking or being in social situations.

- I will learn how to deal with teasing or people who don't know much about stuttering.

- I will stop starting and stopping, trying to say the word perfectly.

- I will learn how to release my words (pullouts) by controlling muscle tension.

- I will learn how to reduce muscle tension when I anticipate stuttering.

- I will look for situations to learn about my stuttering.

- I will not try to stutter less until I become master of the stuttering.

Modification of the Stuttering Moment

Rationale

Most children who are reacting to their stuttering and require desensitization training also need to be considered for exposure to intervention strategies that teach them to stutter without struggle (e.g., Conture, 2001; Dell, 2000; Guitar, 1998; Manning, 2001; Starkweather & Givens-Ackerman, 1997; Shapiro, 1999; Van Riper, 1973; Wall & Myers, 1995). Often it is the child's reaction to the anticipation or moment of stuttering that creates more of the visible abnormality often associated with his attempts to hide, hold back, or force out the uncomfortable stuttering. Further, in his attempts to minimize stuttering through hiding, holding back, or forcing, the child creates tension and actually worsens the stuttering habits. Although such reactions are normal responses seen in many children and most adults who stutter, the reactions must be addressed if the stuttering, associated feelings, and the visible abnormalities are to be reduced. For these reasons, helping the child learn that he can stutter more easily, without concomitant tension and struggle, is necessary for many who show their discomfort with the anticipation or actual moment of stuttering.

Activities and Techniques

Refer to Figure G-12.1 for an outline of the information and activities presented in this section.

Introducing the Topic

1. Model an easier form of stuttering for the child. Suggest to him that when he reacts to the stuttering moment with struggle and tension, the stuttering becomes harder and more difficult to manage. To address this issue, the clinician can contrast hard stuttering with easy stuttering, and then ask the child to imitate the production.

2. Dell's (2000) approach, discussed previously, is an excellent way of teaching the child how to change his speech from hard stuttering to easy stuttering. Playing games in which the child classifies the clinician's production (hard, easy, or regular), and vice versa, provides the child with examples of different speech patterns and empowers him to make choices regarding his stuttering.

Support

The following citations provide support in the literature for our inclusion of this goal and the suggested activities for modification of the stuttering moment.

Conture (1990)	➤ Stuttering patterns will begin to "change as children become more and more objectively aware of where and when in the speech utterance they begin to stutter" (p. 174). Pushing or pulling on speech postures only causes the child to hesitate and stutter even harder.
Dell (2000)	➤ Teach the child that there are essentially three ways of saying a word: the fluent way, the hard-stuttering way, and the easy-stuttering way.
Peters & Guitar (1991)	➤ The concept of "repair" may be used to explain what happens when stuttering behavior is modified at the moment it is occurring, and the concept of "moving forward" may help the school-age child visualize moving from one sound to the next.
Ramig & Bennett (1995)	➤ Intervention can be visualized along a continuum that incorporates both fluency shaping and stuttering modification philosophies.
Shapiro (1999)	➤ Both fluent speech and dysfluent speech are consequences of what the child is doing. Voluntary variations in stuttering help the child understand the connection between behaviors (what he does) and speech results. Discuss, demonstrate and drill to promote fluency.
Starkweather & Givens-Ackerman (1997)	➤ The first goal of stuttering modification treatment for the school-aged child who stutters is to help him reduce the abnormality of his stuttering.
Van Riper (1973)	➤ Immediately make efforts to teach the child who stutters to substitute a new pattern of easy stuttering for the old one of struggle.

continues

Support *continued*

➤ Offers six guiding principles, as recommended for phonology-fluency therapy with four- to seven-year-olds, that include: (1) the use of an indirect phonological approach, (2) the employment of a phonological process approach, (3) the use of direct fluency modification techniques, (4) the concurrent application of phonological and fluency principles, (5) parental involvement, and (6) the use of a group setting. Essentially, the approach taken in this treatment program is to capitalize on the group dynamics of communication by using peer interaction to reduce the focus on actual speech difficulties. This involves facilitating the emergence of new sound patterns through the indirect treatment of phonological processes; giving direct attention to fluency difficulties by reducing rate of speech and encouraging slow, easy speech; and making parental participation a fundamental part of therapy.

Wolk (1998)

demonstrating this involves the clinician clenching her fist at the onset of a moment of stuttering, holding onto the moment, reducing its strength, and slowly opening the fist to direct the child when to gradually release the stuttering moment. Then the child and clinician demonstrate this behavior together, talking about "getting stuck and getting unstuck." The goal is for the child to catch himself during an episode of stuttering and slowly release himself from that moment.

4. Once a child can feel the difference between easy and hard stuttering, he should start to use self-corrections (replacing hard stuttering with easier stuttering). In doing so, when he says something dysfluently, he corrects himself and says it more easily. Initially, if he says something the hard way, the clinician should model use of the easier form and have the child imitate. As described earlier, this can be demonstrated by clenching one's fist when stuttering hard, continuing with the stuttering moment, making it easier, and opening the fist as the stuttering moment is released. The clinician and child should take turns doing this, and eventually the child should start doing it himself when he stutters during natural speech (Ramig et al., 1988; Dell, 2000).

5. A therapy session is the best place to "play" with stuttering, with the intent of being prepared for stuttering moments in public. If the child is stuck on a repetition, have him first slow down the rate. As he slows himself down, have him change the vowel used in the repeated syllable. For example, if the child is stuck on "re-re-re-re," in the beginning of the word "ready," ask him to slow down the repetition while changing the vowel sound to "ra-ra-ra- ri-ri-ri- ro-ro-ro," and so on. Placing the focus on having control over the rate at which the

The use of a counter can demonstrate how many stuttered words can change in a given period of time.

3. During conversational or more unstructured activities, identify instances of hard stuttering for the child and model an easier way of saying the word. He is then asked to imitate the easier, modified form. One way of

---

Introducing the Topic
1. Model an easier form of stuttering
2. Child and clinician practice different ways of stuttering
3. Explore hard vs. easy stuttering
4. Use fist-clenching to show differential tension
5. Play with stuttering
6. Change stuttering
7. Set guidelines for variation
8. Use restimulation

Modification Techniques
1. Pullouts
2. Easing out of blocks
3. Cancellations
4. Preparatory sets

Reinforcing This Component
1. Story generation
2. Prepare and review
3. Delayed auditory feedback
4. "Show and Tell"
5. Role-playing
6. "Musical Mouth" game
7. "Red Light, Green Light" game
8. Continuous practice and analogies
9. "Memory" game
10. Beanbag toss
11. Musical chairs
12. Bowling

Figure G-12.1 Modification of the Stuttering Moment Activities Outline

word is said, as well as the pronunciation of the word, will help give the child a feeling of control over the stuttering moment (Van Riper, 1973).

6. Shapiro (1999) suggests that a child can learn to vary many components of his stuttered speech, including tension, frequency, loudness, rate, and types. A game may be played in which the clinician and child take turns determining how the other should talk; for example:
   * Speaking with more tension
   * Speaking faster (increased rate)
   * Stuttering more often (increasing the frequency by bouncing on every word)
   * Speaking softer (decreased loudness)
   * Varying stuttered events (types) by blocking, then holding/prolonging, or repeating

7. Activities such as singing, varying loudness, and changing pitch are alternate ways a child can vary his speech. Using up and down arrows to determine pitch or loudness can regulate the child's speech volume. For young children, a toy car can also cue the child to increase his noise volume when the car is pushed up a hill.

8. Clinicians can use a technique known as *restimulation*, which involves a casual repetition or paraphrase of the child's particular phrase with the purpose of performing it in a dysfluent manner. This activity is intended to teach the child to stay calm during moments of stuttering.

Modification Techniques

1. Pullouts are used when a child catches himself in a moment of stuttering, freezes the stuttered sound, relaxes the muscles involved in making the sound, and then eases himself through (pulls out of) the rest of the word. Drill activities (single-word to reading levels) are helpful in practicing pullouts. Model for the child examples of appropriate pullouts prior to and during each exercise.

   a. Rather than hurrying through the rest of a stuttered word, the child can say the rest of the word in a slow, prolonged, relaxed manner. Consonants should be produced with light articulatory contacts; the child should not push if he is stuttering, but should be encouraged to release his tension and say the word more easily. Pullouts can be practiced in drill activities, where the clinician and child take turns stuttering hard, freezing on the moment of stuttering, and then easing out of it. Related activities include:

      (1) The clinician taping pictures to the wall; the child shoots them with a squirt gun, and says the word or makes up a sentence about the picture using a pullout.

      (2) The clinician putting pictures of food on the table; the child then uses a pullout while saying what he bought at the store.

      (3) The clinician drawing a picture of a football field; to move down the field to score a touchdown, the players take turns using pullouts. The player who uses the most pullouts gets down the field faster to score.

      (4) The clinician putting together a fake crime scene; the child is the detective who tries to figure out what happened, and must ask the clinician questions about the scene using pullouts (Roth & Worthington, 2000).

      Eventually the two can work up to doing pullouts in conversation.

   b. As the clinician and child become more accustomed to pullouts, practicing them in conversation is important. As the child speaks, the clinician will stop him by using a signal that requires him to use a pullout to recover.

   c. The game of *Outburst Jr.* offers word- and short-phrase-level opportunities to practice pullouts. One person reads a category and the opponent has to name 10 things within the category in a certain time limit. For instance, the category "things you clean the house with" would be answered by "mop," " broom," "duster," and so on. In therapy, the player naming the items in the category would be expected to use a pullout or cancellation during any real stutter. If there are no real stutters, the player must pseudo-stutter and use a pullout or cancellation to earn credit for any answer.

   d. Once the child has learned the best way to use pullouts, invite his parent(s) in to therapy and have him teach them how to successfully perform a pullout in their speech. The child may be allowed to grade the parental performance at the end of the session. Teaching often reinforces what the child knows about pullouts, as well as building his confidence as he shows his parent(s) what it means to successfully pull through a stuttering moment.

2. Wall and Myers (1995) advocate the pullout as being "particularly useful" to help the school-age stutterer learn how to modify unanticipated blocks. For clinicians reluctant to use this technique, they suggest explaining it to the child in this way: "Pushing your way out of a block does not really help. It's a habit and it's uncomfortable. Instead of pushing, ease the word out and move gently onto the rest of the word. You need to loosen up—like a loose contact right there in the middle of the block. But do not forget to get moving and finish the rest of the word."

3. Cancellations are another method used in modification therapy. The child is asked to pause following a moment of stuttering and then say (or stutter) the word again in an easier way. After he stutters, he pauses for a moment, and then repeats the word again using a stretch or easy prolongation, an easy pullout, or a slow bounce. The cancellation allows the frustration and pain of stuttering to be "erased," helping the child increase his awareness of stuttering moments and increase his sense of mastery in modifying his speech.

4. Preparatory sets can be helpful for some children in therapy. Preparatory sets can be used when a child scans ahead for feared words or has specific word or sound fears. He is asked to relax, place his articulators in the position required to form the first sound of the word, and then begin the word in a slow and deliberate, yet relaxed manner, using a light articulatory contact and a gentle onset of phonation.

Reinforcing This Component

1. To provide the child with an opportunity to practice these techniques, the clinician can give him a list of related key words, and invite him to make up a story using the words. When he reads the story back or relates it to the clinician, he can be asked to perform a modification technique every time he uses one of the key words.

2. The child may find it helpful to work on homework from school with his clinician. When preparing a speech or presentation, writing it out on note cards and reviewing it frequently can familiarize him with the difficulties he may have. Together, the therapist and child can practice the difficult words using recommended pullouts and other modification strategies.

3. If the child is having difficulty using the modification techniques, consider using a DAF machine. It should be set to an appropriate delay level to provide success. As he acquires proficiency, the delay level (in milliseconds) can be gradually decreased.

4. To give the child an increased sense of self-efficacy, a "show and tell" activity can be used in the therapy session. Vacation pictures, sports trophies, hobby activities, or toys from home will allow him to describe something in which he is interested and give him the chance to answer questions in a slow and relaxed manner. The clinician could do the same and answer any questions the child might have.

5. Reenact a broadcasted news show on television where the child acts as the reporter and reads a script to his audience. As he "reports," the clinician times the report and then asks the child to repeat the reading, extending the time as long as he can by using a slower rate. As the child works at slowing down his speech, make sure he under-

stands that pauses are not counted; the purpose of the exercise is to concentrate on his speaking rate and fluency.

6. In a game called "Musical Mouth," the child is instructed to hold onto speech sounds or stuttering moments while incorporating music in the therapy session. The clinician and child begin with a conversation while loud music is played on an audiotape. Whenever the clinician stops the tape (often when she hears a stuttering moment), the child holds onto the sound until the music is turned back on. With the help of interruptions in the music, the child is able to increase his ability to prolong his stuttering moment.

7. When working with a child to hold his stuttering moments, play a game of "Red Light, Green Light" in therapy. The clinician uses a traffic light to prompt the child to continue speech with a green light, prolong his speech with a red light, and focus on easy bounces with a yellow light. The child can take his turn in directing stoplight control for the clinician as well.

8. Continuous practice improves the child's chances of producing better prolongations, pullouts, and cancellations, and more effectively using fluency-enhancing techniques. With more mature children, depending on their interest, relating practice in the therapy room to excerpts from either a martial arts text or an athlete's or musical virtuoso's autobiography can be useful. Extensive practice at using modification strategies allows those behaviors to become second nature.

9. A modification of the game "Memory" can be helpful. The player names the picture on the card using three different approaches: the "hard way," then with an easy bounce, and finally with an easy stretch. The player with the most pairs wins the game.

10. A game of beanbag toss or ring toss can be played with younger children. For each ring or beanbag that lands in the bucket, the child names a picture card using an easy bounce, stretch, pullout, or other modification technique. Points are given to the person who sinks the most beanbags or rings.

11. As a group activity, "Musical Chairs" can be played with the intention of using easy bounces or stretches in every round. Each chair in the circle has a different card with a word written on it. Each time the music stops, the children are instructed to read the word using the speech style indicated.

12. Take a trip outside of the therapy room and go bowling. Back in the clinic, a speech version of bowling can be played, with each pin having a different word taped to it. The clinician and child take turns rolling the ball to strike down the pins; for every pin knocked down, the player says the word using hard speech, an easy bounce, and an easy stretch. The player who modifies the most words wins.

Facilitation of Development of Self-Awareness and Self-Monitoring Skills Related to Fluency

Rationale

For older children and adults who stutter, the ability to effectively identify those behavioral elements that interfere with fluency is a crucial prerequisite to making consistent, beneficial changes (e.g., Conture, 2001; Cooper & Cooper, 1985; Ham, 1986; Perkins, 1973; Ramig & Bennett, 1997a; Starkweather & Givens-Ackerman, 1997). In addition, sometimes the most difficult challenge in learning to use pullouts and cancellations is to become actively aware of the onset of stuttering in time to effect the desired change. As the result of improved self-monitoring and self-awareness, a client will be more likely to stutter with less effort and to implement fluency shaping or stuttering modification techniques. Additionally, the same monitoring skills are helpful when he experiences easy, natural fluency so that he may derive positive feedback from the experience.

Activities and Techniques

Refer to Figure G-13.1 for an outline of the information and activities presented in this section.

Facilitating Awareness

Healey and Scott (1995) invite the child to identify imitated stuttering moments from his prerecorded speech. They also ask him to recognize imitations of secondary behaviors he exhibits to avoid or conceal the stuttering. Many of the activities listed in Goal 4, "Determining What Is Interfering with Normal Speech Production," also help to facilitate awareness.

1. The use of audiotaped speech samples is helpful in initial identification of primary or audible secondary behavior(s), as well as continued identification of inappropriate rate and audible tension. Audiotaping is also helpful during the later stages of therapy to improve self-monitoring skills. The child may be asked to assess a sample of his speech for effectiveness of technique use.

2. "Online identification" is an activity in which the clinician begins identifying primary and secondary behaviors, and easy and hard speech, in conversations

Support

The following citations provide support in the literature for our inclusion of this goal and the suggested activities for facilitating development of self-awareness and self-monitoring skills as they relate to fluency.

Conture (1990) ► As children learn more about the "where" as well as the "when" of their stuttering patterns, they begin to learn more about how these behaviors interfere with speech.

Cooper & Cooper (1985) ► The school-age child who stutters must develop self-awareness of stuttering patterns and associated behaviors as part of his intervention program.

Deitrich (2000) ► Dietrich has developed a unique program involving steps to decrease tension and anxiety. Her program also emphasizes proprioceptive and kinesthetic feedback as an essential goal in decreasing stuttering through awareness of existing muscular tension.

Dietrich (2000) ► The client needs to learn to rely less on auditory feedback and more on self-monitoring skills.

Ham (1986) ► "Elements of self-analysis should be available as part of the stutterer's own knowledge and be functional during any situation in which he or she participates" (p. 69).

Healey & Scott (1995) ► For those children who resist open discussions about their stuttering, a basic level of awareness and acceptance of stuttering should precede discussions about normal and dysfluent speech processes.

Healey, Scott, & Ellis (1995) ► Clinicians should not view the goal of therapy as having to 'fix' every child who stutters. Instead, therapy target the child's communicative competence through the pursuit of realistic, functional speech goals.

continues

Support *continued*

Manning (1996)	➤ "During the initial stages of treatment, the client's monitoring is focused on the overt stuttering behavior. Although the focus early in treatment is on monitoring rather than the modification of stuttering events, as the speaker improves his ability to catch his behavior nearer to the initiation of the stuttering event, some instinctive and positive changes in the stuttering often take place" (p. 218).
Perkins (1973)	➤ Awareness of the specific stuttering behaviors to be managed is crucial.
Starkweather & Givens-Ackerman (1997)	➤ Increasing the child's phonological awareness can also help to improve self-awareness and organize the process of speech. School-age children feel a genuine sense of competence when they have learned how each of the sound categories is made.
Van Riper (1973)	➤ Strongly advocates teaching the dysfluent child to identify his own primary and secondary stuttering behaviors.

Facilitating Awareness
1. Audiotaping of stuttering behaviors
2. Apple core and seeds
3. Role reversal
4. Hard versus easy contrast
5. Cueing and describing
6. Benchmarking
7. CSSS software
8. Keeping a journal

Reinforcing This Component
1. Speaking with strangers
2. Support group
3. Self-improvement
4. Long-term follow-up
5. Reading aloud
6. "Hangman"
7. Smiling through stuttering
8. "Touch the talking"
9. Pantomime speech
10. Using tactile cues

Figure G-13.1 Outline of Activities for Facilitation of Development of Self-Awareness and Self-Monitoring Skills Related to Fluency

between her and the child, with the intention that the child learn to identify them in his own speech. It is helpful to contrast the identified behaviors with easier forms of saying the word or describing what made the word hard. For example, Cooper and Cooper (1985) developed the "Apple Core" worksheet that provides a visual demonstration of one's stuttering (the apple core) and what one does because they stutter (the seeds).

3. Giving the child an opportunity to evaluate his clinician's speech is a helpful way to initially increase his awareness of the different ways a person may stutter.

4. In a contrast drill, the child is instructed to produce individual words from a list: one at a time, first hard, then easy. The clinician aids the child in identifying what made each word hard or easy.

5. For the later stages of therapy, the clinician must cue the child to monitor those aspects of his speech that may be interfering with fluency. Gesture cues may be adequate; however, verbal cueing such as "Did that feel hard?," "Is your mouth open enough?," and "Did you feel that you had enough air for relaxed speech?" may be more helpful.

6. Shapiro (1999) recommends building regular, child-initiated benchmarking into therapy. On a weekly basis, the child is required to check his progress in view of his long-term goals. By doing so, he can reassess what adjustments he should try to make to keep on track to achieve those goals. This is similar to checking a road map to see where one is traveling and how many more miles have to be covered. Benchmarking may include taking inventory of current feelings, thoughts, and fluency levels.

7. One way to build awareness is to use a computer program for counting dysfluencies, such as *Computerized Scoring or Stuttering Severity for Windows* (*CSSS*) (Bakker & Riley, 1996). A loud manual counter could also be used. Hearing the click of the mouse or counter each time a stuttered event takes place will focus the child's attention on how often he forgets to use a strategy. To increase success with this activity, the child should be educated in the identifying and counting of voluntary stuttering.

8. For the child to make his stuttering situation personal, with the intention of improving, have him keep a journal that includes topics such as: (1) my most embarrassing experience with stuttering, (2) my funniest experience with stuttering, and (3) my most elaborate avoidance behaviors. Whether attending therapy or not, a stuttering journal is a way the child can document his successes and challenges.

Reinforcing This Component

1. With the help of a friend or clinician, the child can place himself in a public environment where he is asked

to practice speaking with a stranger. The friend or clinician is there to analyze, and help if needed. Afterward, the child should be encouraged to talk to the clinician about the engagement that took place with the stranger, how he was successful, and how he might improve managing his stuttering in future experiences.

2. Seeking advice from children who are successfully managing their stuttering can be inspiring to the child who is beginning this process. Talking with them about past experiences and what strategies worked in improving their stuttering can be motivating. This will also give an opportunity to develop new friendships and resources to go to when questions arise. A support-group system consisting of others who are successfully managing their speech helps one feel that there is hope and that one is not alone.

3. Throughout therapy, an ongoing education in self-improvement should be emphasized and correlated with the many activities practiced (Shapiro, 1999). Informing and educating the family and teacher of the child's progress is required when they are helping the child use fluent speech on a regular basis. The family should also give feedback to the child when helping him improve his fluency (e.g., "I like that you just used slow, gentle speech"). As the child works to improve his speech on his own, the clinician can recommend finding someone he trusts to keep him accountable in the process.

4. For the child to increase his chances to maintain improvements made in therapy, have him return after one year or more for a fluency reevaluation. Parents and teachers can be invited to this session to reinforce his positive changes.

5. Encourage the child to self-correct himself by reading a book of interest to the clinician. The child will be asked to self-correct by moving from a hard stutter to an easy stutter. The clinician can serve as a model in displaying a self-correction method as well.

6. A game of "Hangman" can be played to help a child monitor his own speech and his use of techniques when stuttering. The child is given a small notebook and instructed to draw an additional body part belonging to the stick figure, such as a head, foot, or arm, each time he has a stuttering moment and uses a technique to move through or modify the stutter. Determining whether the child loses or wins when all body parts are placed on the hangman is optional. The main focus of this game is to point out the specific moment of stuttering and assist in demonstrating the importance of modifying a stuttering episode.

7. When the child gets stuck in a difficult stuttering movement, have him smile and then repeat the word in a different, less tense, manner. Show him that by reducing the tension and the inappropriate speech postures, he is able to influence his emotional response to his speech.

8. Give the child a chance to "touch his talking" by placing his hand on his throat as he make the sounds /a/a/a/ and /ga/ga/ga/ and ask him what he feels. Give him different sounds and words to say and have him feel different areas of the body at work, such as the lips, throat, chest, or face. Explain to him that the feeling comes from the movement of specific speech muscles and air moving through the voice box (Goven & Vette, 1966).

9. Instruct the child to pantomime speech. By speaking without a voice, he will be able to focus on the movement of his mouth and how speech is produced for various sounds (Van Riper, 1973).

10. To demonstrate the different ways he can use feeling to change his speech, provide the child with tactile clues. Instruct the child to close his eyes and put out his hands. Place objects, such as a piece of sandpaper, a smooth stone, and a penny, one at a time in his hands. Ask him to name the object and explain how he identified it. Teach him that his brain is capable of identifying objects, regardless of which of the five senses he uses. Most people assume that their ears tell them how to talk; however, in this activity, touch tells the child how to talk. Have him close his eyes again and say a word while he simultaneously touches his lips or jaw. Discuss what happens when he focuses on the movement of a stuttering moment as compared with the feeling of smooth, less tense, speech (Goven & Vette, 1966).

Facilitation of a Positive Attitude toward Communication and Improved Self-Confidence in Communicative Competence

Rationale

It is helpful, and some would say necessary, for the person who stutters to develop a more positive attitude toward himself as a communicator. Experiences that successfully confront difficult speaking situations teach the child to approach communication with less fear and apprehension, and can be an important step toward permanent, positive changes in communicative competence (e.g., Andrews & Cutler, 1974; Daly, 1988; Blood, 1995; Bloodstein, 1995; Ramig & Bennett, 1997a; Craig, 1998; Gregory & Gregory, 1999; Shapiro, 1999).

Activities and Techniques

Refer to Figure G-14.1 for an outline of the information and activities presented in this section.

Facilitating a Positive Attitude

1. Shapiro (1999) highlights the need for a child to learn to view himself in a new, developing role as a successful communicator. The clinician should emphasize to the child a self-perception that is not limited to and defined only by being "a person who stutters." Some roadblocks that may hamper development of a more balanced self-concept may be either a fear that he is deceiving others or that dysfluencies will return, not to mention the added responsibility required by the self-monitoring of fluency skills. A discussion about the cyclical nature of the disorder, as well as realistic, specific goals and objectives, may help to minimize such self-sabotage.

2. Discuss changes, advantages, and possibilities (e.g., what the child wants to do when he grows up or to accomplish in life) that a reduction in dysfluencies may provide. It may be beneficial for the child to compose a "wish list," including an itemized inventory of pros and cons related to changes in speaking. It is important for the child to realize that improved fluency is not meant to change him personally, but to provide him the opportunity to express himself more easily and openly. New internal feedback (e.g., more positive self-talk) should be encouraged to develop alongside expanded, overt communication patterns.

3. Employ hierarchically based therapy activities that provide maximum success with fluency. A well-devised and

Support

The following citations provide support in the literature for our inclusion of this goal and the suggested activities for facilitating a positive attitude toward communication and improved self-confidence in communicative competence

Andrews & Cutler (1974) → Change in the client's self-concept as a speaker is imperative for sustained therapeutic success.

Bennett, Ramig, & Reveles (1993) → At the beginning of a summer fluency camp, children exhibited negative communication attitudes, which consisted of both personal and interpersonal components.

Blood (1995) → "Emphasizing to clients that the acquisition of therapy skills is due to their own efforts, instead of some magic pill" will facilitate client satisfaction (p. 170).

Bloodstein (1995) → "Communicative pressure" related to various components in a child's listening environment, as well as his reactions, are often associated with increased stuttering. To facilitate fluency, parents are encouraged to provide successful speaking situations for children by using nursery rhymes, choral speaking, or singing.

Bray & Kehle (1996) → With adolescent students, Bray and Kehle examined the effects of self-modeling, which promotes positive changes in behavior from observing oneself on video tapes that depict exemplary (i.e., fluent) behaviors.

Craig (1998) → Treatments that include self-control strategies and anti-relapse procedures have long-term advantages. Any experience that "strengthens the association between outcome (e.g., success) and expectation (e.g., 'I have the skills or ability') has potential value" (p. 23).

Daly (1988) → Incorporate both mental imagery and positive self-talk strategies into the treatment paradigm for adolescents and adults who stutter.

DeNil & Brutten (1991) → Communication attitudes of children who stutter were more negative in comparison with their fluent peers.

continues

Support *continued*

Gregory & Gregory (1999)	→ Communicative and interpersonal environmental stresses have been found to increase some children's stuttering. A child's self-esteem is a significant factor in remediation. Clinicians "should model behaviors for parents that will enhance the child's positive self-esteem, feelings of security, and confidence" (p. 52).
Guitar (1976)	→ Pretherapy attitudes may predict therapy outcomes. Subjects who exhibited high pretreatment speech avoidance exhibited significantly higher posttreatment stuttered speech.
Guitar & Bass (1978)	→ Changes in communicative attitudes seem to influence long-term improvements in fluency.
Peck (1978)	→ Peck states that self-esteem is the cornerstone of psychological change.
Ramig & Bennett (1995)	→ Discuss the importance of addressing attitudes and feelings of the school-age child who stutters.
Shapiro (1999)	→ Shapiro reviews personal construct theory, which proposes that "the client's personal experience and understanding of the social world, particularly the clinician-client relationship, are critical to the change process" (p. 120). In particular, we tend to anticipate our future based on our past. Thus, a child's motivation to work in therapy is contingent upon experiencing success and anticipating continued progress.
Starkweather, Gottwald, & Halfond (1990)	→ A child's concern about his speech may result from parental reactions to his stuttering.
Van Riper (1973)	→ Stresses the importance of making speech a pleasant experience. Although persons who stutter do not appear to exhibit significantly lower self-esteem than average, the improvement of self-concept is frequently incorporated within treatment programs.

thought-out hierarchy will help to maintain motivation and increase self-confidence by making therapy more fun, enjoyable, and successful. Doing so increases the likelihood that the child will enjoy attending treatment sessions.

Facilitating a Positive Attitude
1. Developing a new role as a successful communicator
2. Making a wish list
3. Establishing a hierarchy of success
4. Learning "Ways of Becoming a Good Communicator"
5. Overcoming the "conspiracy of silence"
6. Using "global attributions" and self-talk
7. Dealing with shame
8. Using a gymnastics analogy

Reinforcing This Component
1. "All About Me" book
2. "Sometimes I Just Stutter"
3. Modifying the environment
4. Word retrieval
5. Reading aloud
6. Written reaction to feelings

Figure G-14.1 Outline of Activities for Facilitation of a Positive Attitude toward Communication and Improved Self-Confidence in Communicative Competence

4. Activities that explore "Ways of Becoming a Good Communicator" will help the child realize that communication is not only *how* one speaks, but also *what* one says. Discussions about turn-taking, interruptions, pausing, eye contact, and the like. will improve the child's pragmatic speech skills and facilitate the development of speech assertiveness and communicative competence.

5. Always model and encourage open, honest communication regarding stuttering and its impact. The child must trust the clinician's competence and feel unequivocal support from her throughout therapy. To this end, talk openly about stuttering to avoid the "conspiracy of silence" that often surrounds the disorder. The clinician's ability to talk comfortably about stuttering with the child and others will help to create an atmosphere of acceptance in which meaningful changes can be made.

6. Identifying and analyzing the so-called global attributions of a child may lead to important attitudinal changes. In response to the child's "can't" or "never" comments, discuss the negative influence such judgments can have on long-term behavior. For example, changing "negative self-talk" into "positive self-talk," or explaining the differences between opinions, attitudes, and beliefs are both viable topics for the clinician and child to address. The clinician can work with the child to change negative thinking into positive thinking by discouraging words such as "won't," "can't," and "never" (Ramig & Bennett, 1995).

7. Bennett discusses the importance of handling the situational shame that often accompanies stuttering. Bennett points out that feelings of shame are ameliorated by an individual's ability to explain a chance behavior in terms of a logical consequence to one's own habits." As a result, the negative emotions associated with stuttering can be reduced and handled when examined openly and honestly. Figure G-14.2 lists some therapy activities that help resolve shame.

Figure G-14.2 Therapy Activities to Help Resolve Shame

* Provide specific terminology to describe moments of stuttering so that it is demystified.

* Eliminate deficiency messages from the self and significant others.

* Provide possible alternative modes of behavior.

* Reinforce positive self-talk and speech assertiveness.

* Openly talk about stuttering, in contrast to the conspiracy of silence that typically enshrouds the disorder.

8. Reassure the child that his fears about stuttering in public are understandable. However, comparisons with other activities, like gymnastics, can put these fears in perspective. For example, everyone, even a gymnast, initially stumbles and falls when learning how to do a cartwheel. Although gymnastics may come easily to some, others need more time and practice to learn the new movements. Everyone is different, and there is nothing wrong in this. By encouraging the child or adolescent to practice and persevere, he will improve greatly and eventually learn to do cartwheels without fear. Stuttering can be compared with this example or discussed in many other ways for understanding.

Reinforcing This Component

1. Have the child write and illustrate an "All About Me Book," which encourages and reinforces his strengths (e.g., writing, coloring, and artwork). The clinician should emphasize activities in which the child has experienced success. This broader approach may also help those children whose negative attitudes about stuttering eclipse their self-perceptions in other areas.

2. Provide the child with reading materials about other children who stutter. The Stuttering Homepage provides a large list of books related to stuttering in children, (www.stutteringhomepage.com; click on "The Bookstore" link), including *Sometimes I Just Stutter, Ben Has Something to Say: A Story about Stuttering*, and *Jason's Secret*.

3. Zebrowski and Cilek (1997) recommend modifying components in a child's environment to build increased confidence in a variety of situations:
   a. Increase the number of listeners.
   b. Have the child watch the clinician while she pseudostutters when speaking, to study other listeners' reactions to stuttering.
   c. Discuss the child's wish for approval from his listener(s).
   d. Talk about the child's perceptions of time pressure.
   e. Discuss the responsibility shared by speaker and listener during successful communication.
   f. Review the demands that speech places on the cognitive, linguistic, and speech motor systems.

4. Gregory and Gregory (1999) argue that improvements in word retrieval skills have a dual benefit. Improved word retrieval skills not only strengthen word associations and lexical organization, but may also facilitate increases in communicative self-confidence. As described earlier with regard to linguistic stimuli, these word games and activities can facilitate easier descriptions of items that may carry over into the classroom environment. Success in having fun with words may contribute to changes in a child's attitude toward speech in general. Because persons who stutter are usually (and somewhat painfully) aware of the power of words, positive experiences with language may encourage more positive and supportive attitudes about communication.

5. To illustrate how the child can control his own speech, have him stutter on underlined words while reading. The child should continue stuttering on the word until a tactile cue signals him to continue reading. His response to the tactile cue shows that he can control his stuttering as he chooses. This sense of control may boost self-esteem and motivation and help inspire subsequent improvement.

6. An excellent way to demonstrate to the child responsibility for his actions is to record his own speech, review it, and have him write down his feelings and responses. Keep in mind that this activity demands a level of maturity that many younger children lack.

Transfer and Maintenance of Fluency into Everyday Speaking Situations

Rationale

Generally, fluent speech is easily achieved within the clinical environment. However, this fluency is of little value unless the speaker is able to transfer his new skills into his normal, everyday communication environment. As a result, transfer of strategies to facilitate fluency should be encouraged throughout the intervention process (e.g., Adams, 1991; Bennett, 1996; Blood, 1995; Ramig & Bennett, 1997a; Ryan & Van Kirk, 1974; Shapiro, 1999). Before embarking on suggestions for therapy strategies to adopt in accomplishing transfer and maintenance, though, we need a definition of those two terms. In that regard, we quote from the Stuttering Foundation booklet "Stuttering Therapy: Transfer and Maintenance" (1996):

> ***Transfer*** *of behavior change involves the occurrence or acquisition of changes in behavior in situations other than where the previous learning took place. In stuttering therapy, this most frequently refers to communicative responses being made in the natural, real-life environment following changes in the clinical situation. Thus, we speak of transfer from one situation to another. Responses transferred may be overt behavioral, including speech, and more covert attitudinal ones. Stimulus generalization enhances transfer, but clinicians also plan activities in which responses made successfully in one situation are practiced in another.*
>
> ***Maintenance*** *of behavior change refers to the continuation or persistence of speech and attitudinal changes over time. It is the opposite of regression or relapse. Maintenance is related to the effectiveness of therapy in general, but clinicians also plan specific activities aimed toward the retention of therapeutic effects. Continuing the process of transfer is probably important in maintaining gains [and enhancing] transfer.*

Beginning with easier speaking situations, transfer and maintenance should be encouraged throughout the intervention process as the child learns skills in the treatment room.

Support

The following citations provide support in the literature for our inclusion of this goal and the suggested activities for transfer and maintenance of fluency into everyday speaking situations.

Adams (1991) ➤ Transfer activities should be conducted systematically and must involve active participation of the clinician and significant adults in the child's environment.

Bennett (1992) ➤ Consider comparing maintenance to a "roof of fluency," citing the need for a regular maintenance plan, the need to understand the phenomenon of relapse, and the need to revisit earlier stages of therapy to do "touch-up jobs."

Blood (1995) ➤ Management of relapse should include phases that teach the client problem-solving skills.

Brutten (1975) ➤ Self-ratings by individuals who stutter on the "Fear Survey Schedule" indicate that speaking on the telephone elicited much fear.

Craig (1998) ➤ There remains "no known single major cause for failure to maintain treatment gains" in stuttering (p. 22). However there are some trends: (1) the greater the pretreatment severity, the higher the possibility of relapse; (2) combinations of pretreatment severity, personality, speech attitudes, self-management, and locus of control factors are important.

Fraser (2004) ➤ "When using a telephone, a stutterer is forced to communicate, relying on his voice alone. Specific word pressure and time pressure are also present in most telephone conversations" (p. 163).

Georgieva (1996) ➤ Stutterers identified talking on the telephone as the most stressful situation, and the situation most likely to induce stuttering, of all situations examined.

Gregory (1991) ➤ The school environment is an excellent place for extending the use of improved speech. This transfer of speech skills is facilitated early on in the therapy process.

continues

Support *continued*

Healey (2004) → Develop a speech practice contract with the child and negotiate conditions of the transfer assignments.

Hurt (1993) → The swings and cycles between success and relapse should serve to make the clinician more aware of ongoing difficulties and encourage patience and empathy in the clinician.

Leith & Timmons (1983) → Leith and Timmons's results indicated that telephone calling was more feared than telephone answering, and acquisition of fear of the telephone occurred earlier for telephone answering than for telephone calling.

Lincoln & Onslow (1997) → Tracked speech fluency of 43 children who had received therapy between the ages of 2 and 5 years. One to seven years later, *all* children had maintained near-zero levels of dysfluency.

Peters & Guitar (1991) → The goal is to transfer the child's fluency from the therapy environment to a wide variety of other settings and other people.

Ramig & Bennett (1995) → It is the clinician's job to discuss the occurrence of "relapse" in the disorder of stuttering. They assert that comprehending relapse and preparing coping strategies to deal with its occurrence are essential to successful therapy.

Ryan & Van Kirk (1974) → Are convinced that those clients who are enrolled in maintenance programs sustain their fluency better than those clients who are not enrolled.

Santacreu Mas (1984) → Attitudes toward specific words were measured through a semantic differential test. Results did not show significant differences between the stuttering and nonstuttering groups with respect to attitude, except for the word *telephone*.

Shapiro (1999) → Recommends regular maintenance checks of decreasing frequency for at least two years after regular treatment ends. From the initial session, the goal has been to create an environment in which the child assumes ownership for his speech production and communication skills.

Silverman (1997) → The use of the telephone has been acknowledged subjectively by individuals who stutter and their clinicians as one of the most stressful situations encountered in daily living.

Activities and Techniques

Refer to Figure G-15.1 for an outline of the information and activities presented in this section.

Transfer

1. Transfer parameters:
   a. Use ongoing strategies.
   b. Define a hierarchy of situations from easy to difficult.
   c. Use different physical environments.
   d. Increase audience size and encourage "guests" in therapy.
   e. Use appropriate reinforcement systems in which the child is given tokens or prizes to encourage fluent speech.
2. Role-playing of everyday situations can prepare a child to utilize his strategies outside of therapy.
3. Bennett's "House That Jack Built" (Ramig & Bennett, 1995) incorporates fluency shaping and stuttering modification techniques to provide a framework for the transfer and maintenance of more fluent speech. The framework of activities includes:
   a. Laying the foundation of knowledge—Activities designed to increase the child's cognitive awareness of the normal speaking process and stuttering.
   b. Installing the plumbing—Exploring the dynamics of stuttering to increase perceptual awareness and facilitate desensitization. The child identifies the "clogs" that represent the moments of stuttering and learns how to unclog them.
   c. Building rooms and walls—Encouraging the child to build his own "House of Fluency," incorporating various elements and practices that facilitate better speech communication, including "rooms" for self-therapy and the handling of relapse.
   d. Building the roof of fluency—Fluent speech is envisioned as a roof that needs regular maintenance. Continual attention to the foundation, rooms, and walls is required to support the roof.
4. Westbrook (1994) describes a transfer and maintenance activity, called "Jacob's Secret Speech Bracelet," that

Transfer 1. Transfer parameters 2. Role-playing 3. The "House that Jack Built" 4. "Jacob's Secret Speech Bracelet" 5. Challenging the child 6. Semantic maps 7. Strategies in naturalistic environments 8. Involving others 9. Speaking in front of an audience 10. Transfer within the school environment 11. Taking therapy "on the road" 12. Hierarchy of activities **The Telephone** 1. Discussing telephone-related fears 2. Targeting avoidance words during phone calls	3. Testing scripted versus unscripted phone calls 4. Varying the complexity **Maintenance** 1. Maintenance parameters 2. Recording and self-analysis of speech 3. Diary keeping 4. Booster sessions 5. Periodic reevaluation 6. Pseudo-stuttering 7. Volunteering 8. Self-therapy **Relapse** 1. Factors associated with relapse 2. Realistic fluency goals 3. Use of available role models 4. Toastmasters

Figure G-15.1 Outline of Activities for Transfer and Maintenance of Fluency into Everyday Speaking Situations

assists the child's prospective memory (often called "remembering to remember"). The child makes a beaded bracelet, each bead of which represents a particular strategy he has learned that should be transferred. The child decides what each bead represents and shares this with someone else. This reminder, worn throughout the day, serves as a subtle cue to transfer speech skills to different settings. Similarly, other cues, such as stickers placed on the child's notebook, or memos placed on his mirror, in his lunchbox, and in his desk at school, can also be used. A child may also wish to place something in his pocket, such as a lucky stone, to remind him throughout the day to use his strategies.

5. Challenge the child to be daring with his speech. For example, ask him to tell a joke to his friends, make the morning announcement in school, or deliver a spoken message to a teacher (Ramig & Bennett, 1995).

6. Healey, Scott, and Ellis (1995) suggest making a semantic map for each feared situation. The map should describe the feared situation, including the child's usual speech in the situation and the thoughts and feelings the situation evokes. Then the child should include a description of new behaviors and feelings to counteract the old pattern. This type of "map" encourages the child to carefully consider a challenging situation and plan for how he can be more successful in managing his stuttering.

7. Helping the child use therapy techniques in a natural environment is important, as well as required. Many pragmatically appropriate situations can be utilized during intervention. For example, treat the child to a soda

and have him place the order. When taking a trip to a store, have him talk to the cashier and ask appropriate questions. While accompanying the child, support and praise him for going into the situation and confronting his stuttering.

8. Involve important people from the child's environment as much as possible and explain to them what happens in therapy. Important people to include are the parents, teacher, siblings, principals, librarian, and others. To this end, maintain a "speech folder" with information about the child's therapeutic approach to hand out to teachers and parents. The folder should include the child's explanation of stuttering and any additional information he wants to include (Ramig & Bennett, 1995).

9. Bring additional people into the therapy room after a child has mastered a new strategy and have him practice using it in front of his audience. Begin with one outside person, and then gradually increase the number of people invited at one time (Peters & Guitar, 1991). Have the child give a presentation about stuttering to his class or to a student group. This is an excellent activity because it not only lets the child practice his techniques in a stressful situation, but also provides information to others about stuttering.

10. If a clinician and child are working together in a school setting, use the opportunities provided by the school environment to transfer therapy skills. For example, an arrangement can be made to have the child pick up a note from the school secretary and use this situation as an opportunity to use his techniques.

11. Similar to some of the activities described earlier, Healey (as cited in Stuttering Foundation video No. 89) recommends taking therapy "on the road." For example, he accompanies his clients to the school playground, takes them to McDonald's, or visits the secretary's office to practice strategies in different situations where the child is encouraged to use his skills. To facilitate changes across many different environments, the clinician can provide activities and strategies to the family members to incorporate at home.

12. Before the child reduces therapy contact with his clinician and becomes more independent, the clinician should help him create a list of activities to be accomplished. Each activity is then confronted and the results discussed with the clinician before moving on to the next one on the list. This will help the child gradually gain comfort in each situation, whether it be at school, work, or elsewhere. Next, a survey can be used to practice confronting strangers. This survey may contain surprises, such as taking the bus to various destinations to collect pieces of a scavenger hunt. The child is required to converse with many people along his journey. He should log each conversation to permit reflection and feedback when in therapy. Following the survey, the child should be prepared to make phone calls and successfully converse on the telephone with people of interest. The final situation may involve a simulated job interview conducted, for example, by a friend of the clinician. To make this final transfer as realistic as possible, the interview should take place in a different setting from the therapy room.

The Telephone

1. Children who are willing to share their experiences about telephone conversations can encourage communication. Discussing their fears may help them analyze what can be done to reduce feelings of anxiety. When discussing feelings about the phone activity, add a role-playing game for practice with difficult situations. Later, the clinician can take the child to a populated area where he can make phone calls from a cell phone.

2. In a common telephone conversation, the child can be asked to use a list of avoidance words he has previously created. When calling a stranger, he can use at least two of the avoidance words so as to practice these in an unfamiliar setting.

3. The child is asked to make two phone calls, one using a practiced script and the other without. Once accomplished, he is then asked to compare his fluency and feelings during each task.

4. Using role-playing as practice, plan different types of conversations for various phone calls. Give the child (or

develop with him) cards that outline certain types of discussions he will have with different people. For example, calling a friend, the child will have a personal, lengthy, and practiced speech. When calling a stranger, he will try to stimulate a brief and spontaneous discussion. Working through these activities in a group setting can also be helpful.

Maintenance

1. Maintenance parameters:
   a. Weekly or monthly telephone checks with the parents
   b. Sessions reduced to weekly, biweekly, monthly, and so on
   c. Intermittent home practice in structured and unstructured activities
   d. Maintenance form to document information on the child's continued maintenance activities

2. Have the child record several conversations at home. Ask him to grade his performance in terms of speaking rate, soft contacts, stretches, or other planned fluency-enhancing or speech modifications. Have him bring the tape to therapy for feedback and discussion with the clinician. Often, children are surprised to realize that they do not stutter all the time. By listening to an audiotape of himself, he may learn that more of his speech is fluent than he previously thought.

3. Reinforce the child's new self-image as a more fluent speaker. Ask him to keep a diary for a period of time, recording what types of strategies were used each day, along with his associated feelings. This provides a catalyst for future discussions and pinpoints areas for further attention. It also provides the child with a sense of clinical independence. Have him keep a chart on which he rates himself and others on volume, smoothness, tension, and more. This chart increases awareness of various qualities of speech and teaches self-monitoring.

4. To maintain progress, Dell (2000) suggests scheduling "booster sessions" after the child is dismissed from therapy. Session frequency could reduce from every week to two weeks, to every month, to every two months, and so on as appropriate. During these sessions, the child is encouraged to share what has worked for him, how he feels in the classroom, any trouble he is having, and other issues at hand. These booster sessions also remind the child that the clinician remains available and interested in his progress.

5. Guitar (1998) encourages the idea of a periodic reevaluation of the child's fluency across several years after therapy. Guitar suggests that the parents' involvement in this process should be substantial. Clinician examples of how parents can continue to support the child

should be provided at each reevaluation session. Ideally, consistent, daily involvement is necessary for improvement of strategies and self-confidence.

6. Suggest the child speak using pseudo-stuttering to one stranger per day and keep a journal of his experiences in these situations. This activity can be discussed in subsequent therapy sessions to illustrate the benefits of expanding his comfort zone within real-life situations. Once the child is comfortable with the idea of talking to strangers, "compete" to see who can talk to the most strangers in a day while including pseudo-stutters. An alternative assignment could be to talk with strangers on the phone and insert pseudo-stuttering.

7. Encourage the child to become involved in community activities as a way of gaining self-confidence. Organizations provide opportunities for fellowship, provide experiences outside of therapy and school, and give him a chance to meet new people. Involvement in activities can help the child develop a healthy attitude toward stuttering and life in general. Volunteer organizations in particular are likely to appreciate his efforts, and may help the child to see that there are hardships greater than stuttering.

8. It is important to develop a maintenance plan to assist the child in becoming his own therapist. During maintenance, therapy is reduced to weekly, biweekly, and monthly sessions, but the clinician continues to consult with the parents to maintain contact. The child should practice stuttering modification at home, audiotape the practice, grade himself on the different strategies, and bring the tape to therapy so that the clinician can give the child feedback (Ramig & Bennett, 1997a).

Relapse

1. If the child experiences relapse and expresses frustration with his strategies, the clinician should convey her willingness to provide continued support as needed. Work with him to identify potential factors associated with relapse and develop coping strategies. The manifestation of stuttering is usually cyclical in nature, so the child needs to be prepared to respond positively in the face of its variability. Blood (1995) suggests strategies that include helping him express negative emotion, develop appropriate assertiveness responses, and bounce back after stuttering episodes.

2. Clinicians should be careful not to set fluency goals that are too high; likewise, unrealistic goals expected by the parents should be identified and discussed by the clinician. The clinician has the responsibility to follow up with those individuals directly involved in the child's life, such as teachers and caregivers. Periodic visits with these individuals will allow the clinician to observe to what extent the child uses strategies outside of therapy.

3. The clinician can share an image of and information about a well-respected athletic coach to demonstrate how the quest for excellence is a process without an end. Encourage the child to play a new sport, join a new club, or take dance lessons to boost self-esteem.

4. At the appropriate time, the child may be encouraged to enroll in a public speaking class at a community college, to practice his skills under pressure. A Toastmasters group may offer another similar possibility. At first, he may want to practice his speeches with the clinician before each meeting.

Cluttering Therapy

Rationale

Although many of the same techniques that are used for stuttering therapy are used in treating cluttering, several important aspects are different. Unlike the stuttering child, children who clutter often become more fluent as they become aware of their dysfluencies. Therefore, the clinician can progress more rapidly to more complex fluency tasks. In addition, because cluttering sometimes coexists with stuttering, therapy techniques often become diagnostic tools, which reveal the dynamics of this association.

Activities and Techniques

Refer to Figure G-16.1 for an outline of the information and activities presented in this section.

Slowing Very Fast Speaking Rates

1. The child and clinician read word lists or flash cards as rapidly as possible, with the effects of this noted. Then the words are read alternating fast and slow rate. Finally, all words are read using slow-rate speech. During slow-rate speech, the clinician should model easy onsets of phonation and short stretches at the beginning of each word.
2. Word lists or flash cards are read with attention paid to deliberate pronunciation and prolongation of the final sound of each word.

- Slowing rate
- Increasing the use of rhythm, pitch changes, and pauses to reinforce meaning
- Identifying marker behaviors that indicate the presence of disorganized speech
- Increasing word-finding ability and vocabulary enrichment
- Increasing awareness of structure and form in language
- Using delayed auditory feedback activities

Figure G-16.1 Outline of Activities for Cluttering Therapy

Support

The following citations provide support in the literature for our inclusion of this goal and the suggested activities for cluttering therapy.

Craig (1996) ➤ For those who both stutter and clutter, an intensive treatment for stuttering, which contains rate control, can successfully treat cluttering.

Daly & Burnett (1996) ➤ Clinicians must be aware that individuals exhibiting features of cluttering typically do not fit neatly into a single diagnostic category. The assessment process must be comprehensive, with thorough data collection being essential.

Myers (1996) ➤ Cluttering has attracted relatively little interest by speech-language pathologists in the United States until rather recently.

Myers & St. Louis (1996) ➤ Rather than struggling to utter what has already been encoded (like stuttering), the speech disruptions of clutterers appear to reflect attempts to encode sequences of propositions. Cluttering behaviors between individuals differ in terms of severity and diversity; like stutterers, clutterers do not constitute a homogeneous population.

St. Louis & Hinzman (1986) ➤ Most SLPs do not feel adequately trained to manage cluttering. Clutterers also tended to exhibit learning disabilities. Reports of therapy with clutterers were inconsistent and typically pessimistic.

Teigland (1996) ➤ Compared with normal speakers, clutterers frequently manifest pragmatic errors and communication failures. Clutterers often engage in irrelevant and verbose explanations. Pragmatic skills of clutterers should be given higher attention in therapy.

3. The clinician and child select word pairs at random and practice blending the last sound of one word with the first sound of the other, using very slow and deliberate prolongations.
4. An easy card game, such as UNO, is played using short carrier phrases, with each player saying each word distinctly, separated by a short pause from the next word (e.g., "I ... have ... a ... blue ... five"). When this target is

met, the activity is repeated, but with stretches at the beginning and end of each word. Finally, the pauses are eliminated, and the phrases are spoken using continuous phonation, with stretches blending all of the words.

5. The clinician marks up an appropriate text to identify short phrases or selects poetry with short lines. The clinician and child take turns reading the text, inserting one- to two-second pauses at the break points. The preceding activity is performed using the various steps used to play the card game, until the phrases are being spoken with continuous phonation and are separated with easy pauses. Once the breaks are established during the previous activity, the child and clinician take turns stretching the last sound of each word before the breaks and the first sound of the next word.

6. In a speaking or reading activity, the clinician and child take turns cueing each other to pause for at least two seconds after the next word, stretching the last sound of the word and the first sound of the next word.

7. The behaviors practiced in items 4 and 5 may be reinforced by using them in a game such as *Trivial Pursuit* or a board game such as *Payday*. Players can increase their resistance to time pressure by speaking slowly and inserting pauses when playing these games.

8. The child is asked to identify three times during the week when he feels time pressure and to make a note of when it was, who he was talking with, what the subject was, and how he coped with the feeling.

Increasing the Use of Rhythm, Pitch Changes, and Pauses to Reinforce Meaning

1. Spend some time watching and listening to recordings of news and sports announcers, poetry readings, and other dramatic readings and identify places where the speakers are varying rhythm, pitch, and rate and inserting pauses to emphasize what they are saying. Sections of the recordings may be isolated and imitated by both the clinician and child to get the feeling of what it is like to speak this way. Exaggeration of the speech behaviors should be encouraged.

2. Select a number of sentences and ask the child to read each of them twice, using a different rhythmic and stress pattern each time. Gradually increase the number of readings until the child is reading each sentence in five different ways. To illustrate how stress can change meaning, record several of the trials and discuss them, identifying ways that the meaning changed because of the different stress applied.

Identifying Marker Behaviors That Indicate the Presence of Disorganized Speech

The clinician uses the marker behavior (such as a mid-word break) in his own speech while playing a simple game. The child is asked to identify the behavior and then to count the number of times the clinician uses it by placing marbles in a cup or by keeping track with an abacus. The child is asked to use the behavior as many times as possible while playing a game. The clinician counts each use and gives the child a tangible reward for a predetermined number of uses.

Word Finding and Vocabulary Enrichment

Early on in therapy, *Outburst* or a similar game can be used to combine speech targets (such as slowed rate, increased kinesthetic monitoring of articulation and co-articulation, gentle onsets, and easy prolongations) with vocabulary enrichment (e.g., "provide 10 words for emotions") and similar questions.

Increasing Syllable and Word Awareness

1. Use a commercial word game or create cards with common syllables, prefixes, and suffixes on them. Invite the child to make as many words as he can using these cards. Then see how many different words he can make by rearranging the cards.

2. Ask an older child to mark up a text into syllables or edit a document file on a computer to identify the syllable breaks within several paragraphs of text. Alternatively, the clinician and the child can take turns making up a series of nonsense words using the cards. The challenge is then to rearrange the syllables into real words.

3. A good transfer or home activity is to ask the child to mark up into syllables a page in a book or magazine he is reading for enjoyment or at school. The clinician will want to provide feedback on this activity to make sure the divisions are accurate. The child then reads this page with the clinician present, taking care to give equal stress to all the syllables in the passage.

Increasing Awareness of Structure and Form in Language

1. To prepare for the next session, instruct the child to identify and mark all of the adjectives in a reading passage that is interesting to him. During the session, the child reads the passage, placing rhythmic stress or increasing (or reducing) the volume or pitch of each adjective. Subsequent sessions can involve the identification and reading of nouns, pronouns, prepositions, verbs, and other parts of speech. The preceding activity can be conducted for any of the speech behavior changes, including pauses and stretching at the beginning and/or the ending of words.

2. To emphasize the effect of verb tense on language and sentence structure, the clinician can identify (using clinical workbooks intended for language therapy) or develop simple declarative sentences that can then be modified by changing to passive or future tense. If the speaker tends to use a weak or passive voice, the clinician can use this activity to stimulate the child's use of more dynamic expressive language.

3. For children who use circumlocutions when they speak or who are not concise, the clinician can develop her own examples of such language and ask the child to simplify them without changing their meaning. A transcription of the child's own speech may also be used.

4. Language activities can be used to provide another opportunity for practicing slow rate, pause insertion, and other modifications.

Delayed Auditory Feedback Activities

1. Many of the preceding activities can also be accomplished while the child is speaking with a DAF device.

2. Two types of speech targets are commonly used with DAF work: (a) highly exaggerated slow rate (allowing the delay to slow the speech rate) to reinforce kinesthetic awareness of speech gestures, and (b) normal or rapid rate (resisting the delay) to force the child to use kinesthetic monitoring rather than the more automatic auditory monitoring.

   a. Slow-Rate Activities

      (1) Classic slow-rate DAF use involves reading an age-appropriate text or engaging in a descriptive activity in an extremely slow and deliberate manner. Each utterance should be limited to three or four words and every syllable within the utterance should be prolonged.

      (2) Once the child masters a slow rate, his ability to resist the pressure of communication partners can be exercised by asking him to maintain the reduced talking style while the clinician deliberately speaks using a fast rate. Before asking the child to do this, however, it is recommended that the clinician demonstrate that it is possible. To accomplish this, it may be useful to take turns with the child.

   b. Fast-Rate Activities

      (1) The other speech target involves "beating the delay" imposed by the DAF machine. Success in this activity involves resisting the speech breaks that occur when the speaker is "tripped up" by the delayed feedback by focusing on kinesthetic and tactile feedback rather than auditory feedback.

      (2) The clinician may prepare several reading passages with words that are precounted. The child may be encouraged to read several passages as fast as he can without making errors. Errors can be counted and compared with words previously read within a given period to gauge progress.

      (3) All DAF activities should also be performed in an identical way, without use of the device, before the end of a treatment session. This will demonstrate to the child that he is capable of making modifications on his own without the influence of a device, and it will provide experience in what the modification feels like in a real speaking situation.

Please fill out this form as completely as possible and bring to the evaluation. If there are any items you do not fully understand, put a check mark in the left margin and we can discuss them when you come in for your appointment.

Peter R. Ramig, Ph.D., CCC-SLP
Professor & Associate Chair
Board-Recognized Fluency Specialist
Department of Speech, Language, & Hearing Sciences
University of Colorado at Boulder
Boulder, CO 80309

Date _____   Person completing this form _____

Relationship to child _____

I. IDENTIFICATION

Child's name _____ Birth date _____ Sex _____ Age _____

Street address _____ City _____

State _____ ZIP _____ Home phone _____

Mother's name _____

Street address _____ City _____

State _____ ZIP _____ Home phone _____

Mother's employment _____ Work phone _____

Father's name _____

Street address _____ City _____

State _____ ZIP _____ Home phone _____

Father's employment _____ Work phone _____

Referred by _____ Phone _____

Family doctor _____ Phone _____

Child's pediatrician _____

Street address _____ City _____

State _____ ZIP _____ Phone _____

II. STATEMENT OF THE PROBLEM

Describe as completely as possible the child's speech, language, and hearing problem.

_____

_____

_____

_____

When was the problem first noticed? _____

How has the problem changed since you first noticed it? _____
_____

What has been done about it? _____
_____

When your child has this problem, what is your typical response? _____
_____ Has this helped? _____

What do you think caused this problem? _____
_____

Are there any family members or relatives who have or had speech, language, or hearing problems?
_____

Does your child feel that he or she has a problem speaking? _____

Do you feel your child is more sensitive than the average child his or her age? _____
_____

III. SPEECH, LANGUAGE, AND HEARING HISTORY

How much did your child babble and coo during the first six months? _____

When did he or she speak the first words? _____ What were your child's first few words? _____
_____

How many words did your child use at 1½ years? _____ When did he or she begin to use two-word

sentences? _____

Does he or she use speech: Frequently? _____ Occasionally? _____ Never? _____

Does he or she use many gestures? (Give examples, if possible.) _____
_____

Which does the child prefer to use? Complete sentences _____ Phrases _____ One or two words _____

Sounds _____ Gestures _____

Does he or she make sounds incorrectly? _____ If so, which ones? _____

Does he or she hesitate, "get stuck," repeat, or stutter on sounds or words? _____

If so, describe what happens. _____
_____
_____
_____
_____

Please check the following stuttering danger signs you have heard or seen your child use:

DANGER SIGN	Not Observed	Sometimes Observed	Frequently Observed
Multiple part-word repetitions— Repeating the first letter or syllable of a word, such as "t-t-t-table" or "ta-ta-ta-table."	_____	_____	_____
Prolongation— Stretching out a sound, such as rrrr-abbit.	_____	_____	_____
Schwa vowel— Use of the weak ("uh") vowel. For example, instead of saying "bay-bay-bay-baby," the child substitutes "buh-buh-buh-baby."	_____	_____	_____
Struggle and tension— The child struggles and forces in the attempt to say a word.	_____	_____	_____
Pitch and loudness rise— As the child repeats and prolongs, the pitch and loudness of his or her voice increases.	_____	_____	_____
Tremors— Uncontrolled quivering of the lips or tongue may occur as the child repeats or prolongs sounds or syllables.	_____	_____	_____
Avoidance— An unusual number of pauses; substitutions of words; interjection of extraneous sounds, words or phrases; avoidance of talking.	_____	_____	_____
Fear— As the child approaches a sound that gives him or her trouble, he or she may display an expression of fear.	_____	_____	_____
Difficulty in starting or sustaining airflow or voicing speech— This is heard most often when the child begins sentences or phrases. Breathing may be irregular and speech may occur in spurts as the child struggles to keep the voice "on."	_____	_____	_____

How does the child's voice sound? Normal _____ Too high _____ Too low _____ Hoarse _____ Nasal _____

How well can the child be understood? By parents _____ By brothers and sisters _____

By playmates _____ By relatives and strangers _____

Did your child acquire speech and then slow down or stop talking? _____

How well does the child understand what is said to him or her? _____

Does your child hear adequately? _____ Does his or her hearing appear to be constant, or does it

vary? _____ Is his or her hearing poorer when he or she has a cold? _____

IV. GENERAL DEVELOPMENT
A. Pregnancy and Birth History

Total number of pregnancies _____ How many miscarriages, stillbirths? _____

Explain. _____

_____

Which pregnancy was this child? _____ Length of pregnancy? _____ Was it difficult? _____

What illnesses, diseases, and accidents occurred during pregnancy? _____

Was there a blood incompatibility between the father and mother? _____

Age of mother at child's birth _____ Age of father at child's birth _____

What was the length of labor? _____ Were there any unusual problems at birth (breech birth, caesarean

birth, others)? If so, describe _____

What drugs were used? _____ High or low forceps? _____ Weight of child at birth _____

Were there any bruises, scars, or abnormalities of the child's head? _____

Any other abnormalities? _____

Did infant require oxygen? _____ Was the child blue or jaundiced at birth? _____

Was a blood transfusion required at birth? _____

Were there any problems immediately following birth or during the first two weeks of the infant's life (health, swallowing, sucking, feeding, sleeping, others)? If so, describe _____

_____

At what age did the infant regain birth weight? _____

B. Developmental

At what age did the following occur? Held head erect while lying on stomach _____ Rolled over alone _____

Sat alone unsupported _____ Crawled _____ Stood alone _____ Walked unaided _____ Fed self with spoon _____

Had first tooth _____ Bladder trained _____ Bowel trained _____ Completely toilet trained _____

Waking _____ Sleeping _____ Dressed and undressed self_____ What hand does the child prefer? _____

Has handedness ever changed? _____ If so, at what age? _____

How would you describe your child's current physical development? _____

_____

_____

_____

_____

Check these as they apply to your child:

	Yes	No	Explain: Give ages if possible
Cried less than normal amount			
Laughed less than normal amount			
Yelled and screeched to attract attention or express annoyance			
Head banging and foot stamping			
Extremely sensitive to vibration			
Very alert to gesture, facial expression, or movement			
Shuffled feet while walking			
Generally indifferent to sound			
Did not respond when spoken to			
Responded to noises (car horns, telephones) but not to speech			
Difficulty using tongue			
Difficulty swallowing			
Talk through nose			
Mouth breather			
Tongue-tied			
Difficulty chewing			
Drooled a lot			
Food came out nose			
Constant throat clearing			
Difficulty breathing			
Large tongue			
Difficulty moving mouth			

V. MEDICAL HISTORY

Is your child under the care of a doctor? _____ Why? _____

Is your child taking medication? _____ Type/Dosage _____

Why? _____

_____

_____

At what ages did any of the following illnesses, problems, or operations occur? Please indicate how serious they were.

Condition	Age	Mild	Mod	Severe	Condition	Age	Mild	Mod	Severe
Adenoidectomy					Heart problems				
Allergies					High fevers				
Asthma					Influenza				
Blood disease					Mastoidectomy				
Cataracts					Measles				
Chickenpox					Meningitis				
Chronic colds					Mumps				
Convulsions					Muscle disorder				
Cross-eyed					Nerve disorder				
Croup					Orthodontia				
Dental problems					Pneumonia				
Diphtheria					Polio				
Earaches					Rheumatic fever				
Ear infections					Scarlet fever				
Encephalitis					Tonsillectomy				
Headaches					Tonsillitis				
Head injuries					Whooping cough				

Has the child ever fallen or had a severe blow to the head? _____

If so, did he or she lose consciousness? _____ Did the injury cause a concussion?_____

Did the injury cause: Nausea _____ Vomiting _____ Drowsiness _____ Other _____

Describe any other serious illnesses, injuries, operations, or physical problems not mentioned above

_____

_____

What illnesses have been accompanied by an extremely long, high fever? _____

_____

Temperature _____ How long did the fever last? _____

Which of the above required hospitalization? _____

VI. BEHAVIOR

	Yes	No	Explain: Give ages if possible
Eating problems			
Sleeping problems			
Toilet-training problems			
Difficulty concentrating			
Needs a lot of discipline			
Underactive			
Excitable			
Laughs easily			
Cries a lot			
Difficult to manage			
Overactive			
Sensitive			
Personality problem			
Gets along with children			
Gets along with adults			
Emotional			
Stays with an activity			
Makes friends easily			
Happy			
Irritable			
Prefers to play alone			

VII. EDUCATIONAL HISTORY

Did child attend day care or nursery school? _____ Where? _____

Ages _____ Kindergarten? _____ Where? _____ Ages _____

School now attending _____ City _____

Grade he or she is now in _____ Grades skipped _____ Grades failed _____

What are the child's average grades? _____ Best subjects _____ Poorest _____

How do you discipline your child? _____

What are the child's favorite play activities? _____

Is the child frequently absent from school? _____ If so, why? _____

_____

How does the child feel about school and his or her teacher(s)? _____

_____

What is your impression of your child's learning abilities? _____

_____

Describe any speech, language, hearing, psychological, and special education services that have been performed, including where these were obtained. How often was your child seen for this service? _____

_____

_____

VIII. HOME AND FAMILY INFORMATION

Last grade father completed in school _____ Degree(s) _____

Last grade mother completed in school _____ Degree(s) _____

Are parents divorced? _____ Separated? _____ Do both parents live together? _____

Brothers and sisters:

Name	Age	Sex	Grade in school	Speech, hearing, or medical problem (if any)

Are any other languages spoken in the home? _____ If so, what? _____

By whom and how often? _____

Please give any additional information you feel will help us in understanding your child and his or her problem(s):

_____

_____

_____

_____

_____

_____

How do you feel about your child's problem? _____

_____

_____

_____

_____

_____

_____

How would you like us to help? _____

_____

_____

_____

_____

_____

_____

The following questions are provided as possible suggestions for designing an interview session for a particular child. They are organized into the various kinds of information that you need to obtain to conduct a thorough evaluation.

Peter R. Ramig, Ph.D., CCC-SLP
Professor & Associate Chair
Board-Recognized Fluency Specialist
Department of Speech, Language, & Hearing Sciences
University of Colorado at Boulder
Boulder, CO 80309

Darrell M. Dodge, M.A. CCC-SLP
Peter R. Ramig, Ph.D. & Associates
Associated Stuttering Treatment Clinics
6436 South Quebec Street, Building 6, Suite 400
Greenwood Village, CO 80111

Motivation

- Why are you here today?

_____

_____

- What would you like to learn today?

_____

_____

- What would you like to take away from our meeting today?

_____

_____

- What aspect of your child's speech concerns you the most?

_____

_____

Family Background

- Did you or your spouse have speech or language problems at any time? If so, please describe them and what (if anything) was done to help them.

_____

_____

- Do you know of any relatives who have had speech and/or language problems? If so:

  ▪ Who were they?

_____

_____

▪ Are they on the father's side, mother's side, etc.?

_____

_____

• What was the nature of the problem?

_____

_____

• Did they receive treatment?

_____

_____

• What were the results?

_____

_____

• Did you ever notice the same behavior in your other children at any time? In your relative's children? In your neighbor's children?

_____

_____

Characteristics of Present Stuttering

• Describe your child's nonfluencies. Please try to demonstrate some of them for me.

_____

_____

• Are there particular sounds with which your child seems to have more trouble?

_____

_____

• Is your child's speech the same in all situations?

_____

_____

• How is your child's speech in school?

_____

_____

• Is he or she ever fluent? In which situations?

_____

_____

• Is he or she ever more nonfluent?

_____

_____

• Is he or she more nonfluent with specific people?

_____

_____

• Does your child have trouble saying or pronouncing words or sounds? What are these specific sounds?

_____

_____

• How well can you understand your child's speech?

_____

_____

• How typical is your child's everyday speech today?

_____

_____

Development Course

• When did your child's speaking problem start?

_____

_____

• Who first noticed the problem? Under what circumstances?

_____

_____

• Were you worried or concerned about it at the beginning?

_____

_____

- What did you do about it at first?

  _____

  _____

- Did you bring the speaking "problem" to your child's attention? How did you call it to your child's attention? What was his/her reaction to this?

  _____

  _____

- What did you call the problem? (e.g., stuttering, hard speech, getting stuck, etc.)

  _____

  _____

- When did you begin to use the word "stuttering?" If you did not use this term, did anyone?

  _____

  _____

- Is your child's speech the same now as when the problem started?

  _____

  _____

- If it has changed, please describe this. Can you give examples? (Explore the changes in type of dysfluency, duration, frequency, body movements and eye contact, etc.)

  _____

  _____

- Has your child had any speech therapy or counseling? If so,
  - Where?

    _____

    _____

  - What type?

    _____

    _____

  - When?

    _____

    _____

- How long?

  _____

  _____

- What were the results?

  _____

  _____

- Why was the therapy terminated?

  _____

  _____

Communication Abilities and Style

- Would you consider your child a good or poor communicator of his or her needs and wants?

  _____

  _____

- Does your child enjoy talking?

  _____

  _____

- Does your child use other communication methods, such as writing or drawing, to convey information or needs?

  _____

  _____

- Would you consider your child to be a good listener?

  _____

  _____

- Does your child seem to have any difficulty in understanding what other people are saying? If so, do you consider this to be a problem?

  _____

  _____

- What is your child's general behavior in a social situation?

  _____

  _____

• Are there some times when your child seems more likely to communicate or be more willing to speak than others?

_____

_____

• Who does the child talk with the most? Least? Why do you think this is so?

_____

_____

Degree of Awareness, Handicap, or Adjustment

• How does your child react to his or her speech behaviors?

_____

_____

• Is he or she aware of them?

_____

_____

• Does your child show embarrassment or frustration?

_____

_____

• Does he or she ever appear to struggle or become very tense when trying to say a word?

_____

_____

• Does he or she try to improve his speech? What are the results?

_____

_____

• Does your child seem to avoid any situations to keep from speaking?

_____

_____

Environmental Influences

• What is the general atmosphere and pace of the child's home environment?

_____

_____

• Is there tension or conflict in the home? If so, please describe.

_____

_____

• Have your child's dysfluencies ever increased during tension or conflict in the home? If so, please describe.

_____

_____

• What kinds of experiences has your child had in trying to communicate?

_____

_____

  ▪ Are most listeners responsive or unresponsive?

_____

_____

  ▪ Do people give the child enough time to talk?

_____

_____

  ▪ Is the child often interrupted?

_____

_____

  ▪ Is the child often told to be quiet?

_____

_____

  ▪ Is the child asked to explain his or her behavior?

_____

_____

- How does your child get along with his or her siblings? Is there any hostility, jealousy, or rivalries?

  _____

  _____

- How do you and your spouse handle disputes among your children?

  _____

  _____

- Has the school observed your child's speech problem?

  _____

  _____

- If so, when and what did they do?

  _____

  _____

- What is the teacher's attitude and reaction toward your child's speech problem?

  _____

  _____

- How has your child adjusted to school in general?

  _____

  _____

- Does your child have any other problems at school? If so, explain.

  _____

  _____

- Did your child's nonfluencies increase or decrease when he or she started school? How did they change?

  _____

  _____

- How do others (children, friends, relatives, strangers, etc.) react to your child's nonfluencies?

  _____

  _____

- Do they tease him or her?

  _____

• Do they criticize him or her?

_____

_____

• How does your child react to teasing and/or criticism?

_____

_____

Parent/Child Relationship

• How much do you talk with your child? How much does each parent talk, read, or play with the child?

_____

_____

• How much attention does your child require from you?

_____

_____

    ■ More than your other child?

_____

_____

    ■ More from one parent or the other?

_____

_____

• Does your child generally do what you ask and complete his or her chores?

_____

_____

• How do you discipline your child? How does he or she react to this?

_____

_____

• Does your child do anything that particularly annoys you?

_____

_____

- If yes, why does this annoy you?

  _____

  _____

- How do you attempt to resolve this problem?

  _____

  _____

• How do you react to your child's nonfluencies?

  _____

  _____

• Do you attend or not attend when he/she stutters?

  _____

  _____

• Do you look away, grimace, interrupt, punish, or speak for the child?

  _____

  _____

• How do you react when your child speaks to other people?

  _____

  _____

• What have you done to help your child stop stuttering?

  _____

  _____

• Did it help?

  _____

  _____

• What has helped the most? The least?

  _____

  _____

• Who recommended this help?

  _____

- Why did you do it?

  _____

  _____

- How does your child react to your help?

  _____

  _____

- What aspirations and expectations do you have for your child?

  _____

  _____

- If you could wish for three things for your child (the sky's the limit), what would you wish for?

  _____

  _____

Skills, Interests, and Locus of Control

- What are the child's interests and hobbies? What does he or she enjoy the most? The least?

  _____

  _____

- How well does your child adjust to new situations, new environments, or changes in routine?

  _____

  _____

- What is your impression of your child's ability to learn?

  _____

  _____

- Does your child have any strong fears or dislikes?

  _____

  _____

- Is your child left- or right-handed? Was this ever deliberately changed for any reason?

  _____

  _____

Recommended Interview Questions for Older Children

If the child is older and obviously aware to some extent of a speech problem, the clinician may want to ask some direct questions of the child regarding his or her awareness of, and reaction to, the stuttering problem, such as:

• Do you know why you are here today?

_____

_____

• What things seem to make your speech worse (harder)?

_____

_____

• What things seem to make your speech better (easier)?

_____

_____

• How is your speech with your parents and at home?

_____

_____

• How do you talk about your speech with your mom, dad, brother, sister, etc.?

_____

_____

• How are you doing in school? Do you enjoy school?

_____

_____

• How is your speech at school?

_____

_____

• What do your teachers think about your speech? How do they react to your speech?

_____

_____

• What do your friends in school think about your speech? How do they react to your speech?

_____

_____

• Are you ever asked to give oral reports or to read aloud in class? How is your speech at those times?

_____

_____

• Has anyone ever tried to help you speak?

_____

_____

• Are you right-handed, left-handed, or both? Has anyone ever tried to change the hand you use to do anything?

_____

_____

• How is your speech when you:

  ▪ Talk in class?

  _____

  _____

  ▪ Talk to strangers?

  _____

  _____

  ▪ Talk to friends?

  _____

  _____

  ▪ Talk to boys?

  _____

  _____

  ▪ Talk to girls?

  _____

  _____

  ▪ Talk to teachers?

  _____

  _____

- Talk to older people?

_____

_____

- Talk to younger people?

_____

_____

- Talk on the telephone (when you make the call)?

_____

_____

- Talk on the telephone (when someone calls you)?

_____

_____

• Are there any other times when you have trouble, such as:

- When you are angry?

_____

_____

- When you are happy?

_____

_____

- When you are sad?

_____

_____

- When you are excited?

_____

_____

• When did you first notice your speech difficulty?

_____

_____

• Did anyone ever mention it or call your attention to it?

_____

_____

• Have your parents tried to help you? If they did, how did you feel about that? Did it help?

_____

_____

• Have you had help with your speech before from a teacher or speech teacher of any kind?

_____

_____

• What did you do during speech class?

_____

_____

• Do you think speech class helped your speech?

_____

_____

• Are there certain sounds you have trouble with? What are they?

_____

_____

• Do you know you are going to have difficulty before you actually do?

_____

_____

• Have you ever avoided speaking?

_____

_____

• Do you ever slow down when you start to have trouble?

_____

_____

• Do you ever take a big breath to help you?

_____

_____

• Have you ever tried whispering? Did that seem to help?

_____

_____

• Do you ever change a word or leave out a hard word?

_____

_____

• What do you expect to gain from speech class/how do you think speech class will help you?

_____

_____

• Do you think you are willing to work hard to improve your speech?

_____

_____

Handout C:
ASHA ORAL MECHANISM EXAMINATION FOR CHILDREN AND ADULTS

Darrell M. Dodge, M.A., CCC-SLP
Peter R. Ramig, Ph.D. & Associates
Associated Stuttering Treatment Clinics
6436 South Quebec Street, Building 6, Suite 400
Greenwood Village, CO 80111

XII Hypoglossal	**Range of Motion** __ Protrude tongue to midline __ Push out cheeks on both sides using tongue __ Open mouth and raise tongue to roof of mouth = check for symmetry **Strength** __ Push tongue depressor forward with tongue __ Push tongue depressor to each side using tongue __ Push tongue depressor up to roof of mouth (hold chin) **Speed** __ /pa/ __ /ta/ __ /ka/ __ /pa-ta/ __ /pa-ta-ka/ say rapidly = assess speed and accuracy
XI Accessory	__ Shrug shoulders and try to push down = check for strength and symmetry
X Vagus	__ Cover mouth and cough = crispness/sharpness __ Open mouth and say "ahh" = check for soft palate elevation __ Say /mmm/ = check for nasal emission using mirror __ Say /sss/ = check for nasal emission
IX Glossopharyngeal	__ Subjective = wet, hoarse voice or complaint of choking __ Objective = elicit gag reflex bilaterally
VIII Vestibulocochlear	__ Finger rub test = check lateralization
VII Facial	__ Smile big = check for symmetry __ Say "oooh" = check for pursing of the lips __ Bite teeth, close lips; try to open lips with fingers = check lip strength bilaterally __ Close eyes tightly; try to open with fingers = check eye closure bilaterally __ Raise eyebrows = check for symmetry
V Trigeminal	__ Clench teeth/bite hard = feel masseter contract __ Resist jaw opening and closing (hold top of head and chin) = check symmetry
VI Abducent III Occulomotor	__ Visually track finger side-to-side
IV Trochlear	__ Visually track finger to each of the four visual quandrants (upper r, upper l, lower r, lower l) __ Visually track finger to nose
II Optic/I Olfactory	__ Subjective = ask about vision and sense of smell

This form is designed to be filled out by the clinician.

Darrell M. Dodge, M.A., CCC-SLP
Peter R. Ramig, Ph.D. & Associates
Associated Stuttering Treatment Clinics
6436 South Quebec Street, Building 6, Suite 400
Greenwood Village, CO 80111

Clinician _____ Date _____

Name _____

Age ___Yr ____ Mo/Birthdate _____ Grade _____

School _____

Teacher _____

SLP or Counselor _____

Parents/Caregivers _____

Siblings (age) _____(___) _____(___) _____(___)

_____(___) _____ (___) _____ (___)

Previous diagnosis or referral information _____

_____

_____

_____

Made by _____ Date _____

ASSESSMENT RESULTS

1. Articulation _____ Within normal range

Age-appropriate errors: _____

Delayed sounds: _____

Intelligibility: _____ Poor _____ Fair _____ Good _____ Excellent

2. Voice
    _____ Normal   _____ Soft voice

    _____ Hoarse   _____ High/Low voice

    _____ Breathy   _____ Baby talk

3. Oral peripheral
    _____ No structural abnormalities; movement normal

    _____ Structural anomalies: _____

        _____

    _____ /pa^ ta^ ka^/   _____ Normal, rhythmic

        _____ Dysrhythmic

        _____ Abnormal rhythmic pattern

        _____ Difficulty initiating airflow or voicing

        _____ Could not do or abandoned

4. Language tests conducted _____

_____

_____

_____ Age-appropriate expressive language

_____ Age-appropriate receptive language

_____ Other issues: _____

_____

_____

5. Fluency

A. Danger signs of stuttering observed

_____ Multiple part-word repetitions   Average number _____

_____ Schwa vowel

_____ Prolongations   Average length _____

_____ Pitch or loudness rise

_____ Hard onsets

_____ Silent blocks   Average length _____

_____ Mid-word blocks

_____ Distortions: _____

_____ Struggle and tension in:

    _____ mouth

    _____ eyes

    _____ body

_____ Avoidance behaviors: _____

_____

_____ Difficulty initiating airflow/voicing:

_____ Phonemic consistency (sounds): _____

_____ Obvious fear or anticipation

_____ Tremors: __clonic __tonic

B. Secondary characteristics

_____ eye aversion: _____

_____ eye closures or blinking: _____

_____ head movements: _____

_____ hand, arm, or body movements: _____

_____ verbal interjections: _____

_____ revisions: _____

_____ stops talking: _____

_____ audible inhalations: _____

_____ audible exhalations: _____

_____ obvious awareness: _____

_____ obvious response to stuttering: _____

_____ silent posturing

_____ other

6. Response to trial therapy

Fluency shaping

(__ gentle onsets, __ continuous voicing, __ other: _____)

_____

_____

Stuttering modification

(__ initial sound stretches __, other: _____)

_____

_____

Delayed auditory feedback (DAF)

(Delay: _____ m.s.)

_____

_____

7. Caregiver observations:

_____
_____
_____
_____
_____
_____
_____
_____
_____
_____
_____
_____
_____
_____
_____

8. Clinician comments:

_____
_____
_____
_____
_____
_____
_____
_____
_____
_____
_____
_____
_____
_____
_____
_____
_____

Peter R. Ramig, Ph.D., CCC-SLP
Professor & Associate Chair
Board-Recognized Fluency Specialist
Department of Speech, Language, & Hearing Sciences
University of Colorado at Boulder
Boulder, CO 80309

The following pages contain guidelines, suggestions, and general information for parents or other significant adults (e.g., day care providers) who have or know a young child who repeats, blocks, or hesitates when speaking.

Learning to speak is a highly complex task. As a result, children repeat sounds and words, hesitate, and stumble during the early developmental stage of speech and language. For most children, those "errors" are only normal nonfluencies. For some children, however, they can be the beginning signs of stuttering. Below is a list of danger or warning signs to look for in any child's speech. These signs can occur randomly; however, frequent and consistent appearance of one or more of them should be brought to the attention of an SLP.

Stuttering Danger or Warning Signs

(Adapted from *If your child stutters: A guide for parents,* Stuttering Foundation Publication No. 11)

Multiple Part-Word Repetitions
Repeating the first sounds of a word, such as "tuh-tuh-tuh-tuh-table" more than one or two times, faster than normal, or with irregular tempo. Although these have often been distinguished from whole-word repetitions, repetitions of short words such as "I" or "It" or "and" should be noted as well. These may be postponing behaviors where words or sounds later in an utterance are anticipated or feared.

Prolongations
Stretching out a sound at the beginning of or (particularly) within a word, such as "rrrrrrrrrabbit" or "raaaaaa—bit." It is important to distinguish easy stretches (which may be associated with previous ther-apy or—more unlikely—represent a self-calming mechanism) from prolongations associated with tension or struggle.

Use of the Reduced Schwa ("uh") Vowel
Instead of saying "re-re-re-read," the child says "ruh-ruh-ruh-read." This behavior indicates that the speech difficulty has become uncoupled from language and communication and is being felt as a performance struggle. It also indicates that the child has lost a measure of awareness due to the severity of the blocking experience.

Blocking
Stopping or getting stuck before or during the production of a sound or word. Blocks may be anticipated as the person approaches a word, or blocking may be used to close down the system so as to draw less attention to the stuttering moment

Struggle and Tension
Increased muscular tension of the articulators accompanies stuttering that has developed to the point where intervention is indicated. To overcome this tension, the child recruits additional surrounding muscles and muscle groups in an attempt to overcome the feeling of blockage. These behaviors can quickly become classically conditioned (identified with the original feeling of blockage), resulting in the recruitment of even more muscles. Struggle and tension may be seen in the nose, jaw, neck, cheeks, lips, forehead, and upper chest. Given that evidence, the clinician may wonder if they also exist in other body areas that are unseen.

Pitch and Loudness Rise
These phenomena often occur on prolongation of sounds, when the child is struggling to break out of a

block and proceed to the next sound. The child may anticipate or feel that he is going to have difficulty on the sound and uses the pitch or loudness rise as a way to force his way through the block.

Tremors

Quivering of the jaw, lips, and tongue as the person speaks (fluently or dysfluently) should be noted. These observations will assist in defining the loci of tension associated with stuttering. Tremors are viewed by most clinicians as a more advanced coping behavior.

Avoidance of Speaking Situations, Words, or Sounds

The child's reluctance to engage in speaking activities may not indicate avoidance associated with stuttering. There may, however, be other cues that the child is attempting to manage the situation to avoid speaking challenges, such as continually wanting to change activities, wanting to stop an activity during which he is experiencing excessive dysfluencies, and postponing by acting out or creating distractions.

Pauses, Extraneous Sounds, Interjected Words, or Even Repeated Whole Words or Phrases

These may indicate an attempt to postpone speech to avoid stuttering or delay until the child feels that a word can be uttered fluently. More direct avoidance signs are word substitutions, silences, breaking off speech for another activity, or changing the topic.

Disturbed or Irregular Breathing

Upon anticipating stuttering, child may hold his breath, take several breaths, or display other types of erratic or irregular breathing patterns, such as trying to rapidly say lots of words per breath group, and the like.

Movement of Other Body Parts

When experiencing one or more of the danger signs listed earlier, the child may jerk his head forward or back; move his arm, leg, or hand; or attempt other unusual behavior as he expects to stutter or actually experiences the moment of stuttering.

Fear of Speaking

One or more of the behaviors described earlier may indicate that the child is fearful of speaking. The clinician should distinguish between simple speech and performance anxiety and actual stuttering behaviors.

Additional Behaviors

Additional behaviors that tend to be associated with the danger signs (but are not in themselves indicative of stuttering) include hard onsets of phonation, shallow or irregular breathing (gasping or gulping) during speech, aberrant voice quality (such as excessive vocal fry), and dysrhythmic phonation during prolonged sounds. Phonemic consistency of dysfluencies should also be noted; for example, a tendency to become blocked on one or more specific sounds, such as /s/, /f/, /b/, or /d/, or on vowels, voiced sounds, or unvoiced sounds exclusively.

Some Important Facts about Stuttering

We hear many fallacies regarding the *cause(s)* of stuttering in children. Experts on stuttering openly acknowledge that the causes are unknown and are multidimensional and multifaceted in nature. Much of the recent research, however, supports a possible weakness in the neurophysical or neuromuscular systems. Few specialists of stuttering support or subscribe to a totally psychological cause or base for stuttering. However, there is little doubt that stress from feelings of embarrassment, inadequacy, shame, and frustration caused by stuttering may also increase and maintain it. There is no respected research evidence that targets parents as a primary cause of stuttering.

Stuttering can become an embarrassing and frustrating problem for the child and may influence behavior, academic performance, and self-esteem and confidence.

Stuttering can be changed and, in some cases, eliminated in younger children if professional help is sought before excessive struggle and tension develop.

We often hear that children who stutter should not be enrolled in treatment because "they will outgrow it." Is this true? Many very young stuttering children (3½ years and less) do appear to outgrow stuttering; however, many in this age range do not, and far fewer outgrow it who are beyond the age of 5 years.

Characteristics Sometimes Evident in Nonfluent Children

1. The child may exhibit inadequate attending behaviors, such as hyperactivity, distractibility, and difficulty attending to tasks.

2. The child may have oral motor difficulty, as evidenced by misarticulation of sounds or inability to rapidly coordinate the tongue or lips.

3. The child may have perfectionistic tendencies and may appear to be exceptionally sensitive to environmental changes, disruptions, and stresses.

Some Characteristics of the Onset of Stuttering

1. Some children may display nonfluencies or stuttering as soon as they begin combining words, but most do not start until approximately one year later.

2. Stuttering often begins gradually. Its progression can be episodic, containing oscillations in severity across different communicative tasks and periods of time.

3. Repetitions of syllables that occur on the initial words of an utterance are one of the more common types of nonfluency occurring in children who are beginning to stutter.

Suggestions for Talking and Interacting with Young Nonfluent Children

1. Speak slowly. Use the appropriate names or words for objects and events. Use sentences and vocabulary appropriate for your child's age. This is important so that the child is not frustrated because of an inability to repeat or imitate more complex words, phrases, or sentences.

2. Beginning at a very young age, associate talking with pleasant activities. Use a pleasant voice when speaking. For example, while rocking or holding your child, talk about pleasant daily activities or events.

3. Talk about people, objects, and events that are meaningful to your child.

4. Promote spontaneous conversation with your child by waiting silently for him to initiate the conversation during free play. Reinforce your child's responses with smiles and praise.

5. Provide a variety of entertaining language experiences, such as trips to the zoo, amusement park, museum, circus, and so on. Talk with your child about each experience.

6. Read to your child in a relaxed manner that is slightly slower than normal and has a natural rhythm. After you have read a story, discuss what happened. Let him finish sentences in familiar stories or tell them in his own words. Let him do as much talking as he desires. Tell stories about events in your own life and when he was smaller. Using familiar pictures for this activity may be helpful. Avoid frightening stories because they may be disturbing even though he may appear to enjoy them.

7. Help your child express his feelings, both verbally and nonverbally, by acting as a role model.

8. Listen to your child when he is expressing rage, anger, or frustration. Discuss what caused these feelings.

9. Pay attention to his nonverbal communication: Is he asking you something because he really wants to know the answer, or is he really asking for attention?

10. Consider your child's feelings. Neither children nor adults wish to be ridiculed for speaking differently, or frequently to be told "no," or to be reprimanded for something that is insignificant. The following suggestions may help your child deal with his feelings:
    a. You can listen quietly and attentively.
    b. You can acknowledge his feelings with a word: "Oh," "Mmm,"or "I see."
    c. You can give the feelings a name; "That sounds frustrating."
    d. You can give your child his wishes in fantasy; "I wish I could make the cold weather disappear for you right now!"

(Taken from Faber & Mazlish, 1980).

11. When you ask your child a question, use "closed-ended" queries like, "Did you have a good time at school today"? "What did you do that you liked best?" These types of questions are more likely to elicit short, simple responses. Short, simple responses are more desirable on days your child is especially nonfluent, because they are more likely to be produced fluently.

12. When your child wants to talk to you, and you are busy doing something, stop if you can and give him your full attention. If you cannot do this:
  a. Tell him you will listen soon, after you have finished what you are doing.
  b. Try to find a convenient stopping place in whatever you are doing soon so your child does not have to wait longer than one or two minutes.
  c. Give your full attention as much as possible.
  d. If crying, nagging, or temper tantrums occur, explain that you will listen in a minute or two, but try not to engage in an argument.
  e. Try not to pay more attention to your child when he is nonfluent than when he is fluent. The amount of time he must wait for you should depend on what you are doing, not on his fluency.
  f. When you are ready to listen to your child, sit down with him so that you are at the same eye level.

13. Everyone should take turns talking.
  a. If your child interrupts someone who is talking, tell him: 'When ____ is finished, it will be your turn, and no one will interrupt you." This should be applied to everyone (children and adults) in the family.
  b. Minimize your child's interruptions.
  c. Role-play interrupting and take turns with interrupting; the one who interrupts is told to wait.
  d. If one person's turn is lasting for an unusually long time, tell him it is someone else's turn now, and he will have time to talk again later.

14. If possible, avoid using the word stuttering to describe your child's speech when talking to him. Instead, use descriptive words that demonstrate your acknowledgment of the difficulties, such as: "gets stuck," "bumpy speech," "hard talking," and so on. However, if your child is well aware of his nonfluencies and casually refers to them as stuttering, it would be unnatural for other family members to avoid using the word.

15. Do not demand that your child perform in front of people (asking him to say the alphabet, recite nursery rhymes, etc.). If he wishes to and initiates the activity, then it is acceptable.

16. Avoid extensive questioning or interrogation.

17. Do not expect your child to speak excessively on days when he is extremely nonfluent.

18. After a nonfluent utterance, you are encouraged to repeat back the content of what your child said. This will help reduce his memory of the nonfluency. In addition, you show your child that you are listening to him. (Child: "I went I-I-I-I went shopping with a-a-a-aunt Mary." Parent: "Soooo you went shopping today," etc.)

19. Try not to convey a sense of time pressure when talking. Behaviors can purposely be modeled to reduce time pressure by your speaking more slowly. Speech should be evenly paced and not contain fast rushes followed by long pauses. "Brisk" turn-taking and frequent interruptions also convey a sense of time pressure and should be minimized.

20. Talk openly with your child about stuttering if he expresses a desire to do so.

21. A child usually develops his attitudes about talking by observing his parents' behaviors. Take advantage of everyday opportunities to see that your child experiences some form of success and praise.

Specific Do's and Don'ts When Your Child Is Nonfluent

When your child is nonfluent, the following behaviors may only make him feel that you are dissatisfied with his manner of communication. They may make him feel that nonfluencies are "bad" and result in further attempts to avoid being nonfluent. When apprehension and avoidance develops, the problem of stuttering often worsens.

IT IS NOT RECOMMENDED TO:

1. Hit him for stuttering.

2. Tell him to stop stuttering.

3. Threaten to punish him for stuttering.

4. Help him with the word (unless your clinician states otherwise).

5. Tell him to think about what he is going to say.

6. Answer or "fill in" for him.

7. Look concerned or pained.

8. Appear angry or impatient.

9. Tell him to take a deep breath before speaking.

10. Ask him to stop and start over.

11. Suggest changing pitch.

12. Suggest avoiding or substituting words.

INSTEAD:

We suggest the following when your child is nonfluent:

1. Try to act the same as you do when he is fluent.

2. Remain calm and listen to what he is saying.

3. Try to show that you enjoy talking to him.

4. Seem interested in what he is saying.

5. If he seems especially excited or in a hurry, you might say: "Just a moment, I have the time and I want to hear what you have to say." This is different from telling him to speak more slowly. Instead you are telling him to slow down everything—not just speech.

6. Calmly acknowledge the occurrence of any long, effortful, or forceful awareness of obvious disruptions. A simple statement like "That was hard for you, wasn't it?" can defuse some of your child's concern and show him that such lapses do not upset you. If your child states "I can't say it," or "I can't talk," assure him that talking will be easier if he talks softly and says the word with you, in unison, two or three times. (CAUTION: This approach should be used only on those occasions when your child exhibits obvious distress over his speech failures.)

For further information, refer to *Stuttering and Your Child: Questions and Answers* (Stuttering Foundation of America, 1989.)

The Nonfluent Child's Home and School Environment

Your child's home and school environment can have an impact on his stuttering. The following suggestions pertain to both environments.

1. Define rules so your child knows what is expected of him. Consistency in the home and school is important.

2. When talking, your child should feel he will not be interrupted. He should also know that he will not be allowed to interrupt others who are talking.

3. Your child should know that he will receive specific, predictable, and noninjurious punishment when he seriously misbehaves.

4. Your child should know that he will be consistently rewarded for doing his assigned chores.

5. Praise your child for everything he does well.

6. Try to reduce use of the words "no," "can't," "don't" and "stop."

7. Examine your child's schedule. Does he have enough free time? Does he have enough quiet time? Do you spend enough relaxed time with him?

8. Try to allow 15 to 20 minutes every day to spend alone with your child. During this time you might walk with him, play with him, or read to him. Before bed is a good time to be alone with him for a few minutes. During this time together, ask your child how his day went. This will enable you to find out about his feelings, rather than just asking, *"What* did you do today?"

9. Physical fitness is important to good speech. Your child should have adequate rest, and fatigue should be kept to a minimum.

10. Keep your child's intake of sugar to a minimum.

11. Traumatic events such as illness, accidents, and emotional conflicts cannot be avoided. However, be aware that such events may be accompanied by more nonfluency.
    a. Accept this as normal and try not to give your child more to worry about by reacting to his nonfluencies.

b. Try to counteract the traumatic event by providing pleasant experiences and making him feel secure in his relationship with you.

12. Avoid discussing your child's speech difficulty in his presence. If, however, he mentions it, reassure him that everyone finds it difficult to talk at times.

13. Vacations and events, such as Christmas, Chanukah, out-of-town guests, or starting school, can also result in increased nonfluency. Reducing the intensity of those events is encouraged.

14. Be alert not only for events but also people and places that result in increased nonfluency in the child's speech. When possible, change what you can to enhance his fluency.

15. Attempt to alter communicative stress both at home and at school so that more chances for fluency are provided. Try to remove any stigma attached to stuttering which the child may be experiencing. One way to do this is by occasionally modeling easy, unforced stuttering behaviors in your speech so your child begins to realize that everyone is nonfluent sometimes, and that it can be done easily and without tension.

16. Be aware that your child may become frustrated if he experiences a great deal of severe nonfluencies. Try to provide a way to cope with this frustration, such as:
    a. Outdoor exercise.
    b. Allowing him to express his feelings without anyone displaying displeasure.

17. Parental intervention is recommended if brothers or sisters tease the nonfluent child.
    a. Explain patiently and clearly that teasing is impolite and unkind.
    b. Discuss the fact that all people have their weaknesses and strengths. Explain that the nonfluent child sometimes makes mistakes when he talks, and that this is no reason to make fun of him. (If teasing continues, it may be necessary to ask your speech-language pathologist to talk to the siblings.)

18. When your child is experiencing a period of increased nonfluency, try to provide him with successful speaking experiences. Encourage choral speaking, singing, recitation of nursery rhymes, rhythmic speaking, role-playing using puppets, and so on.

19. Remember the power of positive suggestion! You can use it to motivate children by helping them realize they can change.

20. Do not set unrealistic goals for your child. Try to keep your expectations appropriate for his age and level of maturity.

Characteristics of Some Parents of Nonfluent Children

Research indicates that parents of nonfluent children do not cause stuttering, but unrealistic expectations can maintain or increase existing or developing stuttering. For example, some parents may expect their child to:

1. Pronounce words perfectly

2. Use an unusually large vocabulary

3. Perform difficult motor tasks

4. Succeed in advanced academic activities

5. Be involved in too many activities outside of the home

Some parents of nonfluent children speak rapidly or hurriedly. In turn, their children may speak quickly. Because speech and language are very complex and involve complex motor and cognitive acts, rapid speech may cause your child to experience more nonfluencies, such as repeating, hesitating, and the like. Such mistakes may lead to even more mistakes because the child becomes frustrated, tense, self-conscious, or otherwise upset.

If parents speak rapidly or act rushed, the home environment may become more stressful. Hurrying may then become a way of life. A hurried, impatient environment such as this may not be conducive to good speech development, normal parent-child interaction, or normal parent-parent interaction. Parents are encouraged to provide an even-keel home environment, and model a calm, slower speaking rate. This is more effective than telling your child to slow down.

Putting this information into practice may be difficult. Lena Rustin (1991) describes a task called

"Talking Time" in which the parents complete a home assignment involving a commitment to spend three, four, or five minutes, for four, five, or six times per week, playing with their child. "Talking Time" is structured accordingly:

1. Parents are to solicit help from their child with this assignment.

2. Parents should negotiate with their child for a mutually convenient time.

3. The parent asks the child to choose a toy to play with.

4. The parent and child then go into a room and close the door so that they cannot be interrupted by others.

5. During this interaction, the parent should not make any demands on or comments about the child's speech but should listen carefully to what is being said, not how it is said.

6. When the time is completed, the parent should thank the child for helping with this homework, and record in a notebook that the task was completed and make some comments about how they felt doing it. Time limits should be adhered to when participating in "Talking Time" activities (Rustin, pp. 63–64).

When You Have to Discipline: Some Ideas and Suggestions

1. Establish a noninjurious discipline system for your child's misbehaviors. This system should be consistent from day to day and from child to child.

2. When the child unintentionally annoys you:
   a. Try to be tolerant if his behavior is unintentional, is not harmful to people or objects, and occurs infrequently.
   b. Try to remain calm and collected.
   c. Try not to verbally attack your child (refer to his behavior, not to him).
   d. Describe the wrong act (e.g., "You hit your sister.").
   e. State your feeling (e.g., "That makes me angry.").

3. If the same behavior occurs often and apparently carelessly, and if he refuses to correct it, then reasonable, noninjurious punishment may be warranted.

4. When your child intentionally annoys you, and you are sure that he knows his behavior is wrong, we suggest the following:
   a. Tell your child how you feel about what he has done. Be specific about what he has done that is wrong.
   b. Do not argue with him. Ignore any crying, temper tantrums, or nonfluencies. Ignore any negative behavior when he is in his room.

5. When your child wants to do something he is not allowed to do:
   a. Explain to him why he is not allowed to do the activity. For example, "It's too dark to play outside."
   b. After you explain why, do not argue with him.
   c. Acknowledge to him that you realize he is upset.

6. Discipline must be consistent from day to day and from parent to parent. Spanking may stop his behavior, but it can also create mistrust and fear in the child.

Parents and Teachers as Models

When considering the effects the general environment has on your child's speech, it is important to realize that the parents themselves serve as models to the child. Many of the child's behaviors, feelings, and attitudes are directly influenced by the behaviors, feelings, and attitudes of the parent.

1. Some behaviors are modeled directly; however, indirect influences of the parents and other adults important to the child are very powerful.

2. The nonfluent child may adopt the parent's feelings about stuttering. As a result, parents might ask themselves the following:
   a. Do I feel guilty about my child's stuttering?
   b. Do I blame myself for his stuttering?
   c. Do I feel that stuttering is shameful, embarrassing, or bad?
   d. Am I angry at the child because he stutters?

e. Stuttering is one problem for which there is help and a great deal of hope. It can be overcome if dealt with at an early age, before the development of struggle, tension, and the self-concept of a person who stutters.

References and Suggested Resources

Conture, Edward G. (1990). *Stuttering,* Englewood Cliffs, NJ: Prentice-Hall.

Faber, Adele & Mazlish, Elaine. (1980). *How to talk So kids will listen and listen so kids will talk.* New York: Avon Books.

Ramig, Peter. (1993). Parent-clinician-child partnership in the therapeutic process of the preschool- and elementary-aged child who stutters. *Seminars in Speech and Language, 14*(3), 236–237.

Rustin, Lena. (1991). *Parents, families and the stuttering child.* San Diego, CA: Singular Publishing Group.

Stuttering Foundation of America. *The child who stutters at school: Notes to the teacher.* P.O. Box 11749, Memphis, TN, 38111-0749.

Stuttering Foundation of America. (1989). *Stuttering and your child: questions and answers.* P.O. Box 11749, Memphis, TN, 38111-0749.

Zwitman, Daniel H. (1978). *The disfluent child: A management program,* Baltimore, MD: University Park Press.

For more information, the following brochures and video tapes are available through the Stuttering Foundation of America, P.O. Box 11749, Memphis, Tennessee 38111-0749 (800-992-9392):

"The child who stutters at school: Notes to the teacher" (brochure)

"Stuttering and your child: Questions and answers" (booklet)

Stuttering and your child: A video for parents (video)

"Do you stutter: A guide for teens (booklet)

Do you stutter: Straight talk for teens (video)

Peter R. Ramig, Ph.D., CCC-SLP
Professor & Associate Chair
Board-Recognized Fluency Specialist
Department of Speech, Language, & Hearing Sciences
University of Colorado at Boulder
Boulder, CO 80309

The influence of the teacher on the life of the child who stutters can be dramatic. We have developed this short handout to highlight information that we hope is helpful in understanding the impact stuttering can have in the life of the child.

The following pages contain guidelines, suggestions, and general information for classroom teachers who have a child in their class who repeats, prolongs, or hesitates when he or she speaks. The process of learning to speak is a highly complex task. As a result, children may repeat sounds and words, hesitate, and stumble on words during the developmental stage of speech. For most children, such "errors" are only normal nonfluencies. For some children, however, these behaviors can be the beginning signs of stuttering. Below is a list of danger or warning signs to look for in a young child's speech. Some of these signs can occur randomly in any child's speech; however, frequent and consistent appearance of one or more should be brought to the attention of the school SLP.

Important: We hear many fallacies regarding the *cause(s)* of stuttering. Experts on stuttering openly acknowledge that the causes are unknown. However, research on stuttering supports probable neuromotor influences. Few specialists on stuttering support a psychological cause or base for the problem. However, there is little doubt that stuttering can be significantly increased by stress from feelings of embarrassment, inadequacy, shame, and frustration.

Stuttering Danger or Warning Signs

(Adapted from *If your child stutters: A guide for parents,* Stuttering Foundation Publication No. 11)

Multiple Part-Word Repetitions

Repeating the first sounds of a word, such as "tuh-tuh-tuh-tuh-table" more than one or two times, faster than normal, or with irregular tempo. Although these have often been distinguished from whole-word repetitions, repetitions of short words such as "I" or "It" or "and" should be noted as well. These may be postponing behaviors where words or sounds later in an utterance are anticipated or feared.

Prolongations

Stretching out a sound at the beginning of or (particularly) within a word, such as "rrrrrrrrrabbit" or "raaaaaa—bit." It is important to distinguish easy stretches (which may be associated with previous therapy or—more unlikely—represent a self-calming mechanism) from prolongations associated with tension or struggle.

Use of the Reduced Schwa ("uh") Vowel

Instead of saying "re-re-re-read," the child says "ruh-ruh-ruh-read." This behavior indicates that the speech difficulty has become uncoupled from language and communication and is being felt as a performance struggle. It also indicates that the child has lost a measure of awareness due to the severity of the blocking experience.

Blocking

Stopping or getting stuck before or during the production of a sound or word. Blocks may be anticipated as the person approaches a word, or blocking may be used to close down the system so as to draw less attention to the stuttering moment

Struggle and Tension

Increased muscular tension of the articulators accompanies stuttering that has developed to the point where intervention is indicated. To overcome this tension, the child recruits additional surrounding muscles and muscle groups in an attempt to overcome the feeling of blockage. These behaviors can quickly become classically conditioned (identified with the original feeling of blockage), resulting in the recruitment of even more muscles. Struggle and tension may be seen in the nose, jaw, neck, cheeks, lips, forehead, and upper chest. Given that evidence, the clinician may wonder if they also exist in other body areas that are unseen.

Pitch and Loudness Rise

These phenomena often occur on prolongation of sounds, when the child is struggling to break out of a block and proceed to the next sound. The child may anticipate or feel that he is going to have difficulty on the sound and uses the pitch or loudness rise as a way to force his way through the block.

Tremors

Quivering of the jaw, lips, and tongue as the person speaks (fluently or dysfluently) should be noted. These observations will assist in defining the loci of tension associated with stuttering. Tremors are viewed by most clinicians as a more advanced coping behavior.

Avoidance of Speaking Situations, Words, or Sounds

The child's reluctance to engage in speaking activities may not indicate avoidance associated with stuttering. There may, however, be other cues that the child is attempting to manage the situation to avoid speaking challenges, such as continually wanting to change activities, wanting to stop an activity during which he is experiencing excessive dysfluencies, and postponing by acting out or creating distractions.

Pauses, Extraneous Sounds, Interjected Words, or Even Repeated Whole Words or Phrases

These may indicate an attempt to postpone speech to avoid stuttering or delay until the child feels that a word can be uttered fluently. More direct avoidance signs are word substitutions, silences, breaking off speech for another activity, or changing the topic.

Disturbed or Irregular Breathing

Upon anticipating stuttering, child may hold his breath, take several breaths, or display other types of erratic or irregular breathing patterns, such as trying to rapidly say lots of words per breath group, and the like.

Movement of Other Body Parts

When experiencing one or more of the danger signs listed earlier, the child may jerk his head forward or back; move his arm, leg, or hand; or attempt other unusual behavior as he expects to stutter or actually experiences the moment of stuttering.

Fear of Speaking

One or more of the behaviors described earlier may indicate that the child is fearful of speaking. The clinician should distinguish between simple speech and performance anxiety and actual stuttering behaviors.

Additional Behaviors

Additional behaviors that tend to be associated with the danger signs (but are not in themselves indicative of stuttering) include hard onsets of phonation, shallow or irregular breathing (gasping or gulping) during speech, aberrant voice quality (such as excessive vocal fry), and dysrhythmic phonation during prolonged sounds. Phonemic consistency of dysfluencies should also be noted; for example, a tendency to become blocked on one or more specific sounds, such as /s/, /f/, /b/, or /d/, or on vowels, voiced sounds, or unvoiced sounds exclusively.

Characteristics of the Onset of Stuttering

1. Some children begin stuttering as soon as they begin combining words, but most do not start until approximately one year later (2¹/₂ to 3 years old).

2. Stuttering often begins gradually. Its progression can be episodic, containing oscillations in severity across communicative tasks and time.

3. Repetitions of syllables that occur on the initial words or utterances are the most frequent type of nonfluency occurring in children who are beginning to stutter.

4. Stuttering for most children is very frustrating and embarrassing. As a result, the child may begin to act out in class and avoid speaking situations as much as possible.

General Information and Guidelines

1. Teachers can be helpful in providing the speech-language pathologist with a broader picture of the child's classroom speech behavior.

2. Try to treat the child's stuttering casually and matter-of-factly.

3. When the child is experiencing nonfluencies, *PLEASE DO NOT:*
   a. Tell him to stop stuttering.
   b. Tell him to think about what he is going to say.
   c. Answer or fill in for him.
   d. Look concerned or pained.
   e. Appear angry or impatient.
   f. Tell him to take a deep breath before speaking.
   g. Ask him to stop and start over.
   h. Suggest changing pitch.
   i. Suggest avoiding or substituting words.
   j. Reinforce nonfluency by attending more to it than to fluency.
   k. Pretend nonfluencies do not exist.
   l. Express pity.

   INSTEAD:
   a. Try to act the same as you do when the child is fluent.
   b. Remain calm and listen to what the child is saying.

c. Try to show that you enjoy talking with him.
   d. If he seems especially excited or in a hurry, we suggest responding: "I have time and I want to hear what you have to say." This is different from telling him to speak more slowly or to take a deep breath. Instead, you are telling him in a supportive way that it is acceptable to slow down everything, not just speech.

4. If the child has fluent speaking days and nonfluent speaking days, allow more classroom participation on more fluent days and less participation on nonfluent days.

5. If you are unsure whether you should require an older elementary-age child who stutters to give oral reports, we suggest talking to the student about it privately. You might tell him that you realize he sometimes has trouble talking and that you are willing to arrange some options for delivering his report.

6. When the young child is experiencing a period of increased nonfluency, try to provide him with successful speaking experiences by encouraging fluency-enhancing speaking situations such as choral speaking, singing, recitation of nursery rhymes, rhythmic speaking, role-playing using puppets, and so on.

7. To increase the child's fluency during reading group activities, begin the reading passage speaking in unison with the child. If the stuttering child speaks or reads in unison with you, he usually will not stutter. This is called the *choral speaking* (or *reading*) *effect.* We suggest following this procedure with other students as well so the nonfluent child will not be singled out as different.

8. Try to avoid intimidating questioning of the child.

9. Avoid discussing the child's speech differences in his presence. If, however, he broaches the topic, be empathic and try to reassure him that everyone finds it difficult to talk at times.

10. Avoid using the word *stuttering* to describe the child's speech when talking to him. Instead, use descriptive words such as: "gets stuck," "bumpy speech," "hard talking," and the like. However, if the child is well aware of his nonfluencies and refers to them as stuttering, it would be unnatural for everyone else to avoid using the word.

11. After a nonfluent utterance, you might repeat back the content of what the child said. This will help you make sure you are attending to the content of what he said and help to reduce his memory of the nonfluency. In addition, you show the child that you are listening.

12. Be careful not to convey a sense of time pressure while talking. Behaviors can purposely be modeled to reduce this sense of time pressure, such as *speaking more slowly*. Speech should be evenly paced and not contain fast rushes followed by long pauses. Brisk turn-taking and frequent interruptions also convey a sense of time pressure and should be minimized.

13. Talk openly with the child about stuttering if he expresses a desire to do so, but do not make a big issue out of it.

14. A child develops his attitudes about talking by observing others. Take advantage of every opportunity to see that the child experiences some form of success and praise.

15. Try to remove the stigma attached to stuttering which the child may be experiencing. One way to do this is by occasionally modeling unforced stuttering behaviors so that he realizes everyone is nonfluent sometimes and that it can be done easily and without tension.

16. Be aware that the child may become very frustrated if he experiences a great deal of severe nonfluency. Try to provide a way for him to express this frustration.

17. Teachers should intervene if the nonfluent child is teased or harassed by other students. When the nonfluent child is absent, consider using the following discussion strategies with the class:
    a. Explain patiently and clearly that teasing is impolite and unkind.
    b. Discuss the fact that everyone has weaknesses and strengths. Explain that the child sometimes makes mistakes when he talks and this is no reason to make fun of him.
    c. If the teasing continues, it may be necessary for you and the speech-language pathologist to talk to the children responsible.

This form is intended to be given or sent to parents of children who have completed therapy.

Darrell M. Dodge, M.A., CCC-SLP
Peter R. Ramig, Ph.D. & Associates
Associated Stuttering Treatment Clinics
6436 South Quebec Street, Building 6, Suite 400
Greenwood Village, CO 80111

Parent/Child Perceptions

Child _____ Parents _____

Address _____

City _____ State _____ ZIP _____

Dates of therapy _____ to _____

Clinician _____

Please answer the following questions by checking the box that best corresponds to your experience or your perception of the response to therapy:

	Mild							**Severe**		

Stuttering when therapy began

| 1 | 2 | 3 | 4 | 5 | 6 | 7 | 8 | 9 | 10 |

Stuttering when therapy ended

| 1 | 2 | 3 | 4 | 5 | 6 | 7 | 8 | 9 | 10 |

Present stuttering level

| 1 | 2 | 3 | 4 | 5 | 6 | 7 | 8 | 9 | 10 |

	Do Not Agree							**Agree**		

Clinician provided adequate information about stuttering and the maintenance of fluency gains following therapy

| 1 | 2 | 3 | 4 | 5 | 6 | 7 | 8 | 9 | 10 |

Practice is required to maintain fluency

| 1 | 2 | 3 | 4 | 5 | 6 | 7 | 8 | 9 | 10 |

Present level of fluency is acceptable

| 1 | 2 | 3 | 4 | 5 | 6 | 7 | 8 | 9 | 10 |

Do Not Agree   **Agree**

Stuttering is not as important to child as it used to be

1   2   3   4   5   6   7   8   9   10

Stuttering is not a barrier to child's activities and lifestyle

1   2   3   4   5   6   7   8   9   10

Child would benefit from a refresher therapy session from time to time

1   2   3   4   5   6   7   8   9   10

Child is participating in a stuttering support group _____ Yes _____ No

Comments

_____

_____

_____

_____

_____

_____

_____

This form is to be completed by School Personnel based upon observations in the classroom. This form is not to be completed by parents/guardians.

Source: Judith Eckardt, SLP, Board-Recognized Fluency Specialist, USA (August, 2003).

FLUENCY INFORMATION

Student's name _____

Birth date _____ Age _____ Date _____

Teacher/support staff _____

School _____ Grade _____

Your observations of this student's ORAL COMMUNICATION SKILLS will help determine if there is a fluency problem that adversely affects the student's ability to communicate effectively in school learning and/or social situations.

Fluency refers to the typical rate and rhythm of connected speech. When disruption occurs, this is known as dysfluency and/or stuttering.

1. Check any of the following behaviors that you have noticed in this student's speech:

- Revisions (starting and stopping and starting over again). ( )
- Frequent interjections (um, like, you know). ( )
- Phrase repetitions (and then, and then). ( )
- Pauses or hesitations while speaking ("He ... went away.") ( )
- Word repetitions (we-we-we). ( )
- Part-word repetitions (t-t-t-take; mo-mo-mom). ( )
- Prolongations (nooooooo-body). ( )
- Blocks (noticeable tension/no speech comes out). ( )
- Unusual face or body movements (head nods, eye movement). ( )
- Abnormal breathing patterns. ( )

Other _____

_____

2. Answer the following questions with YES or NO.

- Do you listen to HOW the student is speaking rather than WHAT the student is saying? _____
- Does this student avoid speaking in the classroom? _____
- Do classmates react to this student when he or she is stuttering? _____
- If so, does this student have negative responses to the peers' reactions? (stops talking, more stuttering, withdraws, etc.) _____

- Do you feel uncomfortable when you try to communicate with this student? _____
- Do you think this student is aware of his or her fluency problem? _____

3. Information Questions

- How long have you observed the problem?

_____

- How long have you been concerned about the dysfluencies in this student's speech?

_____

- Has the dysfluency been consistent or intermittent?

_____

- Can you recall any unusual event near the onset of the problem? (child, family, environment)

_____

- Have the parent(s)/caregivers ever mentioned the student's fluency problems? If yes, what was discussed?

_____

- Is there a history of stuttering in the biological family?

_____

- Has the student ever talked to you about his or her speech problem? If yes, what was discussed?

_____

- What other information might be helpful in looking at this student's fluency skills?

_____

- Do you have any other concerns regarding this student's speech and language skills, academic functioning, or social appropriateness?

_____

Thank you for taking time to share this helpful information. Please return this form

to _____ SLP by _____ (date).

Books

Books for Speech-Language Pathologists

Clinical Decision Making in Fluency Disorders (W.H. Manning; Singular): 2001.

Clinical Management of Stuttering in Older Children and Adults (R.E. Ham; Aspen): 1999.

Counseling the Communicatively Disabled and Their Families: A Manual for Clinicians (G.H. Shames; Allyn & Bacon): 2000.

Counseling the Communicatively Disordered and Their Families (D.M. Luterman; Pro-Ed): 2001.

Get Out of My Life, But First Could You Drive Me and Cheryl to the Mall? A Parent's Guide to the New Teenager (A.E. Wolfe; Noonday): 2002.

A Handbook on Stuttering (O. Bloodstein; Singular): 1995.

The Lidcombe Program of Early Stuttering Intervention: A Clinician's Guide (M. Onslow, A. Packman, & E. Harrison; Pro-Ed): 2003.

Manual of Stuttering Intervention (P.M. Zebrowski & E.M. Kelly; Singular): 2002.

Nature and Treatment of Stuttering: New Directions (R.F. Curlee & G.M. Siegal, eds.; Allyn & Bacon): 1996.

The Nature of Stuttering (Van Riper, Prentice-Hall): 1982.

Stuttering: An Integrated Approach to Its Nature and Treatment (B. Guitar; Williams & Wilkins): 1998.

Stuttering: Its Nature, Diagnosis and Treatment (E.G. Conture; Allyn & Bacon): 2001.

Stuttering and Other Fluency Disorders (F.H. Silverman; Waveland Press): 2004.

Stuttering Therapy: Rationale and Procedures (H.H. Gregory; Allyn & Bacon): 2003.

Synergistic Stuttering Therapy: A Holistic Approach (C. Bloom & D.K. Cooperman; Butterworth-Heinemann): 1999.

The Treatment of Stuttering (Van Riper, Prentice Hall): 1973.

Working with Parents of Young Children with Disabilities (E.J. Webster & L.M. Ward; Singular): 1993.

Autobiographical Books for Speech-Language Pathologists, Students, and Individuals Who Stutter

Stuttering: A Life Bound Up in Words (M. Jezer; Small Pond Press): 1998.

Living with Stuttering: Stories, Basics, Resources and Hope (K.O. St. Louis; Populore): 2001.

Books Available from the Stuttering Foundation (phone: (800) 992-9392; Web site: www.stutteringhelp.org)

The Child Who Stutters: To the Family Physician

The Child Who Stutters: To the Healthcare Provider

Effective Counseling in Stuttering Therapy

School-Age Child Who Stutters: Working Effectively with Attitudes and Emotions

Straight Talk for Teachers Resource Booklet

Stuttering: Successes and Failures in Therapy

Stuttering Therapy: Prevention and Intervention

Stuttering Therapy: Transfer and Maintenance

Stuttering Words

Therapy for Those Who Stutter

Treating the School Age Child Who Stutters: A Guide

El Niño Que Tartamudea: Para El Pediatra

Books about Childhood Stuttering (for Parents, Child, or Pediatricians)

Books Available from the Stuttering Foundation (phone: (800) 992-9392; Web site: www.stutteringhelp.org)

The Child Who Stutters: To the Pediatrician

If Your Child Stutters: A Guide for Parents

Sometimes I Just Stutter (ages 7–12)

Stuttering: Integration of Contemporary Therapies

Stuttering and Your Child: Q & A

A Veces, Yo Tartamudeo (7 a 12 anos)

La Tartamudez y Su Nino: Preguntas y Respuestas

Mon Enfant Begaie-t-il? Une Guide pour les Parents

Si Su Hijo Tartamudea: Una Guia para los Padres

Books Available from the National Stuttering Association (phone: (800) WE-STUTTER; Web site: www.westutter.org)

Jeremy & the Hippo: A Boy's Struggle with Stuttering

Our Voices: Inspirational Insights from Young People Who Stutter

Preschool Children Who Stutter

Bullying and Teasing: Helping People Who Stutter (J.S. Yaruss, B. Murphy, R.W. Quesal, N.A. Reardon; National Stuttering Association): 2004.

Books Available from Friends: The Association of Young People Who Stutter (phone: 631-499-7504 (NY) or 650-355-0215 (CA); Web site: www.friendswhostutter.org)

The Adventures of Phil Carrot

Away from the Crowd: Essays on the Stuttering Experience

Becoming a Friend: Thoughts from a Stuttering Specialist

Dead Languages

Listen with Your Heart: Reflections on Growing Up Stuttering

Books about Teenage Stuttering (for Parents and Teenagers)

Get Out of My Life, But First Could You Drive Me and Cheryl to the Mall? A Parent's Guide to the New Teenager (A.E. Wolfe; Noonday)

Books Available from the Stuttering Foundation (phone: (800) 992-9392; Web site: www.stutteringhelp.org)

Advice to Those Who Stutter

Do You Stutter: A Guide for Teens

Self-therapy for the Stutterer

A Stutterer's Story: An Autobiography

Auto-terapia para el Tartamudo

Consejos para el Tartamudo

Brochures

Brochures Available from the Stuttering Foundation (phone: (800) 992-9392; Web site: www.stutteringhelp.org)

For Speech-Language Pathologists

Classroom Presentation Packet

Cluttering: Some Guidelines

Down's Syndrome and Stuttering

Neurogenic Stuttering

Stuttering and the Bilingual Child

Brochures for All Ages

15 Famous People Who Stutter: National Stuttering Awareness Week

Did You Know...Fact Sheet

How to React When Speaking with One Who Stutters

Tourette's Syndrome and Stuttering

Como Reaccionar Delante/Persona Que Tartamudea

Brochures about Childhood Stuttering (for Parents or Child)

If You Think Your Child Is Stuttering

Notes to the Teacher: The Child Who Stutters

El Niño Que Tartamudea en la Escuela

Si Usted Cree Que Su Niño Tartamudea

Brochures about Teenage Stuttering (for Parents and Teenagers)

Stuttering: Answers for Employers

Using the Telephone: Guide for People Who Stutter

Why Speech Therapy?

Utilizando el Telefono

Brochures Available from the National Stuttering Association (phone: (800) WE-STUTTER; Web site: www.westutter.org)

18 Ways to Help Your Child Who Stutters

A Classroom Presentation about Stuttering

Being Your Own Best Advocate

Notes to Listeners

The School-Age Child Who Stutters: Information for Educators

Stuttering: So Much Can Be Done

Videos

Videos (VHS Format) Available from the Stuttering Foundation (phone: (800) 992-9392; Web site: www.stutteringhelp.org)

Videos for Speech-Language Pathologists

Note: Many of these videos are helpful for parents and teachers as well.

The Child Who Stutters: School Setting (with Barry Guitar)

Counseling: Listening To and Talking With Parents

Counseling Parents of Children who Stutter (with Patricia Zebrowski)

Making Sound Clinical Decisions (with Charles Healey)

School-Age Child/Stutters: Emotions (with Kristin Chmela)

School-Age Child/Stutters: Guilt & Shame (with Bill Murphy)

School Clinician: Ways to Be More Effective (with Peter Ramig)

Stuttering: Straight Talk for Teachers

Therapy in Action: The School-Age Child Who Stutters

Working with Teachers...for SLPs

Videos about Childhood Stuttering (for Parents or Child)

Kids for Kids

Stuttering and the Preschool Child

Stuttering and Your Child: Videotape for Parents

La Tartamudez y Su Niño: Una Guia para la Familia

Videos about Teenage Stuttering (for Parents and Teenagers)

Stuttering: Straight Talk for Teens

Web sites

Friends: The Association of Young People Who Stutter: www.friendswhostutter.org

National Stuttering Association: www.westutter.org

The Stuttering Foundation: www.stutteringhelp.org

The Stuttering Homepage: www.stutteringhomepage.com

Por favor, complete este cuestionario y tráigalo a la evaluación. Si hay preguntas que no comprende o que no se apliquen a su situación, márquelas al lado izquierdo, y podemos discutirlas cuando venga usted a su cita.

Peter R. Ramig, Ph.D., CCC-SLP
Professor and Associate Chair
Board-Recognized Fluency Specialist
Department of Speech, Language, and Hearing Sciences
University of Colorado at Boulder
Boulder, CO 80309

Fecha _____   Persona que completa este formulario _____

Relación al niño/a _____

I. IDENTIFICACIÓN

Nombre del niño/a _____ Fecha de nacimiento _____ Sexo _____ Edad _____

Domicilio _____ Ciudad _____

Estado _____ Código postal _____ Teléfono (de la casa) _____

Nombre de la madre

Domicilio _____ Ciudad _____

Estado _____ Código postal _____ Teléfono (de la casa) _____

Empleo de la madre _____ Teléfono (del trabajo) _____

Nombre del padre _____

Domicilio _____ Ciudad _____

Estado _____ Código postal _____ Teléfono (de la casa) _____

Empleo del padre _____ Teléfono (del trabajo) _____

Recomendado por _____ Teléfono _____

Médico familiar/particular _____ Teléfono _____

Pediatra del niño/a _____

Dirección _____ Ciudad _____

Estado _____ Código postal _____ Teléfono _____

II. DESCRIPCIÓN DEL PROBLEMA

Describa, de la manera más detallada posible, el problema del habla, lenguaje, y audición.

_____

_____

_____

_____

¿Cuándo se notó el problema por primera vez? _____

¿Cómo ha cambiado el problema desde que usted lo notó por primera vez? _____

_____

¿Qué se ha hecho para resolver el problema? _____

_____

¿Cuando su niño/a presenta este problema, cómo responde usted normalmente? _____

_____ ¿Esto le ha ayudado? _____

¿Qué piensa usted que causó este problema? _____

_____

¿Tiene usted algún familiar que haya tenido o que tenga problemas del habla, lenguaje, o audición?

_____

¿Su hijo/a siente que tiene problemas cuando habla? _____

¿Siente usted que su hijo/a es más sensible que otros niños de su misma edad? _____

_____

III. DESARROLLO DEL HABLA, LENGUAJE, Y AUDICIÓN

¿Cuánto balbuceó y se arrulló su hijo/a en sus primeros seis meses? _____

¿Cuándo dijo sus primeras palabras? _____ ¿Cuáles fueron? _____

_____

¿Cuántas palabras usaba su hijo/a a la edad de un año y medio? _____ ¿Cuándo empezó a usar oraciones

de dos palabras? _____

Usa su hijo/a el habla: ¿Frecuentemente? _____ ¿A veces? _____ ¿Nunca? _____

¿Hace su hijo/a muchos movimientos con las manos o gestos al hablar? (Dé ejemplos, si es posible.) _____

_____

Qué prefiere usar su hijo/a: ¿Oraciones completas? _____ ¿Frases? _____ ¿Una o dos palabras? _____

¿Sonidos _____ ¿Movimientos/Gestos? _____

¿Hace su hijo/a algunos sonidos incorrectos? _____ Si contestó sí, ¿cuáles? _____

¿Hay ocasiones en que su hijo/a titubea, se "atora," repite, o tartamudea sonidos o palabras? _____

Si contestó sí, describa lo que ocurre. _____

_____

_____

_____

Por favor marque cualquiera de las siguientes señales de peligro de tartamudeo que ha observado en su hijo/a:

SEÑAL DE PELIGRO	No Observado	A Veces Observado	Frecuentemente Observado
Repeticiones múltiples de palabras parciales — Repitiendo la primera letra o sílaba de una palabra, como "t-t-t-tabla" or "ta-ta-ta-tabla".	_____	_____	_____
Prolongación — Extendiendo un sonido, como r———atón.	_____	_____	_____
Sonido de la vocal "uh" – Por ejemplo, en vez de decir "ca-ca-ca-carro," el niño dice "cuh-cuh-cuh-carro".	_____	_____	_____
Lucha y tensión — El niño se esfuerza y lucha al intentar decir una palabra.	_____	_____	_____
Tono y volumen aumentan — Al repetir y prolongar el sonido, el tono y volumen de la voz aumentan.	_____	_____	_____
Tremores — Los labios o la lengua pueden temblar descontroladamente a la misma vez que el niño repite o prolonga sonidos o sílabas.	_____	_____	_____
Evitación — Un número inusual de pausas; sustituciones de palabras; interjecciones de palabras, sonidos o frases ajenas; evitando hablar.	_____	_____	_____
Temor — Al llegar a un sonido que le da dificultad, es posible que el niño demuestre una expresión de miedo.	_____	_____	_____
Dificultad en iniciar y/o mantener la respiración o la vocalización al hablar — Esto se oye más a menudo cuando el niño/la niña empieza a decir oraciones o frases. Su respiración puede ser irregular y su habla puede salir en episodios repentinos mientras lucha para mantener su voz.	_____	_____	_____

¿Cómo suena la voz de su hijo/a? Normal _____ Demasiado alta _____ Demasiado baja _____

Ronca _____ Nasal _____

¿Qué tan bien se le puede entender? Por parte de sus padres _____

Por sus hermanos y hermanas _____ Por sus compañeros _____

Por familiares y desconocidos _____

¿Adquirió su hijo/a el habla inicialmente y luego disminuyó su habla o dejó de hablar? _____

¿Qué tan bien entiende su hijo/a lo que se le dice? _____

¿Su niño/a oye adecuadamente? _____ ¿Su capacidad de oír parece ser constante o varía?

_____ ¿Su niño/a oye peor cuando está resfriado/tiene gripa? _____

IV. DESARROLLO EN GENERAL

A. Historial de embarazo y parto

Número total de embarazos _____ ¿Cuántos malogrados? _____

Explique:_____

_____

¿Cuál embarazo fue este niño/a? _____ Duración del embarazo _____ ¿Resultó difícil? _____

¿Qué enfermedades, malestares, y/o accidentes ocurrieron durante este embarazo? _____

¿Hubo incompatibilidad sanguínea entre la madre y el padre? _____

Edad de la madre cuando nació el niño/a _____ Edad del padre cuando nació el niño/a _____

¿Cuánto tiempo duró el parto? _____ ¿Hubo problemas al nacer (parto transverso, por cesárea, otros)? _____

Si contestó sí, describa. _____

¿Qué medicamentos se usaron? _____ ¿Fórceps altos o bajos? _____ Peso del niño al nacer _____

¿Se presentaron moretones, cicatrices, o anormalidades en la cabeza del niño?_____

¿Otras anormalidades? _____

¿El bebé necesitó oxígeno? _____ ¿Estaba el bebé azul o amarillo al nacer? _____

¿Fue necesaria una transfusión de sangre a la hora del parto? _____

¿Hubo problemas inmediatamente después del nacimiento o durante las primeras dos semanas de su vida (salud, habilidad de tragar, mamando, comiendo, durmiendo, otros)? Si contestó sí, describa._____

_____

¿A qué edad recuperó el bebé su peso inicial al nacer? _____

B. Desarrollo

¿A que edad ocurrió lo siguiente? Mantuvo cabeza erguida al estar boca abajo _____ Se volteó solo_____

Se quedó sentado sin apoyo _____ Gateó _____ Se paró _____Caminó sin apoyo_____

Se alimentó usando una cuchara _____ Le brotó el primer diente _____ Control de la vejiga _____

Control intestinal _____ Control completo de vejiga y evacuación intestinal _____ Despertar _____ Dormir _____

Se vistió y desvistió solo _____ ¿Cuál mano prefiere usar? _____ ¿Alguna vez ha cambiado su preferencia

de una mano a la otra? _____ Si contesto sí, ¿a qué edad ocurrió? _____

¿Cómo describiría usted el desarrollo físico actual de su hijo/a? _____

_____

_____

_____

Marque cada descripción que se aplique a su hijo/a:

	Sí	No	Explique: Anote edades si es posible
Lloró menos de lo normal			
Se rió menos de lo normal			
Gritó y chilló para atraer atención o demostrar molestia			
Se golpeaba la cabeza y golpeaba el suelo con los pies			
Extremadamente sensible a la vibración			
Muy alerta a gestos, expresiones faciales, o movimientos			
Arrastraba los pies al caminar			
Por lo general, indiferente a los sonidos			
No respondía cuando se le hablaba			
Respondía a ruidos (bocinas, teléfonos) pero no a voces			
Dificultad usando la lengua			
Dificultad tragando			
Hablaba por la nariz			
Respiraba por la boca			
Tenía la "lengua atada"			
Dificultad al masticar			
Babeó mucho			
Comida salía por su nariz			
Constantemente se despejaba la garganta			
Dificultad respirando			
Lengua grande			
Dificultad en mover la boca			

V. HISTORIAL MÉDICO

¿Está su hijo/a bajo el cuidado de un médico? _____ ¿Por qué? _____

¿Está tomando medicina? _____ ¿Qué tipo/dosificación? _____

¿Por qué? _____

_____

¿A qué edades ocurrieron cualquiera de las siguientes enfermedades, operaciones, o problemas? Por favor, indique la gravedad de cada situación.

	Edad	Leve	Mod.	Grave		Edad	Leve	Mod.	Grave
Adenoidectomía					Problemas cardiacos				
Alergias					Fiebre alta				
Asma					Influenza				
Enfermedad de la sangre					Mastoidectomía				
Cataratas					Viruela				
Varicela					Meningitis				
Resfriados crónicos					Paperas				
Convulsiones					Trastorno muscular				
Ojos cruzados (bizco)					Trastorno nervioso				
Crup					Ortodoncia				
Problemas dentales					Pulmonía				
Difteria					Polio				
Dolor de oído(s)					Fiebre reumática				
Infecciones de oído(s)					Escarlatina				
Encefalitis					Amigdalectomía				
Dolor de cabeza					Amigdalitis				
Lesiones a la cabeza					Tos ferina				

¿Alguna vez se ha caído el niño o recibido un golpe muy fuerte a la cabeza? _____

Si contesto sí, ¿perdió la conciencia? _____ ¿Sufrió una concusión? _____

El accidente le causó: ¿Nauseas? _____ ¿Vómitos? _____ ¿Sueño? _____ ¿Otro síntoma? _____

Describa cualquier otra enfermedad, accidente, operación, o problema grave no mencionado antes.

_____

_____

¿Cuáles enfermedades fueron acompañadas por una fiebre extremadamente alta y de larga duración? _____

_____

Temperatura (grados) _____ ¿Cuánto tiempo duró la fiebre? _____

¿Cuál de las condiciones mencionadas arriba requirió una hospitalización? _____

VI. COMPORTAMIENTO

	Sí	No	Explique: Indique edades si es posible
Problemas comiendo			
Problemas durmiendo			
Problemas para usar el baño			
Dificultad concentrándose			
Necesitó mucha disciplina			
Poco activo			
Excitable			
Se ríe fácilmente			
Lloró mucho			
Difícil de manejar/controlar			
Hiperactivo			
Sensible			
Problema de personalidad			
Se lleva bien con otros niños			
Se lleva bien con adultos			
Emocional			
Se dedica a una actividad			
Hace amigos fácilmente			
Contento			
Irritable			
Prefiere jugar solo			

VII. HISTORIAL ESCOLAR

¿Fue su hijo/a a una guardería o jardín de niños? _____ ¿Dónde? _____ Edades _____

¿A Kinder? _____ ¿Dónde? _____ ¿Edades?_____

Escuela actual _____ Ciudad _____

Año escolar actual _____ Años saltados _____ Años reprobados _____

¿Cuáles son sus calificaciones promedio? _____ ¿Mejores materias? _____ ¿Peores? _____

¿Cómo disciplina usted a su hijo/a? _____

¿Cuáles son las diversiones o los pasatiempos favoritos de su hijo/a? _____

¿Su hijo/a se ausenta de la escuela muchos días? _____ ¿Por qué? _____
_____

¿Qué piensa su hijo/a de la escuela y sus maestros? _____
_____

¿Qué impresión tiene usted de las habilidades de aprendizaje de su hijo/a? _____
_____

Describa los servicios del habla, lenguaje, y audición; psicología; o enseñanza especial que haya recibido
su hijo/a e indique dónde fueron obtenidos. ¿Con qué frecuencia recibió su hijo/a estos servicios? _____
_____
_____

VIII. INFORMACIÓN SOBRE HOGAR Y FAMILIA

Último año escolar que completó el padre _____ Título(s) _____

Último año escolar que completó la madre _____ Título(s) _____

¿Están los padres divorciados? _____ ¿Separados? _____ ¿Viven ambos padres juntos? _____

Hermanos y hermanas:

Nombre	Edad	Sexo	Año escolar	Problema médico del habla o audición (si hay alguno)

¿Se habla más de un idioma en casa? _____ ¿Cuáles? _____

¿Quiénes los hablan y con qué frecuencia? _____

Por favor agregue cualquier información adicional que piense usted que nos ayudaría a entender a su hijo/a y su problema _____

_____

_____

_____

_____

_____

_____

¿Cuáles son sus sentimientos en cuanto al problema de su hijo/a?_____

_____

_____

_____

_____

_____

_____

¿Cómo quisiera que nosotros le ayudemos?_____

_____

_____

_____

_____

_____

_____

Las siguientes preguntas se proponen como sugerencias para diseñar una sesión de entrevista respecto a un niño en particular. Están organizadas según los varios tipos de información que usted necesitará obtener para efectuar una evaluación completa.

Peter R. Ramig, Ph.D., CCC-SLP
Professor and Associate Chair
Board-Recognized Fluency Specialist
Department of Speech, Language, and Hearing Sciences
University of Colorado at Boulder
Boulder, CO 80309

Darrell M. Dodge, M.A. CCC-SLP
Peter R. Ramig, Ph.D. and Associates
Associated Stuttering Treatment Clinics
6436 South Quebec Street, Building 6, Suite 400
Greenwood Village, CO 80111

Motivación

• ¿Por qué vinieron aquí hoy?

_____

_____

• ¿Qué quisieran aprender hoy?

_____

_____

• ¿Qué quisieran recordar después de esta cita?

_____

_____

• ¿Qué aspecto del habla de su hijo/a les preocupa más?

_____

_____

Antecedentes Familiares

• ¿Alguna vez tuvo usted o su esposo/esposa problemas con el habla o lenguaje? Si tuvo algún problema, por favor descríbalo y explique qué (si se hizo algo) se hizo para ayudar a corregir el problema.

_____

_____

• ¿Saben de algún familiar que haya tenido problemas con el habla y/o lenguaje? Si la respuesta es sí:

▪ ¿Quién era?

_____

_____

▪ ¿Es del lado paterno, materno, etc.?

_____

_____

• ¿Cuál fue la naturaleza del problema?

_____

_____

• ¿Recibió tratamiento?

_____

_____

• ¿Cuáles fueron los resultados?

_____

_____

• ¿Alguna vez notaron el mismo comportamiento en sus otros hijos? ¿En los hijos de sus familiares? ¿En los hijos de sus vecinos?

_____

_____

Características del Tartamudeo Actual

• Describan las faltas de fluidez de su hijo/a. Por favor traten de dar ejemplos.

_____

_____

• ¿Hay algunos sonidos en particular que le presentan más dificultad a su hijo/a que a otros?

_____

_____

• ¿Es igual el habla de su hijo/a en cualquier situación?

_____

_____

• ¿Cómo es el habla de su hijo/a en la escuela?

_____

_____

- ¿Habla con mayor fluidez algunas veces? ¿En cuáles situaciones?

_____

_____

- ¿Algunas veces habla con menor fluidez de lo normal?

_____

_____

- ¿Habla con menor fluidez con ciertas personas?

_____

_____

- ¿Su hijo/a tiene dificultades diciendo o pronunciando algunas palabras o sonidos? ¿Cuáles son esos sonidos específicos?

_____

_____

- ¿Qué tan bien pueden entender a su hijo/a cuando habla?

_____

_____

- Si consideran cómo habla su hijo/a normalmente, ¿cómo describirían ustedes su habla en este momento? ¿Dirían que es semejante a la manera en que habla normalmente?

_____

_____

Curso de Desarrollo

- ¿Cuándo empezó el problema del habla de su hijo/a?

_____

_____

- ¿Quién notó el problema por primera vez? ¿Bajo qué circunstancias?

_____

_____

- ¿Estuvieron preocupados por ese problema al principio?

_____

_____

• ¿Qué hicieron para intentar resolver el problema al principio?

_____

_____

• ¿Llamaron la atención de su hijo/a al problema? ¿Cómo llamaron la atención de su hijo/a al problema? ¿Cómo reaccionó él/ella?

_____

_____

• ¿Qué nombre le dieron al problema? (por ejemplo, tartamudeo, habla con dificultad, se atora, etc.)

_____

_____

• ¿Cuándo empezaron a usar la palabra "tartamudeo"? Si no usaron este término, ¿lo usó alguien?

_____

_____

• Desde que empezaron los problemas, ¿sigue igual el habla de su hijo/a?

_____

_____

• Si ha cambiado, por favor descríbalo. ¿Puede dar ejemplos? (Explore los cambios en el tipo de desfluidez, duración, frecuencia, movimientos del cuerpo, miradas a los ojos, etc.)

_____

_____

• ¿Ha tenido su hijo/a terapia del habla o algún tipo de consejo? Si la respuesta es sí,

   ▪ ¿Dónde?

_____

_____

   ▪ ¿Qué tipo?

_____

_____

   ▪ ¿Cuándo?

_____

_____

- ¿Por cuánto tiempo?

_____

_____

- ¿Con qué resultados?

_____

_____

- ¿Por qué terminó la terapia?

_____

_____

Habilidades y Manera de Comunicación

- ¿Ustedes consideran que su hijo/a comunica bien o no tan bien sus necesidades y deseos?

_____

_____

- ¿A su hijo/a le gusta hablar?

_____

_____

- ¿Usa su hijo/a otros métodos de comunicación, como escribir o dibujar, para indicar lo que necesita o para comunicar información?

_____

_____

- ¿Consideran ustedes que su hijo/a escucha bien?

_____

_____

- ¿Parece su hijo/a tener alguna dificultad entendiendo lo que otras personas están diciendo? Si la respuesta es sí, ¿consideran ustedes que es un problema?

_____

_____

- Por lo general, ¿cómo se comporta su hijo/a en una situación social?

_____

_____

- ¿Hay ciertas veces cuando parece más probable que su hijo/a se comunique con alguien o cuando tenga más ganas de hablar?

  _____

  _____

- ¿Con quién habla el niño/la niña más? ¿Menos? ¿Por qué piensa que es así?

  _____

  _____

Grado de Conciencia, Discapacidad, o Ajuste

- ¿Cómo reacciona su hijo/a frente a la eficiencia de su habla?

  _____

  _____

- ¿Está consciente del efecto de su habla?

  _____

  _____

- ¿Demuestra su hijo/a vergüenza, pena, o frustración al hablar?

  _____

  _____

- ¿Hay ocasiones en que parece luchar o se vuelve muy tenso/a cuando trata de decir alguna palabra?

  _____

  _____

- ¿Trata de mejorar su habla? ¿Con qué resultados?

  _____

  _____

- ¿Parece su hijo/a evitar algunas situaciones para no tener que hablar?

  _____

  _____

Influencias Ambientales

• ¿Cuál es el ambiente general y el ritmo del ambiente hogareño?

_____

_____

• ¿Hay tensión o conflicto en casa? Si la respuesta es sí, por favor, describan.

_____

_____

• ¿Han aumentado las desfluideces de su hijo/a alguna vez durante momentos de tensión o conflicto en casa? Si la respuesta es sí, por favor, describan.

_____

_____

• ¿Qué tipo de experiencias ha tenido su hijo/a al tratar de comunicarse?

_____

_____

   ▪ ¿Responden o no responden la mayoría de las personas que lo/la escuchan?

_____

_____

   ▪ ¿Le dan las personas suficiente tiempo para hablar?

_____

_____

   ▪ ¿Lo interrumpen a menudo?

_____

_____

   ▪ ¿A menudo le dicen que se calle?

_____

_____

   ▪ ¿Le piden que explique su comportamiento?

_____

_____

- ¿Cómo se lleva su hijo/a con sus hermanos/as? ¿Hay hostilidad, celos, o rivalidad?

_____

_____

- ¿Cómo manejan usted y su esposo/esposa desacuerdos entre sus hijos?

_____

_____

- ¿En la escuela han notado el problema del habla de su hijo?

_____

_____

- Si la respuesta es sí, ¿cuándo, y qué hicieron?

_____

_____

- ¿Cuáles son las actitudes y reacciones de los maestros hacia el problema del habla de su hijo/a?

_____

_____

- ¿Cómo se ha adaptado su hijo/a a la escuela en general?

_____

_____

- ¿Tiene su hijo/a cualquier otro problema en la escuela? Si la respuesta es sí, explique.

_____

_____

- ¿Aumentaron las desfluideces de su hijo/a o disminuyeron cuando empezó a ir a la escuela? ¿Cómo cambiaron?

_____

_____

- ¿Cómo reaccionan otros (niños, amigos, familiares, desconocidos, etc.) a las desfluideces de su hijo?

_____

_____

- ¿Se burlan de él/ella? _____

_____

• ¿Lo/La critican?

_____

_____

• ¿Cómo reacciona a las burlas y/o críticas?

_____

_____

Relación entre Padres e Hijo/a

• ¿Cuánto hablan ustedes con su hijo/a? ¿Cuánto habla, lee, o juega cada padre individualmente con su hijo/a?

_____

_____

• ¿Cuánta atención requiere su hijo/a de ustedes?

_____

_____

▪ ¿Más que sus otros hijos?

_____

_____

▪ ¿Más de un padre que del otro?

_____

_____

• ¿Su hijo/a generalmente hace lo que le piden y acaba sus quehaceres?

_____

_____

• ¿Cómo disciplinan a su hijo/a? ¿Cómo reacciona?

_____

_____

• ¿Hace su hijo/a algo en particular que los irrita?

_____

_____

- ¿Por qué los irrita?

  _____

  _____

- ¿Cómo han intentado resolver este problema?

  _____

  _____

- ¿Cómo reaccionan a las desfluideces de su hijo/a?

  _____

  _____

- ¿Prestan atención o no cuando tartamudea?

  _____

  _____

- ¿Voltean la cara, hacen gestos, interrumpen, lo/la castigan, o hablan por él/ella?

  _____

  _____

- ¿Cómo reaccionan cuando su hijo/a habla con otra gente?

  _____

  _____

- ¿Qué han hecho para ayudar a su hijo/a a dejar de tartamudear?

  _____

  _____

- ¿Ayudó lo que intentaron?

  _____

  _____

- ¿Qué ha ayudado más? ¿Menos?

  _____

  _____

- ¿Quién recomendó esta ayuda?

  _____

• ¿Por qué lo hicieron?

_____

_____

• ¿Cómo reacciona su hijo/a a su ayuda?

_____

_____

• ¿Qué aspiraciones y expectativas tienen para su hijo/a?

_____

_____

• ¿Si les dieran tres deseos para su hijo/a (sin límite) cuáles serían?

_____

_____

Habilidades, Intereses, y Sitio de Control

• ¿Cuáles son los intereses y pasatiempos de su hijo/a? ¿Qué le gusta más? ¿Menos?

_____

_____

• ¿Qué tan bien se acomoda su hijo/a a nuevas situaciones, nuevos ambientes, o cambios en rutina?

_____

_____

• ¿Cuál es su impresión de la habilidad de su hijo/a para aprender?

_____

_____

• ¿Tiene su hijo/a algunos temores o antipatías fuertes?

_____

_____

• ¿Usa su hijo/a la mano izquierda o la derecha? ¿Alguna vez se cambió esta preferencia a propósito, por cualquier razón?

_____

_____

Preguntas de Entrevista Recomendadas para Niños Mayores

Si el niño/la niña es mayor y obviamente está consciente hasta cierto punto de su problema del habla, el terapeuta tal vez pueda decidir formular unas preguntas directamente al niño/la niña respecto a su conciencia de, y reacciones a, su problema de tartamudeo. Por ejemplo:

• ¿Sabes por qué estás aquí hoy?

_____

_____

• ¿Qué cosas parecen hacer tu habla peor (más difícil)?

_____

_____

• ¿Qué cosas parecen hacer tu habla mejor (más fácil)?

_____

_____

• ¿Cómo sientes que está tu habla cuando hablas con tus padres o en casa?

_____

_____

• ¿Qué le dices a tu mamá, papá, hermano, hermana, etc., sobre tu habla?

_____

_____

• ¿Cómo te va en la escuela? ¿Te gusta la escuela?

_____

_____

• ¿Cómo sientes que está tu habla en la escuela?

_____

_____

• ¿Qué piensan tus maestros de tu habla? ¿Cómo reaccionan a tu habla?

_____

_____

• ¿Qué piensan tus amigos en la escuela de tu habla? ¿Cómo reaccionan a tu habla?

_____

- ¿Alguna vez se te pide que hagas reportes orales en clase, o que leas en voz alta? ¿Cómo sientes que está tu habla en esas ocasiones?

  _____

  _____

- ¿Alguna vez ha tratado alguien de ayudarte a hablar?

  _____

  _____

- ¿Usas la mano derecha, la izquierda o ambas? ¿Alguna vez has tratado alguien de cambiar la mano que usas para hacer algo?

  _____

  _____

- ¿Cómo es tu habla cuando:

  - Hablas en clase?

    _____

    _____

  - Hablas con personas que no conoces?

    _____

    _____

  - Hablas con amigos?

    _____

    _____

  - Hablas con muchachos?

    _____

    _____

  - Hablas con muchachas?

    _____

    _____

  - Hablas con maestros?

    _____

    _____

- Hablas con personas mayores?

  _____

  _____

- Hablas con personas menores?

  _____

  _____

- Hablas por teléfono (cuando tú haces la llamada)?

  _____

  _____

- Hablas por teléfono (cuando alguien te llama)?

  _____

  _____

- ¿Hay otras veces cuando tienes dificultades, como:
  - Cuando estás enojado/a?

    _____

    _____

  - Cuando estás contento/a?

    _____

    _____

  - Cuando estás triste?

    _____

    _____

  - Cuando estás emocionado/a?

    _____

    _____

- ¿Cuándo notaste tu problema del habla por primera vez?

  _____

  _____

• ¿Alguna vez te lo mencionó alguien o te llamó la atención?

_____

_____

• ¿Han tratado tus padres de ayudarte? Si trataron, ¿cómo te sentiste? ¿Te ayudó?

_____

_____

• ¿Has recibido ayuda especial con tu habla de algún maestro o maestra?

_____

_____

• ¿Qué hiciste en la clase de terapia del habla?

_____

_____

• ¿Crees que esa clase te ayudó?

_____

_____

• ¿Hay ciertos sonidos que te dan dificultad? ¿Cuáles son?

_____

_____

• ¿Sabes que vas a tener dificultades antes de que las tengas de verdad?

_____

_____

• ¿Alguna vez has evitado hablar?

_____

_____

• ¿A veces hablas más despacio cuando empiezas a tener problemas?

_____

_____

• ¿A veces respiras profundamente para ayudarte a hablar mejor?

_____

• ¿Has intentado murmullar o hablar quedito? ¿Te pareció que eso te ayudó?

_____

_____

• ¿A veces cambias una palabra o quitas una palabra difícil?

_____

_____

• ¿Qué esperas sacar de la clase del habla/cómo piensas que la clase de terapia del habla te va a ayudar?

_____

_____

• ¿Piensas que tienes ganas de trabajar duro para mejorar tu habla?

_____

_____

Darrell M. Dodge, M.A. CCC-SLP
Peter R. Ramig, Ph.D. and Associates
Associated Stuttering Treatment Clinics
6436 South Quebec Street, Building 6, Suite 400
Greenwood Village, CO 80111

XII Hipoglosal	**Alcance de Movimiento** __ Sacar la lengua hasta posición medial __ Extender las mejillas de los dos lados usando la lengua __ Abrir la boca y levantar la lengua al paladar = verificar simetría **Fuerza** __ Empujar el depresor de lengua hacia adelante con la lengua __ Empujar el depresor de lengua a cada lado usando la lengua __ Empujar el depresor de lengua hacia el paladar (sujetar la barbilla) **Rapidez** __ /pa/ __ /ta/ __ /ka/ __ /pa-ta/ __ /pa-ta-ka/ decir rápidamente = evaluar rapidez y precisión	
XI Accesorio	__ Levantar los hombros y tratar de bajarlos empujando con las manos = determinar fuerza y simetría	
X Nervios Vagos	__ Cubrir la boca y toser = claridad/nitidez __ Abrir la boca y decir "ahh" = determinar la elevación del velo del paladar __ Decir /mmm/ = verificar para emisión nasal usando un espejo __ Decir /sss/ = verificar para emisión nasal	
IX Glosofaríngeo	__ Subjetivo = voz mojada, ronca, o queja de ahogo __ Objetivo = elicitar reflejo de arqueada (nausea) bilateral	
VIII Vestibulococlear	__ Examen de dedos frotando (*finger rub test*) = verificar lateralización	
VII Facial	__ Sonrisa grande = verificar simetría __ Decir "oooh" = verificar aprieto de labios __ Cerrar dientes, cerrar labios; tratar de abrir labios con los dedos = verificar la fuerza de labios en ambos lados __ Cerrar los ojos fuertemente; tratar de abrir con los dedos = verificar cerradura de ojos de ambos lados __ Levantar cejas = verificar simetría	
V Trigeminal	__ Apretar los dientes/Morder duro = para sentir la contracción del masetero __ Resistir el abrir y cerrar de mandíbula (sujetar frente y barbilla) = verificar simetría	
VI Abducens III Oculomotor	__ Habilidad de seguir visualmente el movimiento de un dedo de lado a lado	
IV Troclear	__ Habilidad de seguir visualmente el dedo en cada uno de los cuatro cuadrantes visuales (arriba a lado derecho, arriba a lado izquierdo, debajo a lado derecho, debajo a lado izquierdo) __ Visualmente seguir el dedo hacia la nariz	
II Óptico/I Olfatorio	__ Subjetivo = preguntar acerca de visión y sentido de olfato	

Handout D:
RESULTADOS DE LA EVALUACIÓN DE LA FLUIDEZ

Intenta que ese formulario sea llenado por el/la terapeuta.

Darrell M. Dodge, M.A. CCC-SLP
Peter R. Ramig, Ph.D. and Associates
Associated Stuttering Treatment Clinics
6436 South Quebec Street, Building 6, Suite 400
Greenwood Village, CO 80111

Terapeuta _____ Fecha _____

Nombre _____

Edad _____ Año _____ Mes fecha de nacimiento _____ Año escolar _____

Escuela _____

Maestra/o _____

Terapeuta del habla/lenguaje o consejero _____

Padres/personas encargadas _____

Hermanos/as (edades) _____(__) _____(__) _____ (__) _____

_____(__) _____(__) _____ (__) _____

Diagnóstico previo _____

_____

_____

_____

Realizado por _____ Fecha _____

RESULTADOS DE LA EVALUACIÓN:

1. _____Articulación

_____ Dentro del rango normal

_____Errores aceptables para la edad _____

_____Atraso en el desarrollo de los siguientes sonidos _____

Inteligibilidad _____ Pobre _____ Regular _____ Buena _____ Excelente

2. Voz   _____ Normal   _____ Suave

_____ Ronca   _____ Alta/Baja

_____ Velada   _____ Infantil

3. Periférico oral   _____ No hay anormalidades estructurales; movimiento normal

_____ Anomalías estructurales: _____

_____ /pa^ ta^ ka^/ _____ Normal, rítmico

_____ Disrítmico

_____ Patrón rítmico anormal

_____ Dificultad en iniciar flujo de aire o sonorizando

_____ No pudo hacerlo o rechazó hacerlo

4. Pruebas del lenguaje administradas _____

_____

_____

_____ Lenguaje expresivo apropiado para la edad

_____ Lenguaje receptivo apropiado para la edad

_____ Otros asuntos: _____

_____

_____

5. Fluidez

A. Señales de peligro de tartamudeo observadas

_____ Múltiples repeticiones de porciones de palabras   Número promedio _____

_____ Vocal "uh"

_____ Prolongaciones   Duración promedio _____

_____ Elevación de tono o volumen

_____ Iniciaciones difíciles

_____ Bloqueos silenciosos   Duración promedio _____

_____ Bloqueos a mitad de la palabra

_____ Distorsiones _____

_____ Lucha y tensión en:

_____ la boca

_____ los ojos

_____ el cuerpo

_____ Estrategias usadas para evitar desfluidez:

_____

_____

_____ Dificultad en iniciar flujo de aire/sonorizando

_____ Consistencia fonémica (sonidos): _____

_____ Temor obvio o anticipación

_____ Tremores: _____ clónicos _____ tónicos

B. Características secundarias

_____ desvía los ojos _____

_____ cierra los ojos o parpadea _____

_____ mueve la cabeza _____

_____ mueve mano, brazo o cuerpo _____

_____ hace interjecciones verbales _____

_____ hace revisiones _____

_____ deja de hablar _____

_____ inhalación audible _____

_____ exhalación audible _____

_____ conocimiento obvio _____

_____ respuesta obvia al tartamudeo _____

_____ mantiene una postura silenciosa

_____ otra

6. Respuesta a terapia de prueba

Promulgación de fluidez

(_____ comienzos suaves, _____ sonorización continua, _____ otra: _____)

_____

_____

Modificación de tartamudeo

(_____ extensiones de sonidos iniciales _____ otras: _____)

_____

_____

Reacción auditiva retrasada (*delayed auditory feedback* [DAF])

(Retraso: _____ m.s.)

_____

_____

7. Observaciones de persona encargada:

_____
_____
_____
_____
_____
_____
_____
_____
_____
_____
_____
_____
_____
_____
_____

8. Comentarios del terapeuta:

_____
_____
_____
_____
_____
_____
_____
_____
_____
_____
_____
_____
_____
_____
_____
_____

Peter R. Ramig, Ph.D., CCC-SLP
Professor and Associate Chair
Board-Recognized Fluency Specialist
Department of Speech, Language, and Hearing Sciences
University of Colorado at Boulder
Boulder, CO 80309

Las páginas siguientes contienen direcciones, sugerencias, e información general para padres u otros adultos importantes (por ejemplo, personas encargadas del cuidado de niños) que tienen o conocen a un niño que repite, bloquea, o pausa cuando habla.

Aprender a hablar es una habilidad extremadamente compleja. Como resultado, los niños repiten sonidos y palabras, hacen pausas, y se "atoran" durante la primera etapa de desarrollo del habla y lenguaje. Para la mayoría de niños, estos "errores" sólo forman parte de desfluideces normales. Para algunos niños, sin embargo, pueden constituir las señales principales del tartamudeo. A continuación aparece una lista de señales de peligro o advertencia para las cuales usted tiene que estar alerta respecto al habla de cualquier niño. Estas señales pueden ocurrir al azar; sin embargo, si una o más aparecen con frecuencia, se recomienda llamárselo a la atención de un patólogo del habla y lenguaje.

Señales de Peligro o Advertencia de Tartamudeo

(Adaptación de *If your child stutters: A guide for parents (Si su hijo tartamudea: Una guía para padres)*, Stuttering Foundation Publication No. 11)

Repeticiones Múltiples de Porciones de Palabras
Repitiendo los primeros sonidos de una palabra, como "ta-ta-ta-ta-tabla" más de una o dos veces, más rápido de lo normal o con ritmo irregular. Aunque éstas se han distinguido a menudo de repeticiones de palabras completas, repeticiones de palabras cortas como "yo" o "y" o "mi" también se deben notar. Estos pueden constituir comportamientos que se manifiestan cuando la persona teme o anticipa ciertas palabras o sonidos que ocurren más tarde en la expresión.

Prolongaciones
Extendiendo un sonido al principio, o (particularmente) dentro, de una palabra, como "rrrrrrrrratón" o "raaaaaa—tón". Es importante distinguir extensiones fáciles (que podrán ser asociadas con terapia previa o—menos probable—pueden representar un mecanismo autocalmante) de prolongaciones asociadas con tensión o lucha.

Bloqueo
Un bloqueo ocurre cuando la persona para o se atora antes de, o durante, la producción de un sonido o de una palabra. Pueden anticiparse los bloqueos al momento en que la persona vaya a decir una palabra determinada, o pueden usarse para extinguir el sistema en un esfuerzo para llamar menos atención al momento de tartamudear.

Lucha y Tensión
Una tensión muscular más elevada en los órganos de articulación acompaña el tartamudeo que se ha desarrollado, indicando que algún tipo de intervención es necesario. Para superar esta tensión, el niño usa sus músculos así como otros grupos de músculos para tratar de superar la sensación de bloqueo. Al final, estas reacciones pueden producirse de manera condicionada (al identificarse con la sensación original de bloqueo), y resultan en la utilización de aún más músculos. Pueden notarse rasgos de lucha y tensión en la nariz, mandíbula, cuello, mejillas, labios, frente, y pecho. Al tener este tipo de evidencia, el terapeuta puede preguntarse si esto también existe en otras áreas del cuerpo que no se puedan ver.

Tono y Volumen Aumentan

Estos fenómenos ocurren frecuentemente cuando hay prolongación de sonidos, cuando el niño está luchando para liberarse de un bloqueo y necesita decir el siguiente sonido. El niño puede anticipar o sentir que va a tener dificultades con ese sonido y usa el aumento de tono o volumen como una manera de forzar las palabras cuando siente que va a ocurrir un bloqueo.

Tremores

Tremores de la mandíbula, labios y lengua mientras habla la persona, con o sin desfluideces, deben notarse. Las observaciones hechas ayudarán a identificar la posición de la tensión asociada con el tartamudeo. La mayoría de los terapeutas consideran que los tremores forman parte de un mecanismo avanzado para ayudar a evitar el tartamudeo.

Prevención de Situaciones que Requieran el Uso del Habla, Palabras, o Sonidos

Si el niño tiene pocas ganas de participar en actividades que requieren que hable, no quiere decir necesariamente que las esté evitando porque tiene un problema de tartamudeo. Puede que existan otros indicios que el niño está evitando situaciones en que tendría que hablar. Por ejemplo, el querer cambiar actividades continuamente para evitar aquellas situaciones en que se manifestarían desfluideces, o bien el querer posponer actividades comportándose mal o creando distracciones.

Pausas, Sonidos Adicionales, Palabras Interpuestas, Así Como Palabras o Frases Repetidas

Estas características del habla pueden indicar que el niño está tratando de posponer el hablar para evitar de tartamudear o que está esperando hasta sentir que puede decir una palabra con mayor fluidez. Sustituciones de palabras, silencios, dejar de hablar para participar en otra actividad o cambiar de tema son señales directas para evitar el tartamudeo.

Respiración Alterada o Irregular

Al anticipar que va a tartamudear, el niño puede retener su respiración, tomar varias inhalaciones y/o demostrar otras formas de respiración erráticas o irregulares, como tratar de decir muchas palabras rápidamente con cada grupo de respiraciones, etc.

Movimiento de Otras Partes del Cuerpo

Cuando el niño se enfrenta con una o más de las señales de peligro mencionadas antes (1, 2, o 3), puede observarse que mueve la cabeza para adelante o para atrás, mueve un brazo, una pierna o una mano; o puede adaptar otras reacciones poco comunes cuando piense que va a tartamudear.

Temor de Hablar

Cuando se observan una o más de estas reacciones, eso puede indicar que el niño tiene miedo de hablar. El terapeuta debe distinguir entre ansiedad común asociada con el hablar y comportamientos que verdaderamente indican el tartamudeo.

Comportamientos Adicionales

Estos comportamientos se manifiestan como señales de anticipación (pero no son en sí indicaciones de tartamudeo). Por ejemplo, pueden incluir comienzos difíciles de fonación, respiración poco profunda o irregular (jadeando o tragando) durante la vocalización, calidad de voz aberrante (como excesivo murmullo vocal) y fonación disrítmica durante la producción de sonidos prolongados. También se debe notar la consistencia fonémica de las desfluideces; por ejemplo, una tendencia de bloqueo cuando se dicen palabras que tienen uno o más sonidos como /s/, /f/, /b/ o /d/ o en vocales, sonidos sonorizados o sonidos no sonorizados exclusivamente.

Algunos Hechos Importantes Respecto al Tartamudeo

Con bastante frecuencia escuchamos varias ideas falsas respecto a lo que causa el tartamudeo en los niños. Los expertos en el área del tartamudeo reconocen muy abiertamente que las causas del tartamudeo se desconocen realmente por su naturaleza, que es multidimensional. La mayor parte de las investigaciones recientes indican que se debe a una debilidad en el sistema neurofísico o neuromuscular. Hay muy pocos especialistas en el área del tartamudeo que piensan que el tartamudeo se debe a causas totalmente psicológicas. Sin embargo, cabe poca duda que el estrés que provocan las emociones de vergüenza, inadecuación, humillación o frustración causadas por el tartamudeo también puede aumentar o mantenerse. No hay ninguna evidencia reconocida que implique a los padres como una causa principal del tartamudeo.

El tartamudeo puede volverse un problema vergonzoso y frustrante para el niño y puede influenciar el comportamiento y logros académicos, así como causar problemas de autoestima y confianza en sí mismo.

El tartamudeo se puede modificar y, en algunos casos, puede eliminarse en niños pequeños si se solicita ayuda profesional antes que se desarrollen lucha y tensión excesivas.

Escuchamos frecuentemente que los niños que tartamudean no deben ser inscritos en programas de tratamiento porque "con el tiempo lo superarán". ¿Es acaso verdad? Algunos niños muy pequeños que tartamudean (3½ años de edad o menos) sí parecen superarlo al crecer: sin embargo, un número significativo no lo hacen, y muchos menos pierden el tartamudeo al cumplir los 5 años.

Características que Se Observan en Niños con Desfluideces

1. El niño puede demostrar comportamientos inadecuados cuando debe prestar atención, incluso hiperactividad, distractibilidad y dificultad en poner atención a diferentes tareas.

2. El niño puede tener dificultades orales-motóricas, lo cual puede notarse en la falta de articulación apropiada de sonidos y/o la incapacidad de

coordinar movimientos rápidos entre labios y lengua.

3. El niño puede demostrar tendencias perfeccionistas, y pueda parecer excepcionalmente sensible a cambios en el ambiente interrupciones.

Algunas Características del Comienzo del Tartamudeo

1. Algunos niños pueden demostrar desfluideces o tartamudeo tan pronto como empiezan a combinar palabras, pero la mayoría no empiezan a manifestarlo hasta aproximadamente un año más tarde.

2. A menudo el tartamudeo se manifiesta de manera gradual y puede avanzar episódicamente, así como oscilar en el grado de severidad según distintas tareas que requieren comunicación oral y periodos de tiempo.

3. Unos de los tipos más comunes de falta de fluidez que ocurren en el tartamudeo inicial son repeticiones de sílabas en palabras iniciales de una expresión.

Sugerencias para Hablar e Interactuar con Niños Pequeños con Desfluidez

1. Hable despacio. Use los nombres apropiados para objetos y eventos. Use oraciones y vocabulario apropiados a la edad de su hijo/a. Esto es importante para que no se frustre el niño porque no puede repetir o imitar palabras, frases, u oraciones más complejas.

2. Empezando a muy temprana edad, trate de relacionar el hablar con actividades placenteras. Use una voz agradable cuando hable. Por ejemplo, cuando arrulla o carga a su hijo/a, hable de actividades o eventos agradables que suceden diariamente.

3. Hable de personas, objetos y eventos que tienen un significado especial para su hijo/a.

4. Trate de fomentar una conversación espontánea con su hijo/a esperando (silenciosamente) que él/ella inicie la conversación mientras esté

jugando. Refuerce las respuestas de su hijo/a con sonrisas y alientos.

5. Proporcione una variedad de experiencias que sean divertidas para estimular el lenguaje de su hijo/a. Por ejemplo, éstas pueden ser juegos mecánicos, excursiones al zoológico, museo, circo, etc. Hable con su hijo/a acerca de cada experiencia.

6. Léale a su hijo/a de manera calmada, tal vez un poco más despacio de lo normal y con un ritmo natural. Después de haber leído un cuento, hable de lo que pasó. Permítale que termine cuentos que conoce o que los cuente usando sus propias palabras. Permita que hable tanto como quiera. Cuéntele cosas sobre su propia vida o la de su niño/a cuando era pequeño/a. Retratos pueden ayudar en la realización de esta actividad. Evite historias que produzcan miedo, aunque le parezcan gustar.

7. Ayude a su hijo/a a expresar sus emociones, usando medios verbales o no verbales, demostrándole esas reacciones usted mismo.

8. Escuche a su hijo/a cuando expresa ira, enojo o frustración. Discuta lo que causó estas emociones.

9. Preste atención a la manera en que se comunica en áreas que son de tipo verbal: ¿Le está preguntando algo porque realmente quiere saber la respuesta, o está llamando su atención?

10. Tome en cuenta la manera en la que se siente su hijo/a. Ningún niño o adulto desea ser ridiculizado porque habla de una manera distinta, o que frecuentemente se les diga "no" o ser regañado por haber hecho algo que realmente no significa mucho. A continuación hay sugerencias que pueden ayudarle a su hijo/a a manejar sus emociones:
   a. Puede escucharlo silenciosamente y con atención.
   b. Puede reconocer sus emociones usando unas palabras como "Ajá", "Mmm", "Entiendo".
   c. Puede calificar sus sentimientos. "Eso parece muy frustrante".
   d. Puede formular los deseos que tiene su hijo/a en fantasía. "¡Ojalá que pudiera hacer que el tiempo frío desapareciera para tu bien ahora mismo!"
(Referido en Faber y Mazlish, 1980.

11. Cuando le hace una pregunta a su hijo/a, use preguntas "cerradas", como "¿Tuviste un buen día en la escuela hoy?" "¿Qué hiciste que te gustó más?" Es más probable que este tipo de preguntas resulte en respuestas cortas y sencillas. Respuestas cortas y sencillas son preferibles en días en los cuales su hijo/a se expresa particularmente con falta de fluidez.

12. Cuando su hijo/a quiere hablarle, y usted está ocupado/a con algo, deje lo que está haciendo si puede, y diríjale su atención completa. Si no lo puede hacer:
   a. Dígale que lo escuchará tan pronto como termine lo que está haciendo.
   b. Trate de encontrar una manera apropiada de parar lo que está haciendo para que su hijo/a no tenga que esperar más de 1 ó 2 minutos.
   c. Provea su atención completa tanto como le sea posible.
   d. Si su niño/a empieza a llorar, gritar o a enfadarse, explíquele que lo escuchará en un momento, pero trate de no involucrarse en una discusión.
   e. Trate de no prestarle más atención a su hijo/a cuando tiene desfluideces en comparación de ocasiones cuando habla con mayor fluidez. La cantidad de tiempo que debe esperar puede depender de lo que usted esté haciendo, pero no de la fluidez de su hijo/a.
   f. Cuando usted esté listo/a para escuchar a su hijo/a, siéntese con él/ella para que tengan contacto directo ojo a ojo.

13. Todos deben tomar turnos para hablar.
   a. Si su hijo/a interrumpe a alguien que esté hablando, se le puede decir: "Cuando ____ acabe de hablar, va a ser tu turno, y nadie te va a interrumpir." Esto se debe aplicar a todos los miembros (niños y adultos) de la familia.
   b. Sugerimos minimizar las interrupciones de su hijo/a.
   c. Pueden practicar tomando el papel de interrumpir y tomando turnos; a la persona que interrumpa se le pide que espere.
   d. Si el turno de hablar de una persona determinada toma demasiado tiempo, dígale que ahora le toca a otra persona y que tendrá tiempo de hablar otra vez más tarde.

14. Si es posible, evite usar la palabra "tartamudeo" para describir el habla de su hijo/a cuando habla con él/ella. En vez de esto, use palabras descriptivas que demuestren que reconoce sus dificultades, y pueden ser palabras como: "se atora" "habla de manera irregular", "habla con mucho esfuerzo", etc. Sin embargo, si su hijo/a está consciente de sus desfluideces y se refiere casualmente a ellas usando términos como tartamudeo, no sería natural que otros miembros de la familia evitaran usar esa palabra.

15. No exija que su hijo/a haga presentaciones en frente de otras personas (pedirle que recite el alfabeto, poemas, etc.). Si él/ella quiere hacerlo e inicia esa actividad, entonces está bien.

16. Evite preguntas o interrogaciones extensas.

17. No espere a que su hijo/a hable mucho cuando le falte fluidez.

18. Después de haber dicho algo en que le falte fluidez, se recomienda que repita para su hijo/a el contenido de lo que acaba de decir. Esto le ayudará a olvidar lo que significa la falta de fluidez. Además le está demostrando a su hijo/a que lo está escuchando. (Niño: "Yo fui Yo-Yo-Yo-Yo fui de compras con t-t-t-tía Mari". Padre: "Así que fuiste de compras hoy", etc.)

19. Trate de no impartir un sentido de urgencia cuando hable. Comportamientos adecuados que pueden modelarse para reducir esa urgencia incluyen el hablar más despacio. Su habla debe seguir un paso parejo y no contener porciones dichas rápidamente seguidas por largas pausas. Cuando se toman turnos demasiado cortos y se interrumpe frecuentemente se imparte un sentido de urgencia y esto debe minimizarse.

20. Hable honestamente con su hijo/a sobre su tartamudeo si él/ella expresa deseos de hacerlo.

21. Un niño/a normalmente desarrolla sus reacciones respecto al hablar al observar los comportamientos de sus padres. Tome ventaja de oportunidades que ocurren diariamente para asegurar que su hijo/a sienta alguna forma de éxito y felicitación.

Los "Sí" y "No" Específicos que Deben Usarse cuando Su Hijo/a Tiene Desfluideces

Al tener desfluideces, los siguientes comportamientos pueden darle la impresión a su hijo/a que usted no está satisfecho con la manera en que se comunica. Sus reacciones pueden hacer que sienta que sus desfluideces son "malas", lo cual resulta en un intento para evitar desfluideces. Al desarrollarse la preocupación y el sentimiento de evitarlo, frecuentemente el problema del tartamudeo se empeora.

NO SE RECOMIENDA:

1. Pegarle al niño por haber tartamudeado.

2. Decirle que pare de tartamudear.

3. Amenazarlo con castigos por tartamudear.

4. Ayudarlo con la palabra (a menos que su terapeuta le haya sugerido lo contrario).

5. Decirle que piense sobre lo que va a decir.

6. Contestar o "completar" por él/ella.

7. Poner una cara preocupada o adolorida.

8. Aparecer disgustado o impaciente.

9. Decirle que respire profundamente antes de hablar.

10. Pedirle que pare y empiece de nuevo.

11. Sugerir que cambie su tono de hablar.

12. Sugerir que evite o sustituya palabras.

AL CONTRARIO:

Sugerimos lo siguiente cuando su hijo/a tiene desfluideces:

1. Trate de reaccionar de la misma manera que cuando su habla es normal.

2. Permanezca calmado y escuche lo que está diciendo.

3. Trate de mostrar que le gusta hablar con él/ella.

4. Parezca interesado en lo que está diciendo.

5. Si parece actuar con demasiada emoción o prisa, puede decirle: "Un momento, tengo tiempo y quiero oír lo que quieres decirme". Esto es diferente a decirle que hable más despacio. Al contrario, le está diciendo que vaya más despacio con todo, no sólo su habla.

6. Reconozca con calma que pueden ocurrir interrupciones largas, forzadas o difíciles. Un comentario sencillo como, "¿Eso fue difícil para ti, verdad?", puede disminuir la preocupación de su hijo/a y enseñarle que a usted no le molestan las interrupciones en el habla. Si su hijo/a le dice, "No lo puedo decir", o "No puedo hablar", asegúrele que hablar le será más fácil si habla suavecito y dice la palabra junto con usted 2 ó 3 veces. (ADVERTENCIA: Este método sólo debe usarse en esas ocasiones cuando su hijo/a muestre obvia ansiedad sobre sus fallas de habla.)

(Para más información, refiérase a *La Tartamudez y su Niño: Preguntas y Respuestas,* Stuttering Foundation of America, 1989.)

Ambiente Escolar y Hogareño del Niño con Defluideces

El ambiente que rodea a su hijo tanto en casa como en la escuela puede tener un impacto sobre su tartamudeo. Las siguientes sugerencias se aplican a ambos ambientes.

1. Defina las reglas que debe seguir su hijo/a para que sepa lo que se espera de él/ella. Consistencia en casa y en la escuela es importante.

2. Cuando su hijo/a habla debe sentir que no se le va a interrumpir. También debe saber que no tendrá permiso de interrumpir a otras personas que están hablando.

3. Su hijo/a debe saber que recibirá un castigo específico, que puede esperar pero que no va a causarle ningún daño, cuando se porta muy mal.

4. Su hijo/a debe saber que será premiado de manera consistente por hacer sus tareas asignadas.

5. Felicite a su hijo/a por todo lo que hace bien.

6. Trate de reducir el uso de palabras como "no", "no puedes", "no hagas eso" y "déjalo".

7. Examine el programa diario de su hijo/a. ¿Tiene suficiente tiempo libre? ¿Dedica usted suficiente tiempo para darle un descanso?

8. Trate de dedicarle 15–20 minutos todos los días sólo a su hijo/a y nadie más. Durante este tiempo puede ir de paseo con él, jugar con él o leerle algo. Antes de ir a la cama es un buen tiempo de estar a solas con su hijo/a por algunos minutos. En los momentos en que estén juntos, pregúntele cómo le fue ese día. Esto lo ayudará a averiguar cómo se siente, en vez de preguntar, "¿qué hiciste hoy?"

9. Un buen estado físico es esencial para poder hablar bien. Su hijo/a debe recibir suficiente descanso, y debe minimizarse cualquier tipo de fatiga.

10. Mantenga el consumo de azúcar de su hijo/a al mínimo.

11. No pueden evitarse eventos traumáticos, tales como enfermedades, accidentes y conflictos emocionales. Sin embargo, reconozca que tales eventos pueden causar más desfluidez.
   a. Acepte esto como algo normal y trate de no darle a su hijo/a más cosas que puedan preocuparle al reaccionar a sus desfluideces.
   b. Trate de contrarrestar el evento traumático con experiencias agradables y haciéndolo sentirse seguro en su relación con usted.

12. Evite discutir la dificultad del habla de su hijo/a en su presencia. Sin embargo, si lo menciona, asegúrele que todas las personas tienen problemas al hablar de vez en cuando.

13. Las vacaciones y eventos como la Navidad, Chanukah, invitados, o el comienzo del año escolar también pueden resultar en aumentar el número de desfluideces. Se recomienda reducir la intensidad de estos eventos.

14. Esté alerta no sólo a eventos pero también a personas y lugares que provoquen un aumento de desfluideces. Si es posible, cambie todo lo que pueda para mejorar su fluidez.

15. Intente alterar el estrés asociado con la comunicación tanto en casa como en la escuela para proporcionar más oportunidades de aumentar la fluidez. Trate de deshacer cualquier estigma que esté conectado al tartamudeo por el cual está pasando su hijo/a. Una manera de hacer esto es modelar algunas características del tartamudeo en su propia habla para que su hijo/a empiece a darse cuenta que todas las personas pueden tener desfluideces de vez en cuando, y que eso puede hacerse fácilmente y sin tensión.

16. Reconozca que su hijo/a puede frustrarse si siente que su habla tiene muchas desfluideces severas. Trate de darle maneras de manejar esa frustración, como por ejemplo:
   a. Ejercicio al aire libre.
   b. Permitirle expresar sus emociones sin que nadie muestre ningún disgusto.

17. Cómo pueden intervenir los padres si los hermanos se burlan del niño/a que tartamudea:
   a. Explique de manera calmada y claramente que el burlarse de alguien es malo y demuestra falta de respeto.
   b. Discuta el hecho de que todas las personas tienen algunas cosas que hacen bien y otras que no las hacen tan bien. Explique que el niño que tartamudea a veces se equivoca cuando habla, y que eso no es ninguna razón para burlarse de él. (Si continúa la burla, podrá ser necesario pedir que el patólogo de habla-lenguaje hable con los hermanos.)

18. Cuando su hijo/a esté pasando por un periodo de mayor desfluidez, trate de darle oportunidades de hablar con éxito. Anime a que hable, que cante, recite poemas, hable en ritmo o que actúe tomando distintos papeles usando títeres, etc.

19. ¡Recuerde el gran poder que tienen las sugerencias positivas! Puede usarlas para motivar a niños ayudándolos a reconocer que pueden cambiar.

20. No establezca metas inalcanzables para su hijo/a. Trate de mantener sus expectativas a un nivel apropiado para su edad y madurez.

Características de Algunos Padres de Niños que Tienen Desfluideces

Investigaciones han indicado que los padres de niños que tienen desfluideces no son los que causan el tartamudeo. Sin embargo, expectativas que no sean reales pueden mantener o aumentar el tartamudeo que ya se ha establecido o que se esté desarrollando. Por ejemplo, algunos padres pueden esperar que su hijo/a:

1. Pronuncie palabras perfectamente;

2. Use un vocabulario demasiado amplio para su edad;

3. Haga tareas motóricas demasiado difíciles;

4. Logre actividades académicas avanzadas;

5. Haga demasiadas actividades fuera de la casa.

Algunos padres de niños con desfluideces hablan rápidamente o con prisa. Por lo tanto, sus hijos pueden hablar rápido también. Debido a que el habla y lenguaje es comportamiento muy complejo y cognoscitivo, el hablar rápido puede causar que su hijo/a experimente más desfluideces, como repitiendo, pausando, etc. Estos errores pueden causar aún más errores porque el niño se frustra, se pone tenso o se siente cohibido, etc.

Si los padres hablan rápido o actúan de manera apresurada, el ambiente en casa puede llegar a ser aún más tenso. El estar siempre deprisa puede llegar a ser la forma normal de la vida. Un ambiente apresurado e impaciente como éste no puede ser ideal para un desarrollo óptimo del habla, interacción normal entre padre e hijo o entre los dos padres. Se anima a los padres a que proporcionen un ambiente calmado en casa y que modelen un paso calmado cuando hablan. Esto resulta ser más eficaz que decirle simplemente a su hijo que vaya más despacio.

Poner esta información en práctica puede ser difícil. Lena Rustin (1991) describe una tarea llamada "hora de hablar" en la cual los padres completan una tarea casera que les obliga a pasar tres, cuatro o cinco minutos, cuatro, cinco o seis veces a la semana jugando con su hijo/a. La "hora de hablar" se construye así:

1. Los padres solicitan la ayuda de su hijo/a con esa tarea.

2. Los padres deciden con su hijo/a la hora que más convenga a los dos.

3. El padre le pide al hijo/a que escoja un juguete para jugar.

4. El padre e hijo/a luego entran a un cuarto y cierran la puerta para que nadie pueda interrumpirlos.

5. Durante esta interacción, el padre no deberá pedirle nada al niño o hacer comentarios sobre su habla, pero deberá escuchar con mucha atención lo que dice, no cómo lo dice.

6. Cuando ya ha pasado el tiempo, el padre debe darle las gracias al niño/a por haberle ayudado con su tarea y deberá anotar en un cuaderno que la tarea se completó haciendo algún tipo de comentario sobre cómo se sintió haciéndola. Debe de mantenerse un límite de tiempo cuando participan en las actividades de la "hora de hablar".

(Rustin, págs. 63–64.)

Cuando Hay que Disciplinar: Algunas Ideas y Sugerencias

1. Establezca un sistema de disciplina que no provoque ningún daño para corregir los malos comportamientos de su hijo/a. Este sistema debe ser consistente de día a día y de niño a niño.

2. Cuando el niño lo irrita sin intención:
  a. Trate de ser tolerante si su comportamiento no fue intencional, no hace daño a personas u objetos y ocurre infrecuentemente.
  b. Trate de quedarse calmado.
  c. Trate de no atacar a su hijo/a verbalmente (refiérase a su comportamiento, no a su persona).
  d. Describa lo que no hizo bien (por ejemplo, "Le pegaste a tu hermana.").
  e. Dígale lo que siente usted (por ejemplo, "Eso me enoja.").

3. Si el mismo comportamiento ocurre frecuentemente y aparentemente sin querer, y si el niño se niega a corregirlo, entonces un castigo razonable, que no le cause daño, podría justificarse.

4. Cuando su hijo lo irrita intencionalmente, y usted está seguro que sabe que su comportamiento es malo, sugerimos lo siguiente:
  a. Dígale a su hijo/a cómo se siente sobre lo que ha hecho. Sea específico sobre qué hizo mal.
  b. No discuta el asunto. No haga caso a sus llantos, furia o desfluidez. Tampoco le haga caso a comportamientos negativos cuando está en su cuarto.

5. Cuando su hijo/a quiere hacer algo que no se le permite hacer:
  a. Explíquele la razón por la cual no se le permite hacer la actividad. Por ejemplo: "Está muy oscuro para ir a jugar afuera".
  b. Después de explicar la razón, no lo discuta más.
  c. Reconozca que usted sabe que él está disgustado.

6. La disciplina debe ser consistente de día a día y de padre a padre. Las palmadas pueden parar el comportamiento, pero también pueden crear desconfianza y temor por parte del niño.

Padres y Maestros como Modelos

Se reconoce que los efectos del ambiente general sobre el habla de su hijo/a están relacionados al comportamiento de los padres mismos que sirven como modelos para el niño. Muchos de los comportamientos, emociones y actitudes del niño dependen directamente de los comportamientos, emociones y actitudes del padre.

1. Algunos comportamientos se modelan directamente; sin embargo, las influencias indirectas de los padres y otros adultos en la vida del niño también son muy poderosas.

2. El niño que tiene desfluideces puede adoptar los sentimientos del padre acerca del tartamudeo. Por lo tanto, los padres pueden preguntarse lo siguiente:
  a. ¿Me siento culpable porque tartamudea mi hijo/a?
  b. ¿Me echo la culpa por su tartamudeo?
  c. ¿Siento yo que el tartamudeo es vergonzoso, penoso o malo?
  d. ¿Estoy enojado con el niño porque tartamudea?

e. El tartamudeo es un problema para el cual existe ayuda y mucha esperanza. Se puede superar si se empieza a manejar a una temprana edad, antes que se desarrollen lucha, tensión, y el auto-concepto de una persona que tartamudea.

Referencias

Conture, Edward G. (1990). *Stuttering,* Englewood Cliffs, New Jersey: Prentice-Hall.

Faber, Adele, & Mazlish, Elaine. (1980). *How to Talk So Kids Will Listen and Listen So Kids Will Talk.* New York: Avon Books.

Ramig, Peter. (1993). Parent-clinician-child partnership in the therapeutic process of the preschool- and elementary-aged child who stutters, *Seminars in Speech and Language, 14* (3), 236–237.

Rustin, Lena. (1991). *Parents, families and the stuttering child.* San Diego: Singular Publishing Group.

Stuttering Foundation of America. *The child who stutters at school: Notes to the teacher.* P.O. Box 11749, Memphis, TN, 38111-0749.

Stuttering Foundation of America. (1989). *Stuttering and your child: Questions and answers.* P.O. Box 11749, Memphis, TN, 38111-0749.

Zwitman, Daniel H. (1978). *The disfluent child: A management program.* Baltimore, MD: University Park Press.

Para más información, los siguientes folletos y videos son disponibles a través de la Stuttering Foundation of America, P.O. Box 11749, Memphis, Tennessee 38111-0749 (800 992-9392):

The child who stutters at school: Notes to the teacher (folleto)

La tartamudez y su niño: Preguntas y respuestas (folleto)

Stuttering and your child: A video for parents (video)

Do you stutter? A guide for teens (folleto)

Do you stutter? Straight talk for teens (video)

Peter R. Ramig, Ph.D., CCC-SLP
Professor and Associate Chair
Board-Recognized Fluency Specialist
Department of Speech, Language, and Hearing Sciences
University of Colorado at Boulder
Boulder, CO 80309

La influencia del maestro en la vida del niño que tartamudea puede ser dramática. Hemos desarrollado este folleto para proveer información que esperamos le sea útil para comprender el impacto que el tartamudeo puede tener en la vida de un niño.

Las páginas siguientes contienen direcciones, sugerencias e información general para maestros que tienen un alumno que repite, prolonga, o pausa cuando habla. Aprender a hablar es una habilidad extremadamente compleja. Por consecuencia, niños repiten sonidos y palabras, hacen pausas y se atoran durante la primera etapa de su desarrollo del habla y lenguaje. Para la mayoría de niños, estos "errores" sólo son desfluideces normales. Sin embargo, para algunos niños pueden ser las señales principales del tartamudeo. A continuación aparece una lista de señales de peligro o advertencia para las cuales usted tiene que estar alerta respecto al habla de cualquier niño. Estas señales pueden ocurrir al azar; sin embargo, si una o más aparecen con frecuencia, es recomendable llamarlo a la atención del patólogo del habla y lenguaje de la escuela.

Importante: Escuchamos muchas ideas falsas respecto a las *causas* del tartamudeo en los niños. Los expertos en tartamudeo reconocen abiertamente que se desconocen las causas del tartamudeo. Investigaciones recientes apoyan la idea de influencias neuromotóricas. Pocos especialistas en el área del tartamudeo apoyan o sostienen la idea de que el tartamudeo tiene por base causas psicológicas. Sin embargo, no cabe duda que el estrés que provocan las emociones de vergüenza, inadecuación, humillación y frustración causadas por el tartamudeo puede empeorarlo.

Señales de Peligro o Advertencia de Tartamudeo

(Adaptación de *If your child stutters: A guide for parents (Si su hijo tartamudea: Una guía para padres)*, Stuttering Foundation Publication No. 11)

Repeticiones Múltiples de Porciones de Palabras

Repitiendo los primeros sonidos de una palabra, como "ta-ta-ta-ta-tabla" más de una o dos veces, más rápido de lo normal o con ritmo irregular. Aunque éstas se han distinguido a menudo de repeticiones de palabras completas, repeticiones de palabras cortas como "yo" o "y" o "mi" también se deben notar. Estos pueden constituir comportamientos que se manifiestan cuando la persona teme o anticipa ciertas palabras o sonidos que ocurren más tarde en la expresión.

Prolongaciones

Extendiendo un sonido al principio, o (particularmente) dentro, de una palabra como "rrrrrrrrratón" o "raaaaaa—tón". Es importante distinguir extensiones fáciles (que podrán ser asociadas con terapia previa o—menos probable—pueden representar un mecanismo autocalmante) de prolongaciones asociadas con tensión o lucha.

Bloqueo

Un bloqueo ocurre cuando la persona para o se atora antes de, o durante, la producción de un sonido o de una palabra. Pueden anticiparse los bloqueos al momento en que la persona vaya a decir una palabra determinada, o pueden usarse para extinguir el sistema en un esfuerzo para llamar menos atención al momento de tartamudear.

Lucha y Tensión

Una tensión muscular más elevada en los órganos de articulación acompaña el tartamudeo que se ha desarrollado, indicando que algún tipo de intervención es necesario. Para superar esta tensión, el niño usa sus músculos así como otros grupos de músculos para tratar de superar la sensación de bloqueo. Al final, estas reacciones pueden producirse de manera condicionada (al identificarse con la sensación original de bloqueo), y resultan en la utilización de aún más músculos. Pueden notarse rasgos de lucha y tensión en la nariz, mandíbula, cuello, mejillas, labios, frente, y pecho. Al tener este tipo de evidencia, el terapeuta puede preguntarse si esto también existe en otras áreas del cuerpo que no se puedan ver.

Tono y Volumen Aumentan

Estos fenómenos ocurren frecuentemente cuando hay prolongación de sonidos, cuando el niño está luchando para liberarse de un bloqueo y necesita decir el siguiente sonido. El niño puede anticipar o sentir que va a tener dificultades con ese sonido y usa el aumento de tono o volumen como una manera de forzar las palabras cuando siente que va a ocurrir un bloqueo.

Tremores

Tremores de la mandíbula, labios y lengua mientras habla la persona, con o sin desfluideces, deben notarse. Las observaciones hechas ayudarán a identificar la posición de la tensión asociada con el tartamudeo. La mayoría de los terapeutas consideran que los tremores forman parte de un mecanismo avanzado para ayudar a evitar el tartamudeo.

Prevención de Situaciones que Requieran el Uso del Habla, Palabras o Sonidos

Si el niño tiene pocas ganas de participar en actividades que requieren que hable, no quiere decir necesariamente que las esté evitando porque tiene un problema de tartamudeo. Puede que existan otros indicios que el niño está evitando situaciones en que tendría que hablar. Por ejemplo, el querer cambiar actividades continuamente para evitar aquellas situaciones en que se manifestarían desfluideces, o bien el querer posponer actividades comportándose mal o creando distracciones.

Pausas, Sonidos Adicionales, Palabras Interpuestas, Así Como Palabras o Frases Repetidas

Estas características del habla pueden indicar que el niño está tratando de posponer el hablar para evitar de tartamudear o que está esperando hasta sentir que puede decir una palabra con mayor fluidez. Sustituciones de palabras, silencios, dejar de hablar para participar en otra actividad o cambiar de tema son señales directas para evitar el tartamudeo.

Respiración Alterada o Irregular

Al anticipar que va a tartamudear, el niño puede retener su respiración, tomar varias inhalaciones y/o demostrar otras formas de respiración erráticas o irregulares, como tratar de decir muchas palabras rápidamente con cada grupo de respiraciones, etc.

Movimiento de Otras Partes del Cuerpo

Cuando el niño se enfrenta con una o más de las señales de peligro mencionadas antes (1, 2, o 3), puede observarse que mueve la cabeza para adelante o para atrás, mueve un brazo, una pierna o una mano; o puede adaptar otras reacciones poco comunes cuando piense que va a tartamudear.

Temor de Hablar

Cuando se observan una o más de estas reacciones, eso puede indicar que el niño tiene miedo de hablar. El terapeuta debe distinguir entre ansiedad común asociada con el hablar y comportamientos que verdaderamente indican el tartamudeo.

Comportamientos Adicionales

Estos comportamientos se manifiestan como señales de anticipación (pero no son en sí indicaciones de tartamudeo). Por ejemplo, pueden incluir comienzos difíciles de fonación, respiración poco profunda o irregular (jadeando o tragando) durante la vocalización, calidad de voz aberrante (como excesivo murmullo vocal) y fonación disrítmica durante la producción de sonidos prolongados. También se debe notar la consistencia fonémica de las desfluideces; por ejemplo, una tendencia de bloqueo cuando se dicen palabras que tienen uno o más sonidos como /s/, /f/, /b/ o /d/, o en vocales, sonidos sonorizados o sonidos no sonorizados exclusivamente.

Características del Comienzo del Tartamudeo

1. Algunos niños empiezan a tartamudear tan pronto como empiezan a combinar palabras, pero la mayoría no empiezan hasta aproximadamente un año más tarde (2 años y medio o 3 años).

2. A menudo, el tartamudeo comienza gradualmente y puede avanzar en etapas, cambiando su grado de severidad a través de distintas tareas comunicativas y periodos de tiempo.

3. Unos de los tipos más comunes de falta de fluidez que ocurren en un tartamudeo inicial son repeticiones de sílabas iniciales de una expresión.

4. Para la mayoría de niños el tartamudeo es muy frustrante y vergonzoso. Por lo tanto muchos niños pueden empezar a portarse mal en clase y evitar situaciones en las cuales deben hablar.

Información y Direcciones Generales

1. Los maestros pueden ayudar al patólogo del habla y lenguaje con su perspectiva sobre el comportamiento del niño en el salón de clases respecto a su habla y lenguaje.

2. Intente tratar el tartamudeo del niño sin darle demasiada importancia.

3. Cuando el niño está experimentando desfluideces, *POR FAVOR:*
   a. NO le diga que deje de tartamudear
   b. NO le diga que piense sobre lo que va a decir
   c. NO conteste o complete lo que quiera decir él/ella
   d. NO aparezca preocupado o muestre excesiva empatía
   e. NO aparezca enojado o impaciente
   f. NO le diga que respire profundamente antes de hablar
   g. NO le pida que pare y que empiece a decir lo que iba decir de nuevo
   h. NO sugiera que cambie de tono
   i. NO sugiera evitar o sustituir palabras
   j. NO refuerce su desfluidez prestando más atención a la desfluidez que a la fluidez
   k. NO pretenda que las desfluideces no existen
   l. NO exprese demasiada compasión

AL CONTRARIO:
   a. Trate de actuar de la misma manera que cuando habla con fluidez.
   b. Permanezca calmado y escuche lo que le está diciendo.
   c. Trate de mostrar que le gusta hablar con él/ella.
   d. Si aparece estar particularmente emocionado o apresurado, sugerimos que responda, "Tengo tiempo y quiero oír lo que quieres decir". Esto es distinto a decirle que hable más despacio o respire de manera más profunda. Así, le está diciendo que tiene su apoyo, y que está bien si va más despacio en todo, no sólo en su habla.

4. Si el habla del niño parece ser más fluida en ciertos días pero menos en otros, permita que participe más en la clase en los días cuando su habla es más fluida y menos en días cuando la fluidez es menor.

5. Si no está seguro si debe exigir que el estudiante que tartamudea dé reportes orales, sugerimos que hable en privado con él/ella. Podría decirle que reconoce que algunas veces tiene dificultades hablando y que usted está dispuesto a hacer otros arreglos para que él/ella pueda dar su reporte.

6. Cuando el niño pequeño está pasando por un periodo de desfluidez, trate de darle experiencias en las que puede tener éxito hablando. Promueva actividades tales como hablar en coro, cantar, recitar poemas, hablar usando un ritmo determinado o actuar con títeres, etc.

7. Para aumentar la fluidez del niño durante actividades de una lección en grupo, empiece la lección hablando junto con el niño. Si el niño que tartamudea habla o lee junto con usted, por lo general ya no va a tartamudear. A esto se lo refiere como efecto positivo de poder hablar o leer en coro. Sugerimos que aplique este proceso con otros alumnos para que el niño que tartamudea no se sienta que es diferente a los demás.

8. Trate de evitar que se le hagan preguntas que le causen timidez al niño.

9. Evite discusiones que se refieran a diferencias en el habla del niño en su presencia. Sin embargo, si él introduce el tema, muestre empatía y trate de asegurarle que de vez en cuando todas las personas tienen dificultades cuando hablan.

10. Trate de evitar la palabra "tartamudeo" para describir el habla del niño en su presencia. Para evitarlo, use palabras que demuestren que usted reconoce esas dificultades, como: "se atora" "habla irregular", "habla con mucho esfuerzo", etc. Sin embargo, si el niño está consciente de sus desfluideces y se refiere casualmente a ellas como "tartamudeo", no sería natural que otros evitaran usar la palabra.

11. Después de escuchar una expresión que no sea fluida, puede repetirle al niño lo que hubiera querido decir. Esto le ayudará a usted a asegurarse que está prestándole atención a lo que intentó decir, y al mismo tiempo lo ayudará al niño a olvidarse de sus desfluideces. Además, le está demostrando al niño que lo está escuchando.

12. Tenga cuidado de no transmitir un sentido de apuro cuando habla. Los comportamientos se pueden modelar con propósito de reducir este sentido de apuro simplemente *al hablar más despacio*. El habla debe seguir un paso parejo y no contener pasajes rápidos seguidos por largas pausas. Tomar turnos demasiado cortos e interrumpir con mucha frecuencia también imparten un sentido de apuro y estos deben minimizarse.

13. Hable con franqueza con el niño acerca de su tartamudeo si es que él desea hacerlo, pero no lo convierta en un gran asunto.

14. Un niño desarrolla su actitud respecto al habla cuando observa a otros. Tome ventaja de cada oportunidad para que el niño pueda lograr algún tipo de éxito y logro.

15. Trate de eliminar cualquier estigma que esté ligado al tartamudeo y que podría afectar al niño/a. Para lograrlo, puede ser muy eficiente modelar fácilmente y sin tensión una conducta apropiada con una simulación de tartamudeo en la que el niño empiece a darse cuenta que todas las personas pasan por episodios de desfluidez.

16. Reconozca que el niño se puede frustrar si siente que su habla no es muy fluida. Trate de darle estrategias para manejar esta frustración.

17. Los maestros deben intervenir si otros alumnos se burlan o si molestan al niño porque tiene desfluideces. Si el estudiante que tiene desfluideces está ausente, use las siguientes estrategias en su clase:
    a. De una manera paciente y clara explique que burlarse de alguien es malo y falta de respeto.
    b. Hable de que todas las personas tienen algunas cosas que hacen bien y otras que no hacen tan bien. Explique que a veces el niño que tartamudea se equivoca cuando habla, y que eso no es ninguna razón para burlarse de él.
    c. Si continua la burla, será necesario que el patólogo del habla y lenguaje hable de esto con los compañeros de clase.

Intenta que ese formulario sea dado o mandado a los padres de niños que han completado la terapia.

Darrell M. Dodge, M.A. CCC-SLP
Peter R. Ramig, Ph.D. and Associates
Associated Stuttering Treatment Clinics
6436 South Quebec Street, Building 6, Suite 400
Greenwood Village, CO 80111

Percepciones de Padres/Hijo

Hijo _____ Padres _____

Dirección _____

Ciudad _____ Estado _____ Código Postal _____

Fechas de terapia: de _____ a _____

Terapeuta _____

Por favor conteste las siguientes preguntas marcando las descripciones que mejor correspondan a su experiencia y/o su percepción de los efectos de la terapia.

| **Leve** | | | | | | | **Severo** | | |

Tartamudeo cuando empezó la terapia

| 1 | 2 | 3 | 4 | 5 | 6 | 7 | 8 | 9 | 10 |

Tartamudeo cuando terminó la terapia

| 1 | 2 | 3 | 4 | 5 | 6 | 7 | 8 | 9 | 10 |

Nivel del tartamudeo presente

| 1 | 2 | 3 | 4 | 5 | 6 | 7 | 8 | 9 | 10 |

| **No Estoy de Acuerdo** | | | | | | | **Sí Estoy de Acuerdo** | | |

El terapeuta proporcionó información adecuada sobre el tartamudeo y el mantenimiento de logros de fluidez basado en la terapia.

| 1 | 2 | 3 | 4 | 5 | 6 | 7 | 8 | 9 | 10 |

Se requiere práctica para mantener fluidez.

| 1 | 2 | 3 | 4 | 5 | 6 | 7 | 8 | 9 | 10 |

El nivel actual de fluidez es aceptable.

| 1 | 2 | 3 | 4 | 5 | 6 | 7 | 8 | 9 | 10 |

No Estoy de Acuerdo   **Sí Estoy de Acuerto**

El tartamudeo no es tan importante para el niño
ahora como era antes.

    1   2   3   4   5   6   7   8   9   10

El tartamudeo no presenta un obstáculo para las actividades y
el modo de vida del niño.

    1   2   3   4   5   6   7   8   9   10

El niño podría aprovechar de una sesión de terapia de repaso.

    1   2   3   4   5   6   7   8   9   10

El niño está participando en un grupo de apoyo de tartamudeo. _____ Sí _____ No

Comentarios

_____

_____

_____

_____

_____

_____

_____

Adams, M. R. (1980). The young stutterer: Diagnosis, treatment, and assessment of progress. *Seminars in Speech, Language, and Hearing, 1,* 289–300.

Adams, M. R. (1991). The assessment and treatment of the school-age stutterer. *Seminars in Speech and Language, 12,* 279–290.

Alm, P. A. (2004). Stuttering, emotions, and heart rate during anticipatory anxiety: a critical review. *Journal of Fluency Disorders, 290,* 123–133.

Andrews, G. (1983). Stuttering: A review of research findings and theories circa 1982. *Journal of Speech and Hearing Disorders, 48,* 226–246.

Andrews, G., & Cutler, J. (1974). Stuttering therapy: The relationship between changes in symptom level and attitudes. *Journal of Speech and Hearing Disorders, 34,* 312–319.

Andrews, G., & Harris, M. (1964). *The syndrome of stuttering.* Oxford: Spastics Society Medical Education.

ASHA Special Interest Division 4: Fluency and Fluency Disorders. (2002). Terminology pertaining to fluency and fluency disorders: Guidelines. In *ASHA 2002 desk reference volume 3: Speech-language pathology,* 397–394.

Bakker, K. (1997). Instrumentation for the assessment and treatment of stuttering. In R. F. Curlee & G. M. Siegel (Eds.), *Nature and treatment of stuttering: New directions* (2nd ed., pp. 377–397). Needham Heights, MA: Allyn & Bacon.

Bakker, K., & Riley, G. (1996). *Computerized scoring of stuttering severity for windows.* Austin, TX: Pro-Ed.

Barbara, D. A., Goldart, N., & Oram, C. (1961). Group psychoanalysis with adult stutterers. *American Journal of Psychoanalysis, 21,* 40–57.

Bennett, E. M., Ramig, P. R., & Reveles, V. N. (1993, November). *Speaking attitudes in children: Summer fluency camps.* Poster session presented at the ASHA Convention, Anaheim, CA.

Bennett-Mancha, E. (1990, March). *Parent support groups: For parents of children who stutter.* Paper presented at the Texas Speech-Language-Hearing Association Convention, Dallas, TX.

Bennett-Mancha, E. (1992). The house that Jack built. *Staff.* Aaron's Associates, 6114 Waterway, Garland, TX 75043.

Blood, G. W. (1995). POWER2: Relapse management with adolescents who stutter. *Language, Speech, and Hearing Services in Schools, 26,* 169–179.

Blood, G. W., Ridenour, V. J. Jr., & Qualls, C. D. (2003). Co-occurring disorders in children who stutter. *Journal of Communication Disorders, 36,* 427–448.

Bloodstein, O. (1993). *Stuttering: The search for a cause and cure.* Needham Heights, MA: Allyn & Bacon.

Bloodstein, O. (1995). *A handbook of stuttering* (5th ed.). San Diego: Singular Publishing Group.

Bloom, C., & Cooperman, D. K. (1999). *Synergistic stuttering therapy: A holistic approach.* Boston: Butterworth-Heinemann.

Boberg, E. (Ed.). (1981). *Maintenance of fluency.* New York: Elsevier.

Boberg, E., Yeudall, L., Schlopplocher, D., & Bohassen, P. (1983). The effects of an intensive behavioral program on the distribution of EEG, alpha power in stutterers during the processing of verbal and visiospatial information. *Journal of Fluency Disorders, 8,* 245–263.

Botterill, W., Kelman, E., & Rustin, L. (1991). Parents and their pre-school stuttering child. In L. Rustin (Ed.), *Parents, families, and the stuttering child* (pp. 59–71). San Diego: Singular Publishing Group.

Braun, A. R., Varga, M., Stager, S., Schulz, G., Selbie, S., Maisog, J. M., Carson, R. E., & Ludlow, C. L. (1997). Altered patterns of cerebral activity during speech and language production in developmental stuttering. An $H_2^{15}O$ positron emission tomography study. *Brain, 120,* 761–784.

Bray, M. A., & Kehle, T. J. (1996). Self-modeling as an intervention for stuttering. *School Psychology Review, 25,* 358–369.

Breitenfeldt, D. H., & Lorenz, D. R. (2000). *Successful stuttering management program (SSMP)* (2nd ed.). Cheney, WA: Eastern Washington University.

Brutten, G. J. (1975). Stuttering: Topography, assessment and behavior change strategies. In J. Eisenson (Ed.), *Stuttering: A second symposium* (pp. 199–262). New York: Harper & Row.

Chmela, K. A., & Reardon. N. (2001). *The school-age child who stutters: Working effectively with attitudes and emotions.* Memphis, TN: Stuttering Foundation.

Conture, E. G. (1990). *Stuttering* (2nd ed.). Englewood Cliffs, NJ: Prentice Hall.

Conture, E. G. (1997). Evaluating childhood stuttering. In R. F. Curlee & G. M. Siegel (Eds.), *Nature and treatment of stuttering: New directions* (2d ed., pp. 239–256). Needham Heights, MA: Allyn & Bacon.

Conture, E. G. (2001). *Stuttering: Its nature, diagnosis, and treatment.* Needham Heights, MA: Allyn & Bacon.

Cooper, E. B., & Cooper, C. S. (1985). *Personalized fluency control therapy.* Allen, TX: DLM.

Cosby, B., & Honeywood, V. P. (1997). *The meanest thing to say.* New York: Scholastic.

Costello, J. M. (1983). Current behavioral treatments of children. In D. Prins & R. J. Ingham (Eds.), *Treatment of stuttering in early childhood: Methods and issues* (pp. 69–98). San Diego: College-Hill Press.

Cox, N. J., Seider, R. A., & Kidd, K. K. (1984). Some environmental factors and hypotheses for stuttering in families with several stutterers. *Journal of Speech and Hearing Research, 27,* 543–548.

Craig, A. (1996). Long-term effects of intensive treatment for a child with both a cluttering and stuttering disorder. *Journal of Fluency Disorders, 21,* 329–335.

Craig, A. (1998). Relapse following treatment for stuttering: A critical review and correlative data. *Journal of Fluency Disorders, 23,* 1–30.

Crowe, T. A., & Cooper, E. B. (1977). Parental attitudes towards and knowledge of stuttering. *Journal of Communication Disorders, 10,* 343–357.

Culatta, R. A., & Rubin, H. (1973). A program for the initial stages of fluency therapy. *Journal of Speech and Hearing Research, 16,* 556–568.

Daly, D. A. (1988). *Freedom of fluency.* Tucson, AZ: LinguiSystems.

Daly, D. A., & Burnett, M. L. (1996). Cluttering: Assessment, treatment planning, and case study illustration. *Journal of Fluency Disorders, 21,* 239–248.

Darley, F., & Spriestersbach, D. (1978). *Diagnostic methods in speech pathology* (2d ed.). New York: Harper & Row.

Dell, C. W. Jr,. (1993). Treating school-age stutterers. In R. F. Curlee (Ed.), *Stuttering and related disorders of fluency* (pp. 45–67). New York: Thieme Medical Publishers.

Dell, C. W. Jr. (2000). *Treating the school-age stutterer: A guide for clinicians* (2d ed.). Memphis, TN: Stuttering Foundation.

De Nil, L. F., & Brutten, G. J. (1991). Speech-associated attitudes of stuttering and nonstuttering children. *Journal of Speech and Hearing Research, 34,* 60–66.

De Nil, L. F., Kroll, R. M., Kapur, S., & Houle, S. (2000). A positron emission tomography study of silent and oral single word reading in stuttering and nonstuttering adults. *Journal of Speech, Language, and Hearing Research, 43,* 1038–1053.

Denny, M., & Smith, A. (1997). Respiratory and laryngeal control in stuttering. In R. F. Curlee & G. M. Siegel (Eds.), *Nature and treatment of stuttering: New directions* (2d ed., pp. 128–142). Needham Heights, MA: Allyn & Bacon.

Denny, M., & Smith, A. (2000). Respiratory control in stuttering speakers: Evidence from respiratory high-frequency oscillations. *Journal of Speech, Language, and Hearing Research, 43,* 1024–1037.

Dietrich, S. (2001). *Participant manual.* Stuttering Foundation of America, Eastern Workshop. Greensboro, NC.

Dromey, C., & Ramig, L. (1998). The effect of lung volume level on selected phonatory and articulatory variables. *Journal of Speech, Language, and Hearing Research, 41,* 491–502.

Dunn, L., & Dunn, L. (1997). *Peabody Picture Vocabulary Test* (PPVT-III) (3d ed.). Circle Pines, MN: American Guidance Services.

Fawcus, M. (1970). Intensive treatment and group therapy programme for the child and adult stammerer. *British Journal of Disorders of Communication, 5,* 59–65.

Fawcus, M. (Ed.) (1995). *Stuttering: From theory to practice.* London: Whurr Publishers, Ltd.

Felsenfeld, S. (1997). Epidemiology and genetics of stuttering. In R. F. Curlee & G. M. Siegal (Eds.), *Nature and treatment of stuttering: New directions* (2nd ed., pp. 3–22). Needham Heights, MA: Allyn & Bacon.

Foundas, A. L., Bollich, A. M., & Corey, D. M. (2001). Anomalous anatomy of speech-language areas in adults with persistent developmental stuttering. *Neurology, 57,* 207–215.

Fox, P. T., Ingham, R. J., George, M. S., Mayberg, H., Ingham, J., Roby, J., Martin, C., & Jerabek, P. (1997). Imaging human intra-cerebral connectivity by PET during TMS. *NeuroReport, 8,* 2787–2791.

Fox, P. T., Ingham, R. J., Ingham, J. C., Hirsch, T., Downs, J. H., Martin, C., Jerabek, P., Glass, T., & Lancaster, J. L. (1996). A PET study of the neural systems of stuttering. *Nature, 382,* 158–162.

Fox, P. T., Ingham, R. J., Ingham, J. C., Zamarripa, F., Xiong, J.-H., & Lancaster, J. (2000). Brain correlates of stuttering and syllable production: A PET performance-correlation analysis. *Brain, 123,* 1985–2004.

Fraser, M. (2004). *Self-therapy for the stutterer.* (Rev. 10th ed.). Memphis, TN: Stuttering Foundation.

Frick, J. V. (1970). *Motor planning techniques for the treatment of stuttering.* Unpublished manuscript, Pennsylvania State University.

Gardner, M. F. (2000a). *Expressive one-word picture vocabulary test: 2000 edition.* R. Brownell (Ed.). Minneapolis, MN: Pearson Assessments.

Gardner, M. F. (2000b). *Receptive one-word picture vocabulary test: 2000 edition.* R. Brownell (Ed.). Minneapolis, MN: Pearson Assessments.

Georgieva, D. (1994). Speech situations increasing stuttering by 13–16-year-old persons. In C. W. Starkweather & H. F. M. Peters (Eds.), *Stuttering: Proceedings from the First World Congress on Fluency Disorders* (pp. 259–263). Nijmegen, Netherlands: University Press Nijmegen.

Geschwind, N., & Galaburda, A. M. (1985). Cerebral lateralization: Biological mechanism, associations, and pathology: I. A hypothesis and a program for research. *Archives of Neurology, 42*, 429–459.

Gildston, P. (1967). Stutterers' self-acceptance and perceived parental acceptance. *Journal of Abnormal Psychology, 72*, 59–64.

Ginsberg, A. P. (2000). Shame, self-consciousness, and locus of control in people who stutter. *Journal of Genetic Psychology, 161*, 389–399.

Glasner, P., & Rosenthal, D. (1957). Parental diagnosis of stuttering in young children. *Journal of Speech and Hearing Disorders, 22*, 288–295.

Goldman, R., & Fristoe, M. (2000). *Goldman-Fristoe test of articulation–2.* Austin, TX: Pro-Ed.

Gottwald, S. R., Goldbach, P., & Isack, A. H. (1985). Stuttering: Prevention and detection. *Young Children, 41*, 9–14.

Gottwald, S. R., & Starkweather, C. W. (1995). Fluency intervention for preschoolers and their families in the public schools. *Language, Speech, and Hearing Services in Schools, 26*, 117–126.

Goven, P., & Vette G. (1966). *A manual for stuttering therapy.* Pittsburgh, PA: Stanwix House.

Gray, J. (1987). *The psychology of fear and stress* (2d ed.). Cambridge: Cambridge University Press.

Gregory, H. H. (1989, July). *Stuttering therapy: A workshop for specialists.* Unpublished manuscript, Northwestern University and the Stuttering Foundation, Evanston, IL.

Gregory, H. H. (1991). Therapy for elementary school-age children. *Seminars in Speech and Language, 12*, 323–335.

Gregory, H. H. (2003). *Stuttering therapy: Rationale and procedures.* Boston: Allyn & Bacon.

Gregory, H. H., & Gregory, C. B. (1993). Counseling children who stutter and their parents. In R. F. Curlee (Ed.), *Stuttering and related disorders of fluency.* New York: Thieme Medical Publishers.

Gregory, H. H., & Hill, D. (1980). Stuttering therapy for children. *Seminars in Speech, Language, and Hearing, 1*, 351–364.

Gregory, H. H., & Hill, D. (1993). Differential evaluation—differential therapy for stuttering children. In R. F. Curlee (Ed.), *Stuttering and related disorders of fluency* (pp. 23–44). New York: Thieme Medical Publishers.

Guitar, B. (1976). Pretreatment factors associated with the outcome of stuttering therapy. *Journal of Speech and Hearing Research, 19,* 590–600.

Guitar, B. (1997). Therapy for children's stuttering and emotions. In R. F. Curlee & G. M. Siegel (Eds.), *Nature and treatment of stuttering: New directions* (2nd ed., pp. 280–291). Needham Heights, MA: Allyn & Bacon.

Guitar, B. (1998). *Stuttering: An integrated approach to its nature and treatment* (2d ed.). Baltimore, MD: Williams & Wilkins.

Guitar, B., & Bass, C. (1978). Stuttering therapy: The relation between attitude change and long-term outcome. *Journal of Speech and Hearing Disorders, 15*, 393–400.

Hall, K. D., Amir, O., & Yairi, E. (1999). A longitudinal investigation of speaking rate in preschool children who stutter. *Journal of Speech, Language, and Hearing Research, 42,* 1367–1377.

Hall, B. J., Oyer, H. J., & Haas, W. H. (2001). *Speech, language, and hearing disorders: A guide for the teacher* (3d ed.). Needham Heights, MA: Allyn & Bacon.

Ham, R. (1986). *Techniques of stuttering therapy.* Englewood Cliffs, NJ: Prentice Hall.

Haynes, W., & Pindzola, R. (1998). *Diagnosis and evaluation in speech pathology* (5th ed.). Needham Heights, MA: Allyn & Bacon.

Healey, E. C. (2004). *A multidimensional approach to assessment and treatment of stuttering in school-age children.* Presented at the Stuttering Foundation workshop on Stuttering Therapy: Practical Ideas for the School Clinician, Cincinnati, OH.

Healey, E. C., & Scott, L. A. (1995). Strategies for treating elementary school-age children who stutter: an integrative approach. *Language, Speech, and Hearing Services in Schools, 26*, 151–161.

Healey, E. C., Scott, L. A., & Ellis, G. (1995). Decision making in the treatment of school-age children who stutter. *Journal of Communication Disorders, 28*, 107–124.

Heite, L. (2000). *La petite mort: Dissociation and the subjective experience of stuttering.* Unpublished master's thesis. Temple University, Philadelphia.

Hill, D. (2003). Counseling parents of children who stutter. In *Effective counseling in stuttering therapy* (pp. 37–52). Memphis, TN: Stuttering Foundation.

Hill, D. (1999). Evaluation of child factors related to early stuttering: A descriptive study. In N. B. Ratner & E. C. Healey (Eds.), *Stuttering research and practice: Bridging the gap* (pp. 145–174). Mahwah, NJ: Lawrence Erlbaum Associates.

Hodges, E. V. E., & Perry, D. G. (1996). Victims of peer abuse: An overview. *Journal of Emotional and Behavioral Problems, 5*, 23–28.

Hoit, J. D., Solomon, N. P., & Hixon, T. J. (1993). Effect of lung volume on voice onset time (VOT). *Journal of Speech and Hearing Research, 36*, 516–521.

Hurt, R. D. (1993). Nicotine dependence: Treatment for the 1990s. *Journal of Internal Medicine, 233*, 307–310.

Ingham, R. J. (2003). Brain imaging and stuttering: Some reflections on current and future developments. *Journal of Fluency Disorders, 28*, 411–420.

Ingham, R. J. (2001). Brain imaging studies of developmental stuttering. *Journal of Communication Disorders, 34*, 493–516.

Ingham, R. J., Fox, P. T., Ingham, J. C., Xiong, J., Zamarripa, F., Hardies, L. J., & Lancaster, J. L. (2004). Brain correlates of stuttering and syllable production: Gender comparison and replication. *Journal of Speech, Language, and Hearing Research, 47*, 321–341.

Ingham, R. J. (1984). *Stuttering and behavior therapy: Current status and experimental foundations.* San Diego: College-Hill Press.

Ingham, R. J., Fox, P. T., Ingham, J. C., & Zamarripa, F. (2000). Is overt stuttering a prerequisite for the neural activations associated with chronic developmental stuttering? *Brain and Language, 75*, 163–194.

Ingham, R. J., Fox, P. T., Ingham, J. C., Zamarripa, F., Jerabek, P., & Cotton, J. (1996). A functional lesion investigation of developmental stuttering using positron emission tomography. *Journal of Speech and Hearing Research, 39*, 1208–1227.

Irwin, A. (1980). *Stammering: Practical help for all ages.* Harmondsworth, UK: Penguin.

Johnson, W. (1955). A study of the onset and development of stuttering. In W. Johnson (Ed.), *Stuttering in children and adults.* Minneapolis: University of Minnesota Press.

Johnson, W., Darley, F., & Spriesterbach, D. C. (1952). Stutterer's self-rating of reactions to speech situations. In *Diagnostic manual of speech correction.* New York: Harper & Row.

Johnson, W. (1942). A study of the onset and development of stuttering. *Journal of Speech Disorders, 7*, 251–257.

Johnson, W., Boehmler, R., Dahlstrom, G., Darley, F., Goodstein, L., Kools, J., Neeley, J., Prather, W., Sherman, D., Thurman, C., Trotter, W., Williams, D., & Young, M. (1959). *The onset of stuttering.* Minneapolis: University of Minnesota Press.

Johnston S. J., Watkin K. L., & Macklem, P. T. (1985). Lung volume changes during relatively fluent speech in stutterers. *Journal of Applied Physiology, 75*, 696–703.

Jones, P. H., & Ryan, B. P. (2001). Experimental analysis of the relationship between speaking rate and stuttering during mother-child conversation. *Journal of Developmental and Physical Disabilities, 13*(3), 279–305.

Kagan, J. (1994). *Galen's prophecy.* New York: Basic Books.

Kalinowski, J. S., Armson, J., Roland-Meiszkowski, M., Stuart, A., & Gracco, V. L. (1993). Effect of alterations in auditory feedback and speech rate on stuttering frequency. *Language and Speech, 36*, 1–16.

Kalinowski, J., Armson, J., & Stuart, A. (1995). Effect of normal and fast articulatory rates on stuttering frequency. *Journal of Fluency Disorders, 20*, 293–302.

Kalinowski, J., & Dayalu, V. N. (2002). A common element in the immediate inducement of effortless, natural-sounding, fluent speech in people who stutter: "The second speech signal." *Medical Hypotheses, 58*, 61–66.

Kalinowski, J., Dayalu, V. N., Stuart, A., Rastatter, M., & Rami., M. K. (2000). Stutter-free and stutter-filled speech signals and their role in stuttering amelioration for English-speaking subjects. *Neuroscience Letters, 29*, 115–118.

Kalinowski, J., Noble, S., Armson, J., & Stuart, A. (1994). Pretreatment and post-treatment speech naturalness ratings of adults with mild and severe stuttering. *American Journal of Speech Language-Pathology, 3*, 65–70.

Kasprisin-Burrelli, A., Egolf, D. B., & Shames, G. H. (1972). A comparison of parental verbal behavior with stuttering and nonstuttering children. *Journal of Communicative Disorders, 5*, 334–346.

Kelly, E. M. (1995). Parents as partners: Including mothers and fathers in the treatment of children who stutter. *Journal of Communication Disorders, 28*, 93–105.

Kelly, E. M., & Conture, E. (1991). Intervention with school-age stutterers: A parent-child fluency group approach. *Seminars in Speech and Language, 12*, 310–322.

Kelly, E. M., Smith, A., & Goffman, L. (1995). Orofacial muscle activity of children who stutter: A preliminary study. *Journal of Speech and Hearing Research, 38*, 1025–1036.

Kent, R. D. (1984). Stuttering as a temporal programming disorder. In R. F. Curlee & G. M. Siegal (Eds.), *Nature and treatment of stuttering: New directions.* San Diego: College-Hill Press.

Kidd, K. (1984). Stuttering as a genetic disorder. In R. F. Curlee & G. M. Siegal (Eds.), *Nature and treatment of stuttering: New directions.* San Diego: College-Hill Press.

Kloth, S. A. M., Janssen, P., & Kraaimaat, F. W. (1995). Communicative behavior of mothers of stuttering and nonstuttering high-risk children prior to the onset of stuttering. *Journal of Fluency Disorders, 20*, 365–377.

Langevin, M., Bortnick, K., Hammer, T., & Wiebe, E. (1998). Teasing/Bullying experienced by children who stutter: toward development of a questionnaire. *Contemporary Issues in Communication Science and Disorders, 25*, 12–24.

Langlois, A., Hanrahan, L. L., & Inouye, L. L. (1986). A comparison of interactions between stuttering children, nonstuttering children and their mothers. *Journal of Fluency Disorders, 11*, 263–273.

Lankford, S. D., & Cooper, E. B. (1974). Recovery from stuttering as viewed by parents of self-diagnosed recovered stutterers. *Journal of Communication Disorders, 7*, 171–180.

Lass, N. J., Ruscello, D. M., & Pannbacker, M. D. (1994). School administrators' perceptions of people who stutter. *Language, Speech, and Hearing Services in Schools, 25*, 90–93.

Lass, N. J., Ruscello, D. M., & Schmidt, J. F. (1992). Teachers' perceptions of stutterers. *Language, Speech, and Hearing Services in Schools, 23*, 78–81.

Leahy, M. M. (1994). Attempting to ameliorate student therapists' negative stereotype of the stutterer. *European Journal of Disorders of Communication, 29*, 39–49.

Leahy, M. M., & Collins, G. (1991). Therapy for stuttering: Experimenting with experimenting. *Irish Journal of Psychological Medicine, 8*, 37–39.

LeDoux, J. (2001). *The synaptic self.* New York: Viking.

LeDoux, J. (1996). *The emotional brain.* New York: Simon & Schuster.

Lees, R. M. (1999). Stammering in school children. *Support for Learning, 14*, 22–26.

Leith, W. R., & Timmons, J. L. (1983). The stutterer's reaction to the telephone as a speaking situation. *Journal of Fluency Disorders, 8*, 233–243.

Lew, G. W. (2000). *What parents can do for your child when he is being teased for stuttering.* International Stuttering Awareness Day Online Conference, www.stutteringhomepage.com.

Lincoln, M. A., & Onslow, M. (1997). Long-term outcome of early intervention for stuttering. *American Journal of Speech-Language Pathology, 6*, 51–58.

Logan, K. J., & Caruso, A. J. (1997). Parents as partners in the treatment of childhood stuttering. *Seminars in Speech and Language, 18*, 309–327.

Logan, K. J., & Conture, E. (1997). Selected temporal, grammatical, and phonological characteristics of conversational utterances produced by children who stutter. *Journal of Speech, Language, and Hearing Research, 40*, 107–120.

Maguire, G. A. (2003). Psychopharmacology of stuttering. *Audio–Digest Psychiatry, 32*, May 21.

Mahr, G. C., & Torosian, T. (1999). Anxiety and social phobia in stuttering. *Journal of Fluency Disorders, 24*, 119–126.

Manning, W. (2001). *Clinical decision-making in fluency disorders* (2d ed.). Vancouver: Singular Thompson Learning.

Manning, W. H. (1996). *Clinical decision-making in the diagnosis and treatment of fluency disorders.* Albany: Delmar Publishers.

Max, L., & Caruso, A. J. (1998). Adaptation of stuttering frequency during repeated readings: Associated changes in acoustic parameters of perceptually fluent speech. *Journal of Speech, Language, and Hearing Research, 41*, 1265–1281.

McClean, M. D., & Runyan, C. M. (2000). Variations in the relative speeds of orofacial structures with stuttering severity. *Journal of Speech, Language, and Hearing Research, 43*, 1524–1531.

Meyers, S., & Woodford, L. (1992). *The fluency development system for young children.* Buffalo, NY: United Educational Services.

Miles, S., & Ratner, N. B. (2001). Parental language input to children at stuttering onset. *Journal of Speech, Language, and Hearing Research, 44*, 1116–1130.

Mitchell, H., Hoit, J., & Watson, P. (1996). Cognitive-linguistic demands and speech breathing. *Journal of Speech and Hearing Research, 39*, 93–104.

Moncur, J. P. (1952). Parental domination in stuttering. *Journal of Speech and Hearing Disorders, 17*, 155–165.

Mooney, S., & Smith, P. (1995). Bullying and the child who stammers. *British Journal of Special Education, 22*, 24–27.

Myers, F. L. (1996). Cluttering: A matter of perspective. *Journal of Fluency Disorders, 21*, 175–185.

Myers, F. L., & St. Louis, K. O. (1996). Two youths who clutter, but is that the only similarity? *Journal of Fluency Disorders, 21*, 297–304.

Myers, F. L. & St. Louis, K. O. (1992). Cluttering: Issues and controversies. In F. L. Myers & K. O. St. Louis (Eds.), *Cluttering: A clinical perspective.* Kibworth, UK: Far Communications.

National Stuttering Association. (2000). *A classroom presentation about stuttering.* New York: Author.

Neilson, M. D., & Neilson, P. D. (1987). Speech motor control and stuttering: A computational model of adaptive sensory-motor processing. *Speech Communication, 6*, 325–333.

Nelson, L. A. (1998). Advice for persons who stutter: what you can do to help yourself. In *Advice for those who stutter* (pp. 45–50). Memphis, TN: Stuttering Foundation.

Onslow, M., & Packman, A. (2001). Ambiguity and algorithms in diagnosing early stuttering: Comments on Ambrose and Yairi (1999). *Journal of Speech, Language, and Hearing Research, 44*, 593–594.

Onslow, M., Packman, A., & Harrison, E. (2003). *The Lidcombe program of early stuttering intervention: A clinician's guide.* Austin, TX: Pro-Ed.

Paden, E. P., & Yairi, E. (1996). Phonological characteristics of children whose stuttering persisted or recovered. *Journal of Speech and Hearing Research, 39*, 981–990.

Parker, J. G., & Asher, S. R. (1987). Peer relations and later personal adjustment: Are low accepted children at risk? *Psychological Bulletin, 102*, 357–389.

Perkins, W. H. (1992). *Stuttering prevented.* San Diego: Singular Publishing Group.

Perkins, W. H., (1973). Replacement of stuttering with normal speech: 1. Rationale. *Journal of Speech and Hearing Disorders, 38*, 283–294.

Perkins, W. H., Kent, R. D., & Curlee, R. F. (1991). A theory of neuropsycholinguistic function in stuttering. *Journal of Speech and Hearing Research, 34*, 734–752.

Peters, H. F., & Boves, L. (1988). Coordination of aerodynamic and phonatory processes in fluent speech utterances of stutterers. *Journal of Speech and Hearing Research, 31*, 352–361.

Peters, T. J. (1991). An integration of contemporary therapies with school-age children. *Seminars in Speech and Language, 12*, 301–308.

Peters, T. J., & Guitar, B. (1991). *Stuttering: An integrated approach to its nature and treatment.* Baltimore, MD: Williams & Wilkins.

Pindzola, R. (1985). Classroom teachers: Interacting with stutterers. *Teacher Education, 21*, 2–8.

Pool, K. D., Devous, M. D., Freeman, F. J., Watson, B. C., & Finitzo, T. (1991). Regional cerebral blood flow in developmental stutterers. *Archives of Neurology, 48*, 509–512.

Ramig, P. R. (1998a). Don't ever give up. In *Advice for those who stutter* (pp. 45–50). Memphis, TN: Stuttering Foundation.

Ramig, P. R. (1998b). *The school clinician: Ways to be more effective.* [Videotape No. 0087]. Memphis, TN: Stuttering Foundation.

Ramig, P. R. (1993). Parent-clinician-child partnership in the therapeutic process of the preschool and elementary-aged child who stutters. *Seminars in Speech and Language, 14*, 226–237.

Ramig, P. R. (1984). Rate changes in the speech of stutterers after therapy. *Journal of Fluency Disorders, 9*, 285–294.

Ramig, P. R., & Bennett, E. M. (1997a). Clinical management of children: Direct management strategies. In R. F. Curlee & G. M. Siegel (Eds.), *Nature and treatment of stuttering: New directions* (2d ed.). Needham Heights, MA: Allyn & Bacon.

Ramig, P. R., & Bennett, E. M. (1997b). Considerations for conducting group intervention with adults who stutter. *Seminars in Speech and Language, 18*, 343–356.

Ramig, P. R., & Bennett, E. M. (1995). Working with 7–12-year-old children who stutter: Ideas for intervention in the public schools. *Language, Speech, and Hearing Services in Schools, 26*, 138–150.

Ramig, P. R., & Smith, M. (1999). *Fiberoptic laryngoscopy study on two males who stutter.* [Videotape].

Ramig, P. R., Stewart, P., Ogrodnick, P., Bennett, E., Dodge, D., & Lamy J. (1988). *Treating the school-age child who stutters: Some intervention ideas and resources.* Unpublished manuscript. The University of Colorado, Boulder.

Ratner, N. B. (1995). Treating the child who stutters with concomitant language or phonological impairment. *Language, Speech, and Hearing Services in Schools, 26*, 180–186.

Rentschler, G. J. (2001). *Speech therapy: Group therapy.* www.home.duq.edu/~rentschler/STUTTER/group.htm.

Riley, G. (1994). *Stuttering severity instrument for children and adults* (3d ed.). Austin, TX: Pro-Ed.

Riley, G. (1981). *Stuttering prediction instrument for young children.* Austin, TX: Pro-Ed.

Riley, G., & Riley, J. (1986). Oral motor discoordination among children who stutter, *Journal of Fluency Disorders, 11*, 335–344.

Riley, G. D., & Riley, J. (1983). Evaluation as a basis for intervention. In D. Prins & R. J. Ingham (Eds.), *Treatment of stuttering in early childhood: Methods and issues.* San Diego: College-Hill Press.

Riley, G. D., & Riley, R. (1985). *Oral Motor assessment and treatment: Improving syllable production.* Austin, TX: Pro-Ed.

Roth, I., & Beal, D. (1999). *Teasing and bullying of children who stutter.* www.stutteringhomepage.com.

Roth, F., & Worthington, C. (2000). *Treatment resource manual for speech-language pathology* (2d ed.). San Diego: Singular Publishing Group.

Runyan, C. M., & Runyan, S. E. (1999). Therapy for school-age stutterers: An update on the Fluency Rules Program. In R. F. Curlee (Ed.), *Stuttering and related disorders of fluency* (2d ed., pp. 110–123). New York: Thieme Medical Publishers.

Rustin, L., & Cook, F. (1995). Parental involvement in the treatment of stuttering. *Language, Speech, and Hearing Services in Schools, 26*, 127–137.

Ryan, B. P. (1984) Treatment of stuttering in school children. In W. H. Perkins (Ed.), *Stuttering disorders*. New York: Thieme-Stratton.

Ryan, B. P., & Van Kirk, B. (1974). The establishment, transfer, and maintenance of fluent speech in 50 stutterers using delayed auditory feedback and operant procedures. *Journal of Speech and Hearing Disorders, 39*, 3–10.

Salmelin, R., Schnitzler, A., Schmitz, F., & Freund, H. J. (2000). Single word reading in developmental stutterers and fluent speakers. *Brain, 123,* 1184–1202.

Salmelin, R., Schnitzler, A., Schmitz, F., Jäncke, L., Witte, O. W., & Freund, H. J. (1998). Functional organization of the auditory cortex is different in stutterers and fluent speakers. *NeuroReport, 9*, 2225–2229.

Santacreu Mas, J. (1984). El condicionamiento ante determinadas palabras en la tartamudez. [Conditioning before some words in stuttering]. *Revista de Psicologia General y Aplicada, 39*, 1115–1129.

Schulz, H. (1977). Verleichende Untersuchung von Sprachbehinderten und Nichtsprachbehinderten Schülern des 3. Schuljahres mit dem Rechentest DRE 3 von Samstag, Sander und Schmidt [An investigation comparing primary 3 children with speech/language difficulties using the DRE 3 arithmetic test devised by Samstag, Sander and Schmidt]. *Sprachheilarbeit, 22*, 86–95.

Shames, G. H., & Florance, C. L. (1980). *Stutter-free speech*. Columbus: Merrill.

Shapiro, D. A. (1999). *Stuttering intervention: A collaborative journey to fluency freedom*. Austin, TX: Pro-Ed.

Sharpe, S. (1995). How much does bullying hurt? The effects of bullying on the personal well-being and educational progress of secondary aged students. *Education and Child Psychology, 12*, 81–88.

Sheehan, J. G. (1998). Message to a stutterer. In *Advice for those who stutter* (pp. 45–50). Memphis, TN: Stuttering Foundation.

Sheehan, J. G. (1975). Conflict theory and avoidance-reduction therapy. In J. Eisenson (Ed.), *Stuttering: A second symposium*. New York: Harper & Row.

Sheehan, J. G. (1970). *Stuttering: Research and therapy*. New York: Harper & Row.

Shine, R. E. (1980). *Systematic fluency training for young children*. Tigard, OR: C. C. Publications, Inc.

Silverman, F. H. (1997). Telecommunication relay services: An option for stutterers. *Journal of Fluency Disorders, 22*, 63–64.

Silverman, F. H. (2004). *Stuttering and other fluency disorders* (3d ed.). Long Grove, IL: Waveland Press.

Smith, A., & Kelly, E. (1997). Stuttering: A dynamic, multifactorial disorder. In R. F. Curlee & G. M. Siegal (Eds.), *Nature and treatment of stuttering: New directions* (2d ed.). Needham Heights: Allyn & Bacon.

Smith, A., & Kleinow, J. (2000). Kinematic correlates of speaking rate changes in stuttering and normally fluent adults. *Journal of Speech, Language, and Hearing Research, 43*, 521–536.

Sommer, M., Koch, M. A., Paulus, W., Weiller, C., & Buechel, C. (2002). Disconnection of speech-relevant brain areas in persistent developmental stuttering. *Lancet, 360*, 380–383.

Stager, S. V., Jeffries, K. J., & Braun, A. R. (2003). Common features of fluency-evoking conditions studied in stuttering subjects and controls: an $H_2^{15}O$ PET study. *Journal of Fluency Disorders, 28*, 411–420.

Starkweather, C. W. (1987). *Fluency and stuttering*. Englewood Cliffs, NJ: Prentice Hall.

Starkweather C. W. (1997). Therapy for younger children. In R. F. Curlee & G. M. Siegel (Eds.), *Nature and treatment of stuttering: New directions* (2d ed.). Needham Heights, MA: Allyn & Bacon.

Starkweather, C. W., Gottwald, S. R., & Halfond, M. M. (1990). *Stuttering prevention: A clinical method*. Englewood Cliffs, NJ: Prentice Hall.

Starkweather, C. W., & Givens-Ackerman, J. (1997). *Stuttering*. Austin, TX: Pro-Ed.

St. Louis, K. O., & Hinzman, A. R. (1986). Studies of cluttering: Perceptions of cluttering by speech-language pathologists and educators. *Journal of Fluency Disorders, 11*, 131–149.

St. Louis, K. O. (2002). Office hours: The professor is in, questions and comments (Re: cluttering). International Stuttering Awareness Day Online Conference. www.stutteringhomepage.com

St. Louis, K. O., Raphael, L. J., Myers, F. L., & Bakker, K. (2003, Nov. 18). Cluttering updated. *The ASHA Leader, 4–5*, 20–22.

Stocker, B. (1980). *The stocker probe technique: For diagnosis and treatment of stuttering in young children*. Tulsa, OK: Modern Education Corporation.

Stuttering: Straight talk for teachers. (2002). [Videotape.] Memphis, TN: Stuttering Foundation.

Stuttering Foundation. (2003). *If your child stutters: A guide for parents* (Stuttering Foundation Publication No. 11). Memphis, TN: Author.

Stuttering Foundation. (1996). *Stuttering therapy: Transfer and maintenance.* Memphis, TN: Author.

Swan, A. M. (1993). Helping children who stutter: What teachers need to know. *Childhood Education, 69,* 138–141.

Teigland, A. (1996). A study of pragmatic skills of clutterers and normal speakers. *Journal of Fluency Disorders, 21,* 201–214.

Tiger, R., Irvine, T., & Reis, R. (1980). Cluttering as a complex of learning disabilities. *Language, Speech, and Hearing Services in Schools, 11,* 3–14.

Tunbridge, N. (1994). *The stutterer's survival guide.* Sydney: Addison-Wesley.

Vabiro, K., & Engelmayer, A. (1972). Traumatic fear experience as an etiological factor in the formation of stuttering. *Magyar Pszichologiai Szemle, 29,* 223–238.

van Lieshout, P. H. H. M., Peters, H. F. M., Starkweather, C. W., & Hulstijn, W. (1993). Physiological differences between stutterers and nonstutterers in perceptually fluent speech: EMG amplitude and duration. *Journal of Speech and Hearing Research, 36,* 55–63.

van Lieshout, P. H. H. M., Starkweather, C. W., Hulstijn, W., & Peters, H. F. M. (1995). The effects of linguistic correlates of stuttering on EMG activity in nonstuttering speakers. *Journal of Speech and Hearing Research, 38,* 360–372.

Van Riper, C. (1982). *The nature of stuttering.* Englewood Cliffs, NJ: Prentice Hall.

Van Riper, C. (1973). *The treatment of stuttering.* Englewood Cliffs, NJ: Prentice Hall.

Wall, M. J. (1980). A comparison of syntax in young stutterers and non-stutterers. *Journal of Fluency Disorders, 5,* 321–326.

Wall, M. J. & Myers, F. L. (1995). *Clinical management of childhood stuttering* (2d ed.). Austin, TX: Pro-Ed.

Wall, M. J., Starkweather, C. W., & Cairns, H. S. (1981). Syntactic influences on stuttering in young child stutterers. *Journal of Fluency Disorders, 6,* 283–298.

Watkins, R. V., Yairi, E., & Ambrose, N. G. (1999). Early childhood stuttering III: Initial status of expressive language abilities. *Journal of Speech, Language and Hearing Research, 42,* 1125–1135.

Weiss, D. A. (1964). *Cluttering.* Englewood Cliffs, NJ: Prentice Hall.

Westbrook, J. (1994). Jacob's secret speech bracelet. *Staff.* Aaron's Associates, 6114 Waterway, Garland, TX 75043.

Westbrook, J. (1989). *Staff.* Aaron's Associates, 6114 Waterway, Garland, TX 75043.

Whitney, I., Smith, P. K., & Thompson, D. (1994). Bullying and children with special education needs. In P. K. Smith & S. Sharp (Eds.), *School bullying: Insights and perspectives* (pp. 213–240). London: Routledge.

Wiig, E. H., & Semel, E. M. (1980). Word finding, fluency, and flexibility: Intervention. In *Language assessment and intervention for the learning disabled* (pp. 343–364). Columbus, OH: Charles E. Merrill Publishing.

Williams, D. E. (1971). Stuttering therapy for children. In L. E. Travis (Ed.), *Handbook of speech pathology and audiology.* Englewood Cliffs, NJ: Prentice Hall.

Williams, K. (1997). *Expressive vocabulary test* (EVT). Circle Pines, MN: American Guidance Services.

Wingate, M. E. (2002). *Foundations of stuttering.* San Diego: Academic Press.

Wingate, M. E. (2001). SLD is not stuttering. *Journal of Speech, Language, and Hearing Research, 44,* 381–383.

Wolk, L. (1998). Intervention strategies for children who exhibit coexisting phonological and fluency disorders: A clinical note. *Child Language Teaching and Therapy, 14,* 69–82.

Wood, S. E. (1995). An electropalatographic analysis of stutters' speech. *European Journal of Disorders of Communication, 30,* 226–236.

Wood, F., Stump, D., McKeehan, A., Sheldon, S., & Proctor, J. (1980). Patterns of regional cerebral blood flow during attempted reading aloud by stutterers both on and off haloperidol medication: Evidence for inadequate left frontal activation during stuttering. *Brain and Language, 9,* 141–144.

Woolf, G. (1967). The assessment of stuttering as struggle, avoidance, and expectancy. *British Journal of Disorders of Communication, 2,* 158–171.

World Health Organization. (2001). *The international classification of functioning, disability, and health.* Geneva: Author.

World Health Organization. (1993). *International classification of impairments, disabilities, and handicaps: A manual of classification relating to the consequences of disease.* Geneva: Author.

World Health Organization. (1992). *International statistical classification of diseases and related health problems* (10th rev.). Geneva: Author.

World Health Organization. (1980). *International classification of impairments, disabilities, and handicaps: A manual of classification relating to the consequences of disease.* Geneva: Author.

Yairi, E. (1997a). Disfluency characteristics of childhood stuttering. In R. F. Curlee & G. M. Siegal (Eds.), *Nature and treatment of stuttering: New directions* (2d ed., pp. 49–78). Needham Heights, MA: Allyn & Bacon.

Yairi, E. (1997b). Home environment and parent-child interaction in childhood stuttering. In R. F. Curlee & G. M. Siegal (Eds.), *Nature and treatment of stuttering New directions* (2d ed.). Needham Height MA: Allyn & Bacon.

Yairi, E., & Ambrose, N. G. (1999). Early childhood stuttering I: Persistency and recovery rates. *Journal of Speech and Hearing Research, 35*, 755–760.

Yairi, E., & Ambrose, N. G. (1992). A longitudinal study of stuttering in children: A preliminary report. *Journal of Speech and Hearing Research, 35*, 755–760.

Yairi, E., Ambrose, N., & Niermann R. (1993). The early months of stuttering: A developmental study. *Journal of Speech and Hearing Research, 36*, 521–528.

Yairi, E., Ambrose, N., Paden, E., & Throneburg, R. (1996). Predictive factors of persistence and recovery: Pathways of childhood stuttering. *Journal of Communication Disorders, 29*, 51–77.

Yairi, E., & Williams, D. E. (1971). Reports of parental attitudes by stuttering and by nonstuttering children. *Journal of Speech and Hearing Research, 14*, 596–604.

Yaruss, J. S. (2001). Evaluating treatment outcomes for adults who stutter. *Journal of Communication Disorders, 34*, 163–182.

Yaruss, J. S. (1999). Utterance length, syntactic complexity, and childhood stuttering. *Journal of Speech, Language, and Hearing Research, 42*, 329–344.

Yaruss, J. S. (1   scribing the consequences of dis(ng and the internari   ments, h, 36,

Yaruss, J. S., & Quesal, R. w. (2003). *Overall assessment of the speaker's experience of stuttering (OASES).* Proceedings of the Fourth World Congress on Fluency Disorders, Montreal.

Yaruss, J. S., & Quesal, R. W. (2004). Stuttering and the international classification of functioning, disability, and health (ICF): An update. *Journal of Communication Disorders, 37*, 35–52.

Zebrowski, P. M., & Cilek, T. D. (1997). Stuttering therapy in the elementary school setting: Guidelines for clinician-teacher collaboration. *Seminars in Speech and Language, 18*, 329–341.

Zebrowski, P. M., & Conture, E. G. (1989). Judgments of disfluency by mothers of stuttering and normally dysfluent children. *Journal of Speech and Hearing Research, 32*, 625–634.

Zebrowski, P. M., & Kelly, E. M. (2002). *Therapy for stuttering.* San Diego: Singular Publishing Group.

Zebrowski, P. M., & Schum, R. L. (1993). Counseling parents of children who stutter. *American Journal of Speech-Language Pathology, 2*, 65–73.

Zimmermann, G. N. (1980). Stuttering: A disorder of movement. *Journal of Speech and Hearing Research, 23*, 122–136.

Zimmermann, G. N., & Hanley, J. M. (1983). A cinefluorographic investigation of repeated fluent productions of stutterers in an adaptation procedure. *Journal of Speech and Hearing Research, 26*, 35–42.

Zimmermann, G. N., Smith, A., & Hanley, J. M. (1981). Stuttering: In need of a unifying conceptual framework. *Journal of Speech and Hearing Research, 24*, 25–31.

Zwitman, D. (1978). *The dysfluent child.* Baltimore, MD: University Park Press.